Critical Care Neurology

Blue Books of Practical Neurology
(Volumes 1–14 published as BIMR Neurology)

Critical Care Neurology

Edited by

David H. Miller, M.D., F.R.C.P., F.R.A.C.P.
Professor, Department of Clinical Neurology, Institute of Neurology,
London; Consultant Neurologist, The National Hospital for Neurology and
Neurosurgery, London

and

Eric C. Raps, M.D.
William N. Kelley Associate Professor of Neurology and Director,
Division of Stroke and Neurointensive Care, University of Pennsylvania
Medical Center, Philadelphia

with 24 Contributors

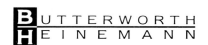

Boston   Oxford   Auckland   Johannesburg   Melbourne   New Delhi

Copyright © 1999 by Butterworth–Heinemann

 A member of the Reed Elsevier group

Every effort has been made to ensure that the drug dosage schedules within this text are accurate and conform to standards accepted at time of publication. However, as treatment recommendations vary in the light of continuing research and clinical experience, the reader is advised to verify drug dosage schedules herein with information found on product information sheets. This is especially true in cases of new or infrequently used drugs.

 Recognizing the importance of preserving what has been written, Butterworth–Heinemann prints its books on acid-free paper whenever possible.

AMERICAN FORESTS
GLOBAL
RELEAF
2000
Butterworth–Heinemann supports the efforts of American Forests and the Global ReLeaf program in its campaign for the betterment of trees, forests, and our environment.

Library of Congress Cataloging-in-Publication Data
Critical care neurology / edited by David H. Miller and Eric C. Raps.
   p.   cm. -- (Blue books of practical neurology ; 22)
   Includes bibliographical references and index.
   ISBN 0-7506-9968-X
   1. Neurological intensive care. I. Miller, David H. (David Hugh)
II. Raps, Eric C. III. Series.
   [DNLM: 1. Nervous System Diseases. 2. Critical Care. W1 BU9749
v.22 1999 / WL 140 C934 1999]
RC350.N49C75   1999
616.8'0428--dc21
for Library of Congress   98-54233
                                                                         CIP

British Library Cataloguing-in-Publication Data
A catalogue record for this book is available from the British Library.

The publisher offers special discounts on bulk orders of this book.
For information, please contact:

Manager of Special Sales
Butterworth–Heinemann
225 Wildwood Avenue
Woburn, MA 01801-2041
Tel: 781-904-2500
Fax: 781-904-2620

For information on all Butterworth–Heinemann publications available,
contact our World Wide Web home page at: http://www.bh.com

10 9 8 7 6 5 4 3 2 1

Printed in the United States of America

Contents

Contributing Authors

Gary L. Bernardini, M.D., Ph.D.
Assistant Professor, Department of Clinical Neurology, Columbia University College of Physicians and Surgeons, New York; Assistant Attending Neurologist, Neurological Intensive Care Unit, Columbia-Presbyterian Medical Center, New York

Shawn J. Bird, M.D.
Assistant Professor, Department of Neurology, University of Pennsylvania School of Medicine, Philadelphia; Director, Electromyography Laboratory, University of Pennsylvania Medical Center, Philadelphia

Thomas P. Bleck, M.D.
Louise Nerancy Professor of Neurology and Professor, Departments of Neurological Surgery and Internal Medicine, University of Virginia School of Medicine, Charlottesville; Director, Neuroscience Intensive Care Unit, University of Virginia Health Sciences Center, Charlottesville

Cecil O. Borel, M.D.
Associate Professor, Department of Surgery, Division of Neurosurgery, and Department of Anesthesiology, Duke University Medical Center, Durham, North Carolina

David P. D'Cruz, M.B.B.S., M.D., M.R.C.P.
Senior Lecturer in Rheumatology, Bone and Joint Research Unit, and Consultant Rheumatologist, Royal London Hospital

Nicholas P. Hirsch, M.B.B.S., F.R.C.A.
Honorary Senior Lecturer, Institute of Neurology, London; Consultant Anaesthetist, The National Hospital for Neurology and Neurosurgery, London

Robin S. Howard, Ph.D., F.R.C.P.
Senior Lecturer in Neurology, Institute of Neurology, London; Consultant Neurologist, The National Hospital for Neurology and Neurosurgery, London

Kenneth G. Jordan, M.D., F.A.C.P.
Director, Neurodiagnostic Laboratories, and Attending Neurointensivist, St. Bernadine's Medical Center, Arrowhead Regional Medical Center, and Jordan NeuroScience, San Bernardino, California

Scott E. Kasner, M.D.
Assistant Professor, Department of Neurology, University of Pennsylvania Medical Center, Philadelphia; Co-Director, Comprehensive Stroke Center, Hospital of the University of Pennsylvania, Philadelphia

Fenella Kirkham, F.R.C.P.
Senior Lecturer in Neurosciences, Institute of Child Health, London; Honorary Consultant in Neurology, Great Ormond Street National Health Service Trust, London

Mariko Kita, M.D.
Neurology Resident, Hospital of the University of Pennsylvania, Philadelphia

Dennis L. Kolson, M.D., Ph.D.
Assistant Professor, Department of Neurology, University of Pennsylvania School of Medicine and Hospital of the University of Pennsylvania, Philadelphia

Daniel T. Laskowitz, M.D.
Assistant Professor, Department of Medicine, Division of Neurology, Duke University Medical Center, Durham, North Carolina

Laurence Loh, F.R.C.A.
Consultant Anaesthetist, Nuffield Department of Anaesthetics, The Radcliffe Infirmary National Health Service Trust, Oxford, United Kingdom

Stephan A. Mayer, M.D.
Assistant Professor, Department of Neurology, Columbia University College of Physicians and Surgeons, New York; Director, Neurologic Intensive Care Unit, Presbyterian Hospital, New York

David H. Miller, M.D., F.R.C.P., F.R.A.C.P.
Professor, Department of Clinical Neurology, Institute of Neurology, London; Consultant Neurologist, The National Hospital for Neurology and Neurosurgery, London

Barnett R. Nathan, M.D.
Clinical Instructor, Department of Neurology, Division of Neurocritical Care and Neuroinfectious Disease, University of Virginia Health Sciences Center, Charlottesville

Eric C. Raps, M.D.
William N. Kelley Associate Professor of Neurology and Director, Division of Stroke and Neurointensive Care, University of Pennsylvania Medical Center, Philadelphia

Mark M. Rich, M.D., Ph.D.
Assistant Professor, Department of Neurology, Emory University School of Medicine, Atlanta

R. W. Ross Russell, M.D., F.R.C.P.
Emeritus Consultant in Neurology, The National Hospital for Neurology and Neurosurgery and St. Thomas' Hospital, London

Robert A. Solomon, M.D.
Byron Stookey Professor, Department of Neurological Surgery, Columbia University College of Physicians and Surgeons, New York; Chairman and Director of Service, Columbia-Presbyterian Medical Center, New York

James W. Teener, M.D.
Director, Stroke Center, St. Mary's Duluth Clinic Health System, Duluth, Minnesota

Adrian J. Williams, M.B.
Honorary Senior Lecturer in Medicine, Guy's, King's, and St. Thomas' Schools of Medicine, London; Director, Lane-Fox Respiratory Unit, St. Thomas' Hospital, London

John B. Winer, M.Sc., M.D., F.R.C.P.
Senior Lecturer in Neurology, University of Birmingham, United Kingdom; Honorary Consultant Neurologist, Queen Elizabeth Hospital, Birmingham

Series Preface

The *Blue Books of Practical Neurology* series is the new name for the *BIMR Neurology* series, which was itself the successor of the *Modern Trends in Neurology* series. As before, the volumes are intended for use by physicians who grapple with the problems of neurological disorders on a daily basis, be they neurologists, neurologists in training, or those in related fields such as neurosurgery, internal medicine, psychiatry, and rehabilitation medicine.

Our purpose is to produce monographs on topics in clinical neurology in which progress through research has brought about new concepts of patient management. The subject of each monograph is selected by the Series Editors using two criteria: first, that there has been significant advance in knowledge in that area and, second, that such advances have been incorporated into new ways of managing patients with the disorders in question. This has been the guiding spirit behind each volume, and we expect it to continue. In effect, we emphasize research, in the clinic and in the experimental laboratory, but principally to the extent that it changes our collective attitudes and practices in caring for those who are neurologically afflicted.

C. David Marsden
Arthur K. Asbury
Series Editors

Preface

Modern critical care neurology is rooted in the iron lung units created during the polio epidemics of the 1940s and 1950s. Since that time, the need for discrete intensive care units specializing in the care of neuromedical and neurosurgical patients has paralleled tremendous advances in therapies. As the "salvage rate" of the critically ill neurologic population improved with new therapies and technologies, the number of trained neurointensive care specialists grew. Acute ischemic stroke, Guillain-Barré syndrome, myasthenic crisis, status epilepticus, meningitis, and viral encephalitis patients are among those with neuromedical conditions who have benefited from the flurry of therapeutic advances.

This monograph offers an updated review of the tactics and techniques used in critical care neurology, with special emphasis on the incremental advances born of scientific investigations. Critical care neurology is a truly multidisciplinary field formed by the intersection of neurology, neurosurgery, neuroradiology, anesthesiology, and pulmonary medicine. Consistent with this mindset, the contributors are a diverse and distinguished group of trans-Atlantic experts.

As well as reviewing primary neurologic disorders that frequently require intensive care unit management, this book deals with a variety of neurologic complications that characteristically or commonly occur in critically ill patients. Some sections also provide a more general discussion of disorders that, although frequent causes of critical illness, may often present to neurologists outside the intensive care unit setting.

Although disease etiology and pathophysiologic mechanisms are discussed, patient management is emphasized throughout. The book is intended primarily for clinicians who encounter patients with neurologic problems in critical care settings.

Eric C. Raps
David H. Miller

1
Respiratory and Bulbar Dysfunction in Neurologic Disease

Daniel T. Laskowitz and Cecil O. Borel

The role of neuromuscular disease in contributing to respiratory dysfunction in the intensive care unit (ICU) is often under-recognized. Not a great deal of literature systematically examines respiratory function after stroke or other primary central nervous system (CNS) disorders, although respiratory complications are certainly not uncommon in this setting. In contrast, respiratory failure is a well-known complication of disorders such as Guillain-Barré syndrome (GBS) and myasthenia gravis, which are often treated in specialized neurologic ICUs. Awareness of critical illness polyneuropathy (CIP) and the myopathy associated with the administration of steroids and nondepolarizing paralytic agents—two entities that occur primarily in the intensive care setting—has grown. Respiratory failure is also the most common proximal cause of death in a number of progressive neuromuscular disorders such as amyotrophic lateral sclerosis (ALS) and muscular dystrophy.

FUNCTIONAL NEUROANATOMY OF BREATHING

Anatomic Basis of Respiratory Control

Much of the information regarding neural control of respiration is based on the work of Thomas Lumsden [1,2]. He worked with brain stem transection of cats and laid the basis for much of the current knowledge of the origin of respiration and ventilatory activity. He described the various patterns of abnormal breathing from his models and localized much of the basic neuroanatomic information of brain stem generation of respiratory drive.

One of the first anatomic brain areas described in relation to respiratory control is known as the *pontine pneumotaxic center*. Later authors have identified this area as the median parabrachial nucleus [3]. This nucleus is located in the brachium pontis or superior cerebellar peduncle. Three patterns of neuronal firing are found: inspiratory, expiratory, and phase spanning. Because respiratory rhythm has been generated from the medulla alone, the pneumotaxic center is no longer thought to be the primary respiratory pacemaker. It appears to play a role in the modification and fine control of respiratory rhythm (e.g., setting lung volume for inspiration) [4]. This center, however, is not necessary for the control and regulation of eupnea.

A second physiologically related area is the so-called apneustic center. Although presumably located in the mid- or caudal pons, this center has not been precisely characterized [5,6]. Apneustic breathing (i.e., breathing with sustained inspiration) is rarely seen in humans. Some authors have suggested that the apneustic center is responsible for suppressing the inspiratory neurons found in the medulla. Thus, it is possible that it functions as a normal inspiratory cutoff switch [5,6].

Respiratory rhythm results from complex interactions between two functional groups of neurons in the medulla known as the *dorsal* (DRG) and *ventral respiratory groups* (VRG). The DRG is located in the dorsolateral portion of the nucleus of the solitary tract. It primarily receives inputs from cranial nerves IX and X, and specifically from the carotid body. The DRG sends fibers to the inspiratory spinal motor neurons and to the VRG, which it modulates [7,8]. The VRG is split into two parts. The rostral portion, primarily part of the nucleus ambiguus, innervates the larynx and has both inspiratory and expiratory functions. The larger caudal part, also known as the *nucleus retroambiguus*, has both inspiratory and expiratory neurons for the diaphragm and the intercostals.

In addition, a large number of cells, often termed *propriobulbar neurons*, appear to arise and terminate almost solely within the medulla, providing interconnections between neurons in the DRG and VRG [8,9]. Finally, a putative gasping center is found in the rostral medulla, in the lateral tegmental field, which may be critical for the neurogenesis of the gasp response. This area seems to have a minimal role in the generation of eupneic ventilatory patterns. Its activity is normally suppressed by pontine, and occasionally medullary, breathing centers. However, in the presence of hypoxia, significant stress, or severe brain stem damage, the activity of the gasping center may become unmasked, giving rise to recognizable clinical patterns [10].

The descending axons of neurons contained in the DRG and VRG cross the midline at the obex, and descend in the ventrolateral columns of the spinal cord, anterior to the corticospinal tract [11]. Although forebrain impulses via the corticospinal tract can alter ventilation, the normal involuntary eupneic activity, which depends on the activity of DRG and VRG neurons, generally suppresses them. Both inspiratory and expiratory axons appear to descend in somewhat different parts of the ventral portion of the cord [12,13].

Pathways for nonrhythmic reflexes that involve respiratory muscles (e.g., coughing) also descend in the ventral part of the spinal cord. These descending pathways, however, do not originate in either the DRG or VRG but rather in closely related medullary nuclei. They are also located in diffuse fiber bundles in the ventral part of the spinal cord. These pathways interact only at the level of the motor neurons [12,13].

The role of spinal motor neurons in respiratory function is similar to the role they play in any other voluntary movements. The muscles involved in respiration include both intra- and extrafusal muscle fibers. The latter are innervated by gamma motor neurons and are part of normal proprioceptive mechanisms, which regulate muscle tone. The muscles of inspiration are actively inhibited during expiration, and vice versa, via this proprioceptive mechanism, which also appears to have some role in regulating diaphragmatic contractions. The major difference in the role of spinal innervation of respiratory muscles and that exerted on other striated muscles is the reciprocal inhibition of the internal and external intercostals, which is not mediated through the usual spinal mechanisms but arises centrally. Descending neurons with inspiratory activity excite the external intercostal motor neurons and also inhibit internal intercostal motor neurons, and vice versa [14].

Mechanism of Action of the Chemoreceptors

Two groups of peripheral chemoreceptors are responsible for the regulation of respiratory function: the carotid body and the aortic bodies. These structures are uniquely sensitive to changes in the partial pressure of oxygen. Neuronal activity appears to increase as the Pao_2 falls below 500 mm Hg and is especially active as it falls below 100 mm Hg. At approximately 30 mm Hg, the chemoreceptor's impulse activity is no longer sustained and may actually decrease [15,16]. Carotid body receptors are also responsive to changes in the Pco_2 and arterial pH [17]. This information is transmitted via myelinated and unmyelinated fibers contained in the glossopharyngeal nerve. It eventually makes its way into the neurons near the VRG. In addition, chemoreceptors are stimulated by a variety of other stimuli, including blood pressure changes and variations in sympathetic activity, which change these areas' markedly high blood flow. The carotid bodies are the primary peripheral chemoreceptors [17].

Despite the apparent sensitivity of the carotid body to carbon dioxide, ventilatory response to increases in CO_2 remains unaltered after denervation of the peripheral chemoreceptors, such as it would when a carotid body is resected during endarterectomy [17]. The ventilatory response to stepwise changes in alveolar carbon dioxide has a slow component with a time constant of 60 seconds [18]. It has been suggested this delay is caused by a central carbon dioxide chemoreceptor.

Several distinct central chemoreceptors are present on the medulla. They appear to be located primarily in the ventral surface of the medulla, close to the origin of the glossopharyngeal and vagus nerves. Other chemosensitive areas, also in the ventral medulla, lie somewhat more posteriorly. They are interconnected with a so-called intermediate zone between the existing nuclei of IX and X and cranial nerve XII. Together, these areas are called the *ventral medullary shell* and act as pH sensors. Because carbon dioxide penetrates the blood-brain barrier, as tissue carbon dioxide increases, it changes the pH of the cerebrospinal fluid and brain extracellular fluid [18].

The ventral medullary shell is also sensitive to changes in local blood flow and metabolism. Pathways from this intermediate area extend upward into the medulla to the DRG and VRG. Overall integration of central peripheral chemoreceptor inputs occurs in the lateral medullary tegmentum. Temporary disruption of the central chemoreceptors does not alter peripheral chemoreceptor function. In addition, the central chemoreceptors have significant effects on the responses to stimulation of the pulmonary mechanoreceptors. It appears that disruption of the ventral medullary shell can decrease irritant responses [19].

Mechanism of Action of Afferent Receptors

The upper airways in the lungs possess a number of receptors that give feedback and can affect breathing. Airways of the nose and pharynx have a variety of receptors that are sensitive to chemical agents and mechanical stimulation. From the nose, these afferent pathways ascend via the trigeminal and olfactory nerves. From the pharynx, they travel primarily through the pharyngeal branch of the glossopharyngeal nerve. Stimulation of the receptors in the nose can result in apnea and bradycardia, as well as sneezing. Mechanical stimulation of nasal mucosa has also been shown to lead to excitation of medullary expiratory neurons [20]. Stimulation in the pharynx excites medullary inspiratory neurons and external intercostal and phrenic motor neurons [21]. This has been associated with a sniff or aspiration reflex that can also trigger bronchodilation and hypertension [22].

Receptors in the larynx are primarily irritant receptors and respond to both chemical and mechanical stimulation. Afferent fibers for these receptors are found in the internal branch of the superior laryngeal nerve and include multiple different fiber types within the superior laryngeal nerve, all capable of stimulating respiratory neurons in the dorsal respiratory group. Respiratory reflex effects from stimulation of these receptors are variable and can include coughing, slow deep breathing, and apnea. They can trigger responses of bronchoconstriction and hypertension [22]. The tracheal irritant receptors are similar to the laryngeal irritant receptors in terms of responses [22].

Three major classes of lung receptors exist: (1) pulmonary stretch receptors, (2) irritant receptors, and (3) type J receptors. Stimulation of these three receptors produces markedly different effects.

Pulmonary stretch receptors are found within the airway's smooth muscle. They are activated by distention of the lungs. The afferent impulses are carried by large myelinated fibers of the vagus nerve. Activation of these receptors causes a slowing of the respiratory frequency as a result of an increase in the expiratory phase, called the *classic Hering-Breuer inspiratory inhibitory reflex*. Other reflex responses include bronchodilation, tachycardia, and vasoconstriction. Central integration of this information is thought to be important in determining the depth of respiration. A species difference exists in the threshold for phasic vagal regulation of the respiratory pattern. In cats, this appears to be at the eupneic level, whereas in humans it appears to be at tidal volumes of approximately 1.5–2.0 times normal eupneic values [23,24].

Irritant receptors lie between airway epithelial cells. They are excited by chemical (e.g., ammonia) and mechanical (particulate matter) irritants [25]. Irritant receptors can be stimulated by histamine release during allergic asthmatic attacks [26]. The vagal afferent fibers from these receptors are myelinated. Reflex effects from irritant receptor stimulation are bronchoconstriction and hyperpnea [27].

Another type of pulmonary neuroreceptor is called a *type J* or *juxtapulmonary capillary* receptor. The name comes from the receptor's purported location. It is excited by an increase in pulmonary interstitial fluid volume. Animal studies have also shown stimulation of these receptors by lung hyperinflation, but the same has not yet been found in humans. Stimulation of type J receptors can cause apnea, hypertension, or bradycardia. Their role in the regulation of ventilation is controversial at this time [27].

Afferent receptors to muscle tension, proprioception, and noxious stimuli can also affect breathing. The phrenic and intercostal nerves contain a full array of afferent fibers [28]. However, data on their effect on central inspiratory motor drive are conflicting. Numerous thin-fiber (groups III and IV) afferents are located in the diaphragm [29]. They have been classified into two groups: mechanoreceptors, which consist mainly of group III fibers and are activated by muscle contraction in the presence or absence of muscle ischemia, and metaboreceptors or nociceptors, which consist mainly of group IV fibers that are activated by muscle ischemia or noxious chemicals such as lactic acid and potassium chloride [30,31]. Activation of these fibers by electrical or chemical methods or by diaphragmatic ischemia elicits a significant increase in the ventilatory drive and arterial pressure [32,33].

Phrenic nerves contain only a few large-fiber afferents. These fibers innervate muscle spindles and Golgi tendon organs. Golgi tendon organs respond to changes in muscle tension, whereas muscle spindles respond to changes in muscle length. Large fibers seem to have an inhibitory effect on diaphragmatic motor output via both supraspinal and spinal mechanisms. Banzett and associates [34] studied the effect of lower body negative pressure on diaphragmatic activity in quadriplegic men. They found an increase in diaphragmatic activity that they thought was likely caused by phrenic afferents. Fryman and Frazier [35] found a significant change in ventilation mediated by alterations in diaphragmatic length that were in turn mediated by phrenic nerve afferents. Cheeseman and Revelette [36] found a significant reduction in ventilatory drive in response to an increase in length. Spinal inhibitory phrenic-to-phrenic reflex has been described by Speck and Revelette [37].

Diaphragmatic weakness, by reducing muscle tension and to a lesser extent muscle length, leads to a fall in the inhibitory activity of large-fiber afferents without a change in small-fiber activation. The subsequent decrease in large-fiber inhibitory activity results in a reflex rise in inspiratory motor activity. A central reflex activity initiates a coordinated response in ventilatory muscles and breathing rate [38].

CENTRAL NERVOUS SYSTEM LESIONS AND DISORDERS OF RESPIRATION

Central disorders of respiration are not uncommon in the neurologic ICU, and understanding the respiratory disturbances caused by specific CNS lesions plays an important role in guiding ventilatory management of these patients. Before considering the specific role of CNS pathology on respiratory dysfunction, it is important to consider the general metabolic and endocrine disturbances that can influence central respiratory control. For example, myxedema can cause chronic hypoventilation, and even mild to moderate hypothyroidism can contribute to decreased central drive that is responsive to thyroid replacement. This is of particular importance in patients who may be at risk for panhypopituitary states caused by parasellar lesions. Often, central hypothyroidism is difficult to differentiate from the sick euthyroid syndrome in the critically ill patient, and an empiric trial of low-dose thyroid replacement may be indicated in selected patients in whom a high clinical suspicion of pituitary insufficiency exists. Metabolic alkalosis causes functional depression of central respiratory neurons and may also contribute to respiratory insufficiency. In particular, the hypochloremic alkalosis associated with intravascular depletion can depress respiratory drive and commonly occurs after the injudicious use of loop diuretics. In these situations, intravascular repletion or the use of acetazolamide to encourage renal wasting of bicarbonate may correct the metabolic alkalosis and improve ventilatory function.

Respiratory Abnormalities after Stroke

Cerebral ischemia can disrupt breathing by damaging any of the supratentorial or infratentorial structures that are normally integrated in the control of automatic and volitional respirations. In humans, cortical control of respirations has been localized to the anterior hippocampus, ventral and medial temporal lobe, and insula [39,40]. Cortical stimulation or seizures that originate from these areas inhibit respiratory drive and result in apnea [41,42]. Although unilateral lesions resulting from ischemia in the anterior circulation may reduce the contralateral diaphragmatic excursion and chest wall movement, hemispheric stroke rarely results in clinically significant respiratory disturbances [43]. Bilateral hemispheric disease has been associated with Cheyne-Stokes breathing, a syndrome of cyclic hyperventilation followed by hypoventilation and apnea. This pattern is not specific for infarction, and can be seen in many models of bihemispheric dysfunction, including uremia, diabetic ketoacidosis, and altitude sickness [39,44]. Although most commonly associated with bilateral hemispheric disease, Cheyne-Stokes respirations have been described with unilateral lesions in the distribution of the anterior circulation, especially when coexistent pulmonary or cardiac disease is present [45]. Experimental evidence exists that this pattern of respiration is caused by interruption of normal cortical inhibition, resulting in abnormally increased reactivity to carbon dioxide [44]. Bilateral hemispheric disease can also interrupt descending corticobulbar projections and cause pseudobulbar palsy, a condition characterized by emotional lability, dysarthria, and dysphagia. Although the disease has not been directly implicated in respiratory disturbance, these patients may have difficulty protecting their airway and experience recurrent aspirations. Respiratory apraxia, which is defined as the inability to voluntarily control respirations in the setting of normal automatic respiratory function (the reverse of Ondine's curse, described in the following paragraph) has been observed after a unilateral stroke. This lesion is most commonly placed in the nondominant internal capsule or subcortical middle cerebral artery distribution [46]. More commonly, this occurs with patients who are "locked-in" secondary to pontine infarction.

Brain stem disease resulting from ischemia in the distribution of the posterior circulation can lead to several well-defined disorders of respiration. The dorsolateral medulla is primarily responsible for the integration of effective rhythmic breathing, and as long as this area, which includes the nucleus ambiguus and solitarius, is not affected, central respiratory control may be relatively normal. Thus, even locked-in patients with rostral brain stem infarction may be left with a relatively normal respiratory drive [47]. Disruption of automatic breathing can result from damage to the lateral medulla and pontine tegmentum caudal to trigeminal outflow. Lateral medullary stroke is most commonly caused by occlusion of the distal vertebral or posterior inferior cerebellar artery, and large infarcts involving the dorsolateral medulla may be associated with fatal apnea [48]. The total loss of automatic respirations has been termed *Ondine's curse*, after the water nymph of German legend who took away autonomic function from her unfaithful knight, Hans. These patients may experience mild hypoventilation while awake, which can be reversed on request. Respirations may cease entirely during sleep, causing convulsions or death. Several cases of Ondine's curse have been described after lateral medullary infarction [48,49]. The majority of these lesions have been unilateral on the left, suggesting laterality of medullary respiratory control [45,49,50]. Ondine's curse has also been described after bilateral cervical tractotomy for refractory pain [51]. Respiratory disturbances have also been reported after pontine hemorrhage, including central hypoventilation, Cheyne-Stokes breathing, and ataxic respirations [52,53]. Apneustic respiration, defined as an inspiratory pause, has also been described in pontine stroke, a finding that corresponds to a model of experimental apneusis induced by transection of the dorsolateral pons in vagotomized animals [54,55]. This is presumably caused by bilateral interruption of the spinoreticular tracts with preservation of the corticospinal tracts subserving volitional respirations. Uncommonly, hemorrhagic or ischemic lesions near the pontomesencephalic junction may result in neurogenic hyperventilation, a condition that may also be seen after severe global insult from anoxia, hypoglycemia, or metabolic encephalopathy (especially hepatic encephalopathy) [56]. When a stroke is associated with a significant spontaneous respiratory alkalosis (pH >7.46, P_{CO_2} <35), prognosis for survival is poor [57].

Although less dramatic than examples of central apnea such as Ondine's curse, brain stem infarction is more likely to cause obstructive or mixed apnea. In obstructive sleep apnea, the tongue and soft palate fall posteriorly during sleep, occluding the pharynx. Respiratory effort intensifies despite the pharyngeal obstruction to airflow, and the patient partially arouses. This has the effect of activating the musculature of the upper airway, relieving the obstruction. Obstructive sleep apnea does not usually present with any respiratory abnormalities while patients are awake and alert, but they often complain of excessive daytime somnolence and morning headache. This condition is of particular significance in the management of patients with primary CNS disease, as nocturnal hypercapnia can cause transient elevation of intracranial pressure. Clinical suspicion of sleep apnea is heightened in the patient with obese habitus who snores. Snoring, which is caused by the vibration of the soft palate when air is inspired through a partially narrowed upper airway, is usually continuous during inspiration; in the patient with obstructive sleep apnea, it is loud and intermittent. Apnea is often position-dependent, being exacerbated by lying supine or on the paretic side. Occasionally, polysomnography is necessary to define the pattern of apnea. In central apnea, no respiratory efforts are made, whereas in obstructive apnea, respiratory effort continues despite pharyngeal obstruction to airflow. Often, a mixed pattern is found in which respiratory effort is initially absent but starts before airflow. In acute cases, patients with obstructive apnea and a reduced level of consciousness may require endotracheal intubation or tracheostomy, although nocturnal continuous positive airway pressure or bilevel positive airway pressure usually suffice in the alert patient. Occasionally, surgical removal of the tonsils, uvula, or soft palate may be of benefit. Patients with central apnea syndromes require longer-term assisted ventilation. There has been no rigorous study demonstrating efficacy of medical therapy with agents such as theophylline or medroxyprogesterone acetate, although these have often been used empirically in this setting.

Parkinson's Disease

Although Parkinson's disease is usually not the primary cause of respiratory failure in the neurologic ICU, it is relatively common with advancing age and a frequent comorbid factor that can complicate respiratory management. Several abnormalities of pulmonary function and respiration have been described with Parkinson's disease and other extrapyramidal syndromes. These patients often have a restrictive pattern of pulmonary function, which may improve after the administration of levodopa (L-dopa) [58–61]. Experimental evidence suggests that this is caused by impaired chest wall compliance secondary to abnormal tonic activity of the intercostal muscles during expiration, when these muscles are normally electrically silent [62]. Growing evidence also exists that, in a subset of patients with Parkinson's disease, symptoms of upper airway obstruction may develop at the supraglottic and laryngeal levels [14]. Pulmonary function tests may reveal a characteristic "sawtooth" pattern of both the inspiratory and expiratory portion of the flow-volume loop, suggesting instability of upper airway caliber [63]. Symptomatic stridor and subsequent respiratory failure may be related to rhythmic involuntary movements of the glottic and supraglottic musculature, which have been visualized by bronchoscopy [64]. Administration of L-dopa may ameliorate symptoms in some patients [65]. In addition to extrathoracic airway obstruction and reduced chest wall compliance, patients with Parkinson's disease may experience abnormalities of central respiratory drive, the most common pattern of which is tachypnea at rest [66,67]. Although the reasons for this are not entirely clear, it has been suggested that denervation hypersensitivity of medullary dopaminergic neurons in patients with advanced Parkinson's disease can result in exaggerated response to hypercapnic and hypoxic stimulation.

In addition to the primary respiratory disturbances that accompany Parkinson's disease, treatment with L-dopa can affect respiration. Numerous case reports have documented tachypnea and ataxic respirations after L-dopa administration [68,69]. Although this phenomenon was initially believed to represent "respiratory dyskinesias," one study suggests that this may not be the case. Instead of the paradoxical chest and abdominal excursions that might be expected with dyskinesia, a decrement in forced vital capacity (FVC) and 1-second forced expiratory volume (FEV_1) was seen that might be more consistent with the "off" phenomenon of Parkinson's disease [70]. In critically ill patients with Parkinson's disease and respiratory disturbance, it is also important to consider the possibility that a continuous high-protein parenteral feeding may be impairing absorption of L-dopa. In these patients, it is often helpful to suspend feedings for 30 minutes before administration of carbidopa-levodopa (Sinemet).

Spinal Cord Injury

Spinal cord injury represents a significant source of morbidity in the United States, with approximately 10,000 new spinal cord injuries occurring yearly [71]. Of these, the majority involve the cervical cord, and 5–10% result in complete quadriplegia [71,72]. The phrenic nerve outflow originates from C3–C5, and patients who sustain cord injuries above this level have complete diaphragmatic paralysis and require immediate respiratory support for survival. Patients with injuries at the level of C3–C5 may retain varying degrees of diaphragmatic function. In these cases, an immediate dramatic reduction in vital capacity and expiratory flow rates still exists, and patients usually require ventilatory support acutely [73]. Immediately after spinal cord trauma, a period of spinal shock often occurs when the intercostals are flaccid, resulting in chest wall distortion and inefficient ventilation. This is often compounded by weakness in the accessory muscles of respiration and ineffective coughing caused by paralysis of the abdominal musculature. Over time, upper motor neuron signs prevail, and the chest wall is stabilized as the musculature of the chest and abdomen change from a flaccid to spastic paresis. Initial flaccid paralysis of the intercostals may also contribute to postural hypoxemia, which is secondary to relative hyperventilation of the upper lung fields [74]. Improved diaphragmatic conditioning, recruitment of accessory muscles, and proper pulmonary toilet may ultimately allow 50–80% of patients with C3–C5 lesions to be weaned from the ventilator [75]. The majority of patients with thoracic cord injury initially have a marked reduction in vital capacity for many of these same reasons, but usually have adequate diaphragmatic function and rarely require long-term ventilatory support.

The immediate concern in the setting of suspected spinal cord injury is securing and protecting the patient's airway. A variety of techniques can be used to accomplish this in patients with suspected cervical injuries. The method chosen should avoid secondary cord injury, prevent aspiration of gastric contents, and protect against massive release of potassium from skeletal muscle caused by extrajunctional chemosensitivity to succinylcholine. The relative efficacy and safety of the various techniques are controversial.

Topical local anesthesia followed by blind or fiberoptic-assisted nasotracheal intubation is an acceptable choice. Alternatively, a rapid-sequence technique using a short-acting barbiturate and a neuromuscular blocking agent with simultaneous application of cricoid pressure is acceptable. No conclusive evidence exists for increased neurologic morbidity with any particular technique [76,77]. Manual in-line neck traction was once believed to reduce cervical dislocation during tracheal intubation. This practice has been discouraged, however, because it can result in dislocation of the unstable neck [78]. Despite worries about in-line traction, in-line head immobilization by an assistant continues to be recommended [76].

Aspiration pneumonitis can be avoided by considering all patients with spinal cord injuries as having full stomachs. Reduction of stomach contents with nasogastric suction decreases the volume and severity of a potential aspirate. Awake or rapid-sequence intubation techniques can reduce the occurrence of aspiration.

If a depolarizing relaxant such as succinylcholine is used to assist intubation, it can generally be given safely within 48 hours of the cord injury. Thereafter, massive release of skeletal muscle potassium can occur after succinylcholine administration [79]. This sudden hyperkalemic response has produced cardiac arrest in some patients. The response is believed to be caused by the proliferation of extrajunctional acetylcholine receptors at the motor end plate, which results from denervation. Although the precise duration of this response is unknown, it is thought to last at least 3–6 months. Hyperkalemic cardiac arrest can be avoided by substituting a nondepolarizing neuromuscular blocker instead of succinylcholine. However, nondepolarizers have a slower onset of action than succinylcholine (3 minutes vs. 1 minute). A shorter onset is desirable in a patient with a full stomach and potential for aspiration. If a nondepolarizer is used, at least 3 minutes of preoxygenation via face mask with 100% inspired oxygen should be given to prevent oxygen desaturation.

Respiratory complications, including pneumonia, acute respiratory distress syndrome, atelectasis, and pulmonary embolism, are common in the initial management of spinal cord injury and head trauma and should be managed supportively. Bronchial mucous hypersecretion, which presumably occurs on a neural basis, is present in 20% of quadriplegic patients and can further complicate acute respiratory management [80].

After initial stabilization, every effort should be made to wean patients with injuries that are located midcervically or below from invasive mechanical ventilation. Although no rigorous systematic study has compared different modes of weaning in this setting, a T-piece is commonly used and appears to be effective. Normally, most individuals show a modest decrease in vital capacity when they move from the upright to the supine position. This effect is often reversed in quadriplegic patients owing to paralysis of the abdominal musculature. An abdominal binder may be effective in increasing the efficacy of cough and promoting rib cage expansion during inspiration [73,81]. Thus, it is often helpful to wean quadriplegic patients from the supine position if the need for a long period of ventilatory dependence is suspected; tracheostomy is indicated to minimize laryngeal trauma and to aid in suctioning. Pulmonary rehabilitation is effective in decreasing ventilator dependence in many cases. In patients who still require ventilatory support, noninvasive positive pressure ventilation may be well tolerated.

Head Injury

Respiratory complications are an important source of morbidity and mortality after closed and penetrating head injury. Hypoxemia and abnormalities of central respiratory drive are fairly common sequelae to head injury, and abnormal pulmonary mechanics can result from thoracic injuries. Trauma patients are also at significant risk for primary pulmonary abnormalities, including pulmonary embolism and aspiration pneumonia. Neurogenic pulmonary edema is a less common but well-described entity of unclear pathogenesis.

Hypoxemia is an early complication of head injury, affecting approximately 30% of trauma patients [82]. Even in the absence of obvious parenchymal injury, pulmonary edema, atelectasis, or infiltrate, hypoxemia is common after head injury. This is believed to be secondary to ventilation-perfusion mismatch and is usually associated with a high alveolar-arterial gradient [83]. In this setting, arterial hypoxemia is usually self-limited and easily managed with supplemental oxygen. Hypoxemia that is prolonged or refractory to treatment is associated with poor outcome [83]. Disturbances of central respiratory drive are also not uncommon after head injury. The most common abnormality in this regard is tachypnea. When associated with a significant spontaneous respiratory alkalosis ($Paco_2$ <30 or respiratory frequency >25), this is also associated with a poor outcome [82].

A number of pulmonary complications frequently occur in head-injured patients. Aspiration is common early in the first week after hospitalization and is even more likely to occur if barbiturates were used to manage refractory increased intracranial pressure [84]. In this setting, initial antibiotic coverage should include gram-positive respiratory flora, anaerobes, and gram-negative nosocomial bacteria. Initial empiric coverage is then narrowed based on culture sensitivities. Deep venous thrombosis and pulmonary embolism also commonly occur in the trauma patient, and this diagnosis may be easily missed by physical examination. Respiratory care can also be compromised by the development of thick, tenacious secretions. Bronchial mucous hypersecretion is relatively common after significant head or cervical cord injury. This takes place too acutely to be explained by glandular hypertrophy and is believed to be caused by changes in autonomic tone. A management dilemma is often posed by the patient with documented venous thrombosis or pulmonary embolism. Anticoagulation is relatively contraindicated for the first several days after significant head injury, and these patients may be candidates for placement of a vena cava filter.

Occasionally, neurogenic pulmonary edema is seen acutely after acute head injury [85]. Although this is a diagnosis of exclusion, and not particularly common, it may be potentially life-threatening. This syndrome was first recognized in an autopsy series of 100 soldiers who died in combat during the Vietnam War. Regardless of thoracic injury, pulmonary edema and thoracic hemorrhage were present in 89% of these soldiers [86]. Neurogenic pulmonary edema is believed to arise from massive sympathetic overflow, leading to increased peripheral and pulmonary vascular resistance [87]. Initially, increased hydrostatic forces caused by abnormally high pulmonary artery pressures force transudate into the alveolar space. Over time, pulmonary capillary endothelial damage can occur, leading to persistent pulmonary edema with high protein content. This diagnosis is one of exclusion and can only be made in the presence of normal cardiac function and left ventricular filling pressures. A 1992 case report has documented a medullary demyelinating lesion as the presumptive etiology of acute pulmonary hypertension, supporting the contention that bilateral injury to the nucleus solitarius may be responsible for this phenomenon [84]. In addition to trauma, neurogenic pulmonary edema has been associated with a variety of neurologic conditions, including subarachnoid hemorrhage, electroconvulsive therapy, seizures, and meningitis [88,89].

Disorders of Respiration Caused by Disease of the Anterior Horn and Peripheral Nerve

Peripheral neuropathy and neuronopathy can also contribute to respiratory insufficiency in the ICU. With the control of poliomyelitis in the United States, ALS has become the disease that most commonly affects the anterior horn cell. Although this disease may begin in the extremity or bulbar musculature, it inexorably progresses to involve the muscles of respiration. Thus, management of respiratory complications of ALS and end-of-life decisions associated with respiratory failure become extremely important factors in the management of this disease. Acute neuropathy can also contribute to respiratory insufficiency, which may be precipitous and potentially fatal if not appropriately managed. These complications are well recognized in the setting of acute inflammatory polyradiculopathy (GBS). Attention has also been paid to the entity of critical illness neuropathy, which can contribute to ventilator dependence in the patient recovering from bacteremia and multiorgan system failure.

Amyotrophic Lateral Sclerosis

ALS is a chronic progressive neurodegenerative disorder with an incidence of 1 to 2 per 100,000 population. Typically, pathology includes degeneration of upper and lower motor neurons, accounting for symptoms of spasticity, hyper-reflexia, wasting, and fasciculations. The clinical presentation of ALS may be quite varied, however, and some patients have preferential involvement of upper motor neuron, lower motor neuron, or bulbar weakness. Progression of weakness is the rule and invariably leads to involvement of the respiratory muscles. Most commonly, slowly progressive respiratory failure occurs in patients with significant pre-existing limb and bulbar weakness who already carry an established diagnosis of ALS. In this setting, progressive weakness of diaphragmatic and accessory muscles of respiration inexorably leads to respiratory failure. Occasionally, precipitous respiratory failure occurs in the patient with established ALS when pneumonia or other pulmonary compromise leads to acute decompensation. Rarely, respiratory failure is the presenting symptom in a patient without the prior diagnosis of ALS. These patients usually have progressive exertional dyspnea and orthopnea caused by diaphragmatic weakness. Pulmonary function tests are generally consistent with neuromuscular disease, displaying a restrictive pattern and decrease in maximal voluntary ventilation and negative inspiratory force. In these cases when the patient has no other symptoms or signs of ALS, the diagnosis becomes largely one of exclusion and is established only after ruling out pulmonary or cardiac dysfunction or other neuromuscular causes of respiratory insufficiency [90,91].

Respiratory failure is the proximal cause of death for most patients with ALS, and the monitoring of respiratory status and management of respiratory complications are extremely important in the comprehensive care of these patients. Weakness of the diaphragm and accessory muscles of respiration leads to a decrease in vital capacity, which may present as exertional dyspnea. Patients with significant diaphragmatic involvement often complain of orthopnea, owing to diaphragm elevation from increased abdominal pressure when they lie in the supine position. As weakness of the respiratory muscles advances, the patient may become progressively tachypneic and hypoxemic. Hypoxemia is often more pronounced when the patient is sleeping, especially when skeletal muscle tone is inhibited during rapid eye movement sleep. Patients may experience frequent nocturnal arousals caused by hypoxemia and complain of excessive daytime somnolence and morning headache. On clinical examination, reduced diaphragmatic excursion may be felt by deep palpation, and paradoxical respiratory movements may be noted. Fluoroscopic evaluation may be helpful in assessing diaphragmatic function, although in the sitting position, even severely weakened diaphragms may appear to move down as a result of passive relaxation of the abdominal musculature. For this reason, measurement of transdiaphragmatic pressures via the simultaneous measurement of gastric and esophageal balloon pressures remains the gold standard in evaluating function of the diaphragm [92].

Serial pulmonary function testing may also be helpful in evaluating respiratory weakness. The earliest and most sensitive sign of respiratory compromise on standard pulmonary function testing is a reduced maximal voluntary ventilation. Serial vital capacities may also be helpful in following respiratory status. Routine blood gas analysis is usually not helpful, as gas exchange is relatively well preserved until late in the disease, when FVC is near 20% of predicted. Measurements of the maximal negative inspiratory force and maximal expiratory force correlate well with subjective symptoms of dyspnea [93] and also give an indication of whether the patient is able to cough and effectively clear secretions, which usually require a maximal expiratory pressure of greater than 40 cm H_2O.

The most important principle in the management of patients with respiratory compromise caused by ALS is prevention of further pulmonary compromise that can lead to acute decompensation. It is often difficult or impossible to wean patients with advanced ALS from mechanical ventilation, even when a potentially reversible component to the respiratory failure exists. Thus, it is imperative that pneumonia be recognized early and treated aggressively. Pneumococcal and yearly influenza vaccines should be administered. Patients with advanced ALS often have bulbar weakness and are prone to aspiration. This can be minimized by having the patient eat in an upright position with his or her neck flexed. Mechanically soft and pureed foods are usually fairly well tolerated in this position until bulbar weakness is severe. Ultimately, these aspiration precautions become insufficient and patients may require a gastrostomy or jejunostomy to minimize risk of aspiration. Therapy with supplemental oxygen can relieve dyspnea and associated air hunger, and home oxygen usually begun at 2 liters via nasal cannula may be helpful. Administration of theophylline has been demonstrated to improve diaphragmatic function and may be of modest benefit to some patients [94].

Ultimately, as respiratory weakness progresses, patients need some form of ventilatory assistance. The decision to undergo tracheostomy and institute positive pressure ventilation should not be made lightly, as patients are usually ventilator-dependent for the remainder of their lives, even if some component of potentially reversible pulmonary disease exists. Several options can forestall this decision, as both positive- and negative-pressure noninvasive modes of ventilatory support exist. Negative pressure devices include the wrap ventilator and shell ventilator [95,96]. Other options such as the rocker bed or abdominal binder rely on abdominal displacement and are relatively inefficient. These devices may be indicated for patients in whom maximal negative inspiratory force has dropped below 30 mm H_2O or in those who are retaining carbon dioxide [97]. Extrapolating from data on patients with severe chronic obstructive pulmonary disease, intermittently resting the diaphragm may improve respiratory function sufficiently to prolong the decision as to whether to perform tracheostomy [98]. Noninvasive devices that deliver positive pressure ventilatory assistance also exist, and nasal intermittent positive pressure ventilators have the advantage of being less cumbersome and are usually relatively well tolerated. Although most patients opt against tracheostomy and long-term mechanical ventilation, this remains a final option and can be provided at home, given a motivated family and adequate financial resources.

Guillain-Barré Syndrome

GBS is an autoimmune, mediated, acute monophasic demyelinating polyneuropathy with an incidence of approximately 0.5–2.0 cases per 100,000 population per year [99,100]. It is the most common peripheral neuropathy to cause respiratory failure, and approximately 15–20% of all affected patients require mechanical ventilation [101], although in tertiary centers, this may reach 40–80%. The overall mortality varies between 2.4% and 6.4%, although outcome is considerably worse in patients who require mechanical ventilation [101,102]. The diagnosis of GBS should be entertained in any patient with a rapidly progressing polyneuropathy. Symptoms are usually symmetric and associated with areflexia. Patients often give a history of recent viral-like gastrointestinal or pulmonary illness, and GBS has been associated with *Campylobacter* infection [103,104]. The diagnosis is supported by compatible cerebrospinal fluid findings (elevated protein with a paucity of cells) and electrodiagnostic studies suggestive of demyelination (reduction in nerve conduction velocity, partial motor conduction block, abnormal temporal dispersion, absent F-response). Occasionally, evidence of axonal involvement is seen as well, and when the compound muscle action potential amplitude is less than 20% of normal, patients have a poor prognosis.

Complications of respiratory failure remain a significant source of morbidity in patients with GBS. Essentially, three ways in which an acute polyneuropathy can lead to acute respiratory insufficiency exist: lack of airway protection, inability to maintain adequate ventilation because of weakness of the muscles of respiration, and pulmonary complications that arise from weakness.

The initial symptoms of classic GBS are distal paresthesias followed by ascending weakness. Cranial nerve paresis may develop with advanced disease. This usually evolves over 1 to 3 weeks after initial symptom onset. Variants of GBS have also been described in which bulbar muscles are the first to be involved. Progressive denervation and weakness of the laryngeal and glottic muscles lead to difficulty in swallowing and coughing and predispose the patient to aspiration [105]. It is important to recognize that patients may be at risk for aspiration before the gag reflex is affected noticeably. Weakness of the tongue and retropharyngeal muscles can cause positional airway obstruction. Onset of nasal speech or difficulty with swallowing or tongue protrusion may herald imminent ventilatory failure [106]. Even in patients with adequate respiratory function, intubation may be justified in those with compromised protection of the upper airway. In any event, intubation may be warranted for airway protection.

Acute respiratory failure is the major life-threatening complication in GBS. Serial assessment of respiratory muscle parameters is crucial in the patient with recently diagnosed GBS, as ventilatory muscle insufficiency may not correlate well with the general neuromuscular examination, and respiratory function may be compromised before clinical signs of ventilatory insufficiency are obvious. Measurement of maximum inspiratory force is often helpful in the assessment of respiratory status. Normally, inspiratory force should exceed 50 cm H_2O; patients who generate less than 20 cm H_2O are at high risk for ventilatory insufficiency [107,108]. FVC, which can be measured at bedside, may also be a useful assessment, as an FVC of less than 15 ml/kg is associated with an increased risk of ventilatory failure. Chest radiographs may reveal subsegmental atelectasis or infiltrate as respiratory insufficiency evolves. Serial blood gas determinations may be of only marginal usefulness in evaluating early respiratory insufficiency, as hypoxemia, hypercarbia, and respiratory acidosis are relatively late findings.

Even in the absence of formal ventilatory parameters, much can be learned at the bedside by clinical examination. Tachypnea, decreased tidal volumes, and paradoxical diaphragmatic excursions are early signs of respiratory compromise. Vital capacity can be approximated by having the patient count as high as possible on a single exhalation. The patient's ability to count rapidly on one breath from 1 to 25 reflects a vital capacity of greater than 20 ml/kg [109]. Patients can alternate between the use of major and accessory respiratory muscles or activate accessory muscles during quiet breathing. A bedside assessment of the strength of the cough can be performed by simply observing the patient cough on command.

In the patient who has evolving symptoms of respiratory insufficiency or requires repeated nocturnal assessments, early intubation is usually indicated. This strategy often minimizes pulmonary complications and avoids the inherent risk of emergency intubation. This is of particular importance in GBS, as the use of succinylcholine can cause hyperkalemia owing to extrajunctional chemosensitivity of denervated muscles [110,111]. Ideally, intubation of patients with GBS should be performed by topically anesthetizing the airway and administering a short-acting benzodiazepine and atropine. If the patient cannot be prepared adequately or the intubation is emergent, laryngoscopy and endotracheal intubation can be performed safely using rapid-sequence techniques. After the decision is made to intubate, both synchronized intermittent mandatory ventilation and pressure support are appropriate modes of mechanical ventilation. In patients with electromyographic (EMG) evidence of axonal involvement or a reduction of the compound muscle action potential of less than 20% of normal, prognosis is poor, and early tracheostomy may be indicated [112]. Approximately one-third of patients no longer need ventilatory assistance after 2 weeks, and some patients may be better served by forestalling the decision for tracheostomy until after the second week of intubation [107,113]. At this time, any therapeutic intervention (i.e., plasmapheresis or intravenous gamma globulin [IVIG]) has been completed and the disease course can be predicted with greater accuracy.

Weaning from mechanical ventilation is usually considered when ventilatory muscle strength begins to improve, as evidenced by an FVC of greater than 15 ml/kg and a maximum inspiratory force of greater than 20 cm H_2O. Oxygenation should also be satisfactory, and the chest radiograph should be free of atelectasis or infiltrate. Weaning can be accomplished satisfactorily either by decreasing the pressure support or by reducing the synchronized intermittent mandatory ventilations, depending on the ventilatory mode used. A small percentage of patients with GBS fail to wean despite satisfactory measurements of respiratory strength and after exclusion of factors such as malnutrition, electrolyte abnormality, or infection. This may be caused by unappreciated residual diaphragmatic weakness or a "discoordination syndrome" of the respiratory muscles, leading to ineffective breathing [109]. Although the exact etiology of the latter syndrome is unclear, it has been attributed to residual autonomic neuropathy.

In addition to acute respiratory failure, many deaths in GBS are attributable to pulmonary complications. This is especially unfortunate because most respiratory complications are preventable or treatable. Postural drainage and chest physiotherapy are the mainstays of treatment. Caution must be exercised during therapy, as patients with GBS often have autonomic hypersensitivity, and reports that chest percussion and airway suctioning can result in dangerous arrhythmias or hypotension exist [114,115]. Subcutaneous low-dose heparin or pneumatic calf compression decreases the risk of deep vein thrombosis, and warfarin (Coumadin) anticoagulation should be considered in patients with prolonged quadriparesis. In addition to supportive care, plasmapheresis and IVIG have been proved effective in reducing time to recovery when they are administered in the acute setting.

Critical Illness Polyneuropathy

Since the 1980s, CIP has become recognized as a major cause of failure to wean and weakness in the ICU. Although the pathogenesis of CIP has never been clearly defined, it is probably caused by nerve ischemia and is related to the septic syndrome. The diagnosis should be considered in any patient with sepsis, prolonged stay in the ICU, weakness, or failure to wean after other causes of neuromuscular weakness such as electrolyte abnormality, GBS, or prolonged neuromuscular blockade have been ruled out.

CIP is fairly prevalent in the ICU, and electrodiagnostic evidence of this disorder may be present in as many as 3% of all patients in the medical or surgical ICU [115]. It is highly associated with length of ICU stay and has never been reported in a patient hospitalized for less than 7 days. It is also associated with bacteremia, multiorgan system failure, hyperglycemia, and hypoalbuminemia, although it is likely that the latter two criteria are just markers for the critically ill patient. In a subgroup of patients with sepsis, multiorgan system failure, and prolonged ICU stay, as many as 70% exhibit clinical or electrodiagnostic evidence of CIP [116]. It is usually associated with metabolic ("septic") encephalopathy and should be suspected in the patient with sepsis and improving encephalopathy in whom multiple attempts to wean from mechanical ventilation have failed.

Clinically, CIP usually presents with symmetric, primarily distal weakness. Disproportionate motor involvement is present, although the patient may report sensory symptoms, and the latter may be difficult to evaluate in the ICU setting. Involvement of the muscles of respiration is common, although the severity of the neuropathy does not necessarily predict the degree of respiratory insufficiency. Involvement of the bulbar musculature is distinctly unusual, and when present should suggest an alternative diagnosis, such as GBS or myasthenia gravis. There have been no reports of autonomic abnormalities, although this has not been systematically studied. On neurologic examination, patients usually display distal motor weakness and hyporeflexia. In severe cases, patients may have areflexia, quadriplegia, and paralysis of the muscles of respiration, with relative sparing of the cranial musculature. Fasciculations and wasting may be present [117].

The clinical diagnosis of CIP may be supported by electrodiagnostic testing, which is consistent with a primary axonopathy. Nerve conduction studies commonly reveal reduced compound motor and sensory amplitudes without evidence of significant slowing or conduction block. F-response latencies are usually normal, as are repetitive stimulation studies. Needle EMG may reveal increased recruitment ratio and duration of motor units. Fibrillation potentials and positive sharp waves may also be present, suggesting partial denervation. Patients often have electrodiagnostic evidence of diaphragmatic involvement, as measured by phrenic nerve stimulation and diaphragmatic compound muscle action potential. This may be helpful in establishing the cause of failure to wean. Only 50% of patients with electrodiagnostic evidence of CIP have clinical features of this entity, suggesting a broad spectrum of clinical severity.

The pathogenesis of CIP remains unclear but is likely associated with the septic syndrome and the release of histamine and inflammatory cytokines that impair the microcirculation, causing nerve ischemia and endoneural edema. Alternatively, the primarily distal nature of the axonopathy associated with CIP has prompted speculation that this entity is caused by a defect in axonal transport. Pathology reveals a noninflammatory axonal degeneration. Chromatolysis of anterior horn cells and dorsal root ganglia has been reported [117].

No specific therapy for CIP exists except supportive care. Because some of CIP's clinical manifestations may overlap with those of GBS, a small uncontrolled trial of plasmapheresis was attempted without evidence of benefit [118]. Although the prognosis for improvement of neuropathy is good, the pool of patients in whom CIP develops is quite sick, and approximately 50% die owing to underlying causes such as sepsis or multiorgan system failure [117]. Those with mild to moderate neuropathy may improve over weeks to months, although occasional patients with severe polyneuropathy may not improve.

Disorders of the Neuromuscular Junction

Disorders of neuromuscular transmission may also contribute to ventilatory insufficiency in the ICU. Although most patients have an established diagnosis of myasthenia gravis before their first respiratory crisis, this condition can be induced by drugs given during hospitalization or unmasked by illness or drugs that further impair neuromuscular transmission. Botulism is another disorder that affects cholinergic transmission and may be associated with respiratory compromise. Probably the most common cause of neuromuscular junction abnormalities in the ICU is iatrogenic secondary to injudicious use of paralytic agents. This may be especially troublesome in patients with renal disease, who may have impaired clearance of these agents. For this reason, it is helpful to intermittently stop administration of all paralytic agents and to monitor patients with a "train-of-four" stimulator.

Myasthenia Gravis

Myasthenia gravis is an autoimmune disease characterized by fluctuating weakness caused by impaired cholinergic transmission at the neuromuscular junction.

This is believed to be caused by binding of circulating antibodies to postsynaptic receptors. Myasthenia has a prevalence rate of approximately 1 to 10,000 and is associated with a bimodal pattern of onset, with peak incidence in women between the ages of 20 and 30 years and men between the sixth and seventh decade of life [119,120]. Systemic myasthenia (as opposed to isolated involvement of the extraocular muscles) usually involves the shoulder and pelvic girdles and neck flexors. In approximately 30% of all patients with myasthenia, weakness of the muscles of respiration develops at some point. Profound weakness of the diaphragm and accessory muscles of respiration may evolve rapidly, leading to acute respiratory insufficiency or "myasthenic crisis" in 15–20% of patients with this disorder [121,122]. When this occurs, the patient may experience dramatic respiratory compromise that necessitates emergent ventilatory support. Several studies have suggested that the danger of death is greatest in the first year after diagnosis [123].

The presentation of fluctuating ocular, bulbar, and facial weakness should immediately raise the clinical suspicion of myasthenia gravis. Isolated respiratory involvement has been reported but is rare. If a consistent deficit or easily fatigable muscle group is found, prompt and dramatic improvement with intravenous administration of edrophonium is also strongly suggestive of the diagnosis. Antibodies directed against the acetylcholine receptor are present in 85–90% of patients with generalized myasthenia. Electrodiagnostic studies may also be of value in confirming the diagnosis. Characteristically, a decremental response in the amplitude of the compound muscle action potential is seen during stimulation at 3 Hz per second. The finding of jitter, or variability of successive discharges from a single fiber, is sensitive for disease at the neuromuscular junction but is not specific for myasthenia gravis.

Acute exacerbations of myasthenia may be associated with precipitous compromise in respiratory muscle strength, and it is imperative that patients be kept under extremely close observation. Although static inspiratory and expiratory mouth pressures are more sensitive to early respiratory weakness, serial measurements of FVC are indicated in the acute setting [92]. In general, FVC of less than 10–15 ml/kg is suggestive of impending ventilatory failure and is an indication for elective intubation. As the vital capacity falls, basilar atelectasis often develops, resulting in a mild ventilation-perfusion mismatch, as blood is shunted through a poorly ventilated lung. Thus, one of the earliest blood gas abnormalities is mild hypoxemia. As with many of the progressive neuromuscular disorders, elective intubation may be most appropriately performed on the clinical grounds of tachypnea or discomfort, as significant blood gas abnormalities of hypercarbia or hypoxemia are usually late findings.

After the decision is made to initiate mechanical ventilation, cholinergic medication is usually temporarily discontinued. In theory, overtreatment with cholinergic agents and subsequent cholinergic crisis can precipitate respiratory failure in myasthenic patients, although this is a distinctly uncommon clinical presentation. After patients have been stabilized on mechanical ventilation, therapy is aimed at optimizing respiratory status by instituting pulmonary toilet and aggressively treating underlying infection. It should be remembered that a long list of medications can unmask or exacerbate myasthenic symptoms, including procainamide, quinine, quinidine, and many beta blockers. Far and away the most common offending agents are aminoglycoside antibiotics, and the possibility that latent myasthenia is being unmasked should be considered in the ICU patient with progressive bulbar and respiratory weakness on these agents. Successful weaning is best correlated with maximal inspiratory and expiratory pressures rather than vital capacity.

Myasthenic crisis is usually treated acutely with plasmapheresis, IVIG, or a combination of plasma exchange followed by IVIG. Plasmapheresis has historically been the mainstay of treatment for myasthenic crisis and preoperative care. Although regimens vary from institution to institution, it is usually performed as a series of five to eight exchanges (1.5–2.0 liters/exchange) on a daily or every-other-day basis. Growing evidence exists that IVIG (usually given in a dosage of 0.4 g/kg for 5 days) is beneficial as well, although the mechanism of action has never been clearly defined.

Anticholinesterase agents remain the mainstay of long-term treatment in myasthenia. When response to anticholinesterase agents is inadequate, a trial of corticosteroids is warranted. It should be kept in mind that prednisone may initially exacerbate the symptoms of myasthenia, and all patients in unstable condition should be hospitalized and closely monitored for evidence of respiratory decompensation when treatment is initiated. In severe cases with inadequate response to steroids and anticholinesterase agents, immunosuppression with azathioprine or cyclophosphamide may be attempted. Thymectomy may also be beneficial and is recommended in the 10% of patients with thymoma and, by some authorities, in all postpubescent patients under the age of 60 with inadequate response to medical therapy. Approximately one-third of patients have a remission with thymectomy, and another 45% show some degree of clinical response.

Eaton-Lambert Myasthenic Syndrome

Eaton-Lambert myasthenic syndrome is a disease of neuromuscular transmission caused by circulating antibodies directed against the presynaptic calcium channels. Eaton-Lambert syndrome is relatively uncommon, with an incidence of approximately 1 in 1,000,000; in more than one-half of cases it is associated with neoplasia, usually small cell carcinoma of the lung [124]. Initial symptoms often include proximal muscle weakness and dry mouth, a sign of autonomic dysfunction. Bulbar weakness and progressive respiratory failure may occur as well [125,126]. The diagnosis of Eaton-Lambert myasthenic syndrome can be confirmed by electrodiagnostic testing, which reveals facilitation on high-frequency stimulation. Symptomatic treatment with pyridostigmine or 3,4-diaminopyrimidine (where available) may benefit some patients.

Botulism

Botulism is a disorder of neuromuscular transmission caused by the exotoxin *Clostridium botulinum*. Disease is food borne, and usually associated with home-preserved vegetables. Although outbreaks have been reported throughout the United States, botulism is much more common in the western portion of the country. Botulism toxin is believed to interfere with the presynaptic release of acetylcholine, although the exact mechanism remains incompletely understood.

In the typical course of botulism, symptoms appear during the first several days after ingestion of contaminated food. Prodromal gastrointestinal symptoms, including nausea, vomiting, and anorexia, may be present, but this is not always the case. Clinical findings include mydriasis, ileus, and dry mouth. Eye findings are usually the first sign of neurologic involvement and include intermittent extraocular muscle weakness, ptosis, and poorly reactive pupils. Other signs of defective cholinergic transmission, including dry mouth, urinary retention, orthostatic hypotension, and constipation may occur as well. Neurologic deterioration usually takes place over the first 48–72 hours and may include progressive bulbar and extremity weakness. The muscles of respiration may become involved as well, and before supportive care was readily available, mortality of greater than 50% was usually caused by respiratory compromise.

The initial symptoms of diplopia and ptosis with signs of intermittent extraocular muscle and bulbar weakness can cause the misdiagnosis of myasthenia gravis. One helpful distinction is that the pupils are poorly reactive in botulism. The diagnosis of botulism can be confirmed by nerve conduction studies, which reveal an increase in amplitude with rapid repetitive stimulation (similar to the findings of Eaton-Lambert myasthenic syndrome). Treatment of patients with botulism is largely supportive and directed toward the prevention of secondary complications such as pulmonary embolism or pneumonia. Respiratory involvement usually occurs during the first week of illness, and patients with progressive neurologic symptoms should be placed under close observation during this period. Trivalent antiserum should also be administered as soon as the diagnosis is suspected. Full recovery may take weeks or months, with ocular motility usually showing the first signs of improvement.

Respiratory Failure Associated with Inherited and Acquired Myopathies

Renewed attention has been paid to the diagnosis of critical illness myopathy, a fulminant noninflammatory myopathy associated with the use of intravenous steroids and paralytic agents, as a cause of weakness and failure to wean in the ICU. Although this entity may be the most dramatic, a variety of inherited and acquired myopathies may contribute to ventilatory dysfunction. Usually, this occurs in the setting of established disease, as with muscular dystrophy. Occasionally, a diagnostic dilemma arises when respiratory dysfunction is the presenting symptom of inherited myopathy, as can occur with the adult variant of acid maltase deficiency. Inflammatory myopathies are the most common form of primary acquired muscle disease and may contribute to respiratory compromise, although frank respiratory failure is distinctly uncommon. Finally, metabolic and endocrine disturbances, such as hypokalemia, hypophosphatemia, and hypothyroidism, can directly affect respiratory muscle function and contribute to respiratory compromise.

Myopathy of Critical Illness

There has been increasing recognition of a syndrome of acute fulminant myopathy in critically ill patients [127,128]. This syndrome, which was first reported in 1977, is usually but not invariably associated with the coadministration of steroids and nondepolarizing neuromuscular blockers [129]. A common clinical scenario is a relatively young patient in the ICU who receives a several-day course of vecuronium or pancuronium bromide in conjunction with intravenous steroids for status asthmaticus. When the neuromuscular blockade is discontinued, the patient is noted to be quadriparetic and reliant on ventilatory support. The acute and fulminant nature of this syndrome may help to distinguish it from steroid myopathy.

The pathogenesis of critical care myopathy is unclear. A similar myopathy has been reproduced in experimental animals given dexamethasone after surgical denervation [130]. Steroid receptors are upregulated in denervated or immobilized muscle, which has been postulated to account for the severe toxicity of steroids in this setting [131]. On examination by electron microscopy, affected muscle may reveal a loss of myosin, a finding that has also been described in patients with acute quadriparetic myopathy [132,133]. It has been speculated that neuromuscular blockade may create a functionally denervated state, rendering the muscle more vulnerable to the effects of steroids. It is unclear to what extent pre-existing neuropathy or neuropathy of critical illness may play a role in contributing to this disorder, although it is worth noting that occasional patients have been described who have not received paralytic agents [132,134,135].

The diagnosis of critical illness myopathy should be entertained in the acutely weak patient with failure to wean, especially after the recent administration of steroids and nondepolarizing neuromuscular blockade. Clinical examination usually reveals muscle wasting and moderate to severe diffuse flaccid paresis. Creatine phosphokinase levels may be normal or elevated. Electrodiagnostic testing usually reveals myopathic changes, but one-third of patients may have neuropathic changes as well [128,131]. Diagnosis is aided by muscle biopsy, which usually indicates the loss of myosin fibers with relative preservation of actin filaments and Z disks. Adenosine triphosphatase stain often reveals central pallor of muscle fibers [132].

Treatment of acute myopathy associated with steroids and nondepolarizing agents is largely supportive, and prognosis is excellent. It is hoped that recognition of this entity will lead to a more judicious use of prolonged neuromuscular blockade with nondepolarizing agents in the setting of high-dose steroids and close monitoring of at-risk patients.

Muscular Dystrophy

Duchenne's and Becker's muscular dystrophy are X-linked diseases caused by mutation of the gene that codes for dystrophin, a cytoskeletal protein. Patients with Duchenne's muscular dystrophy present in childhood with progressive proximal muscle weakness, which inexorably progresses to respiratory failure during the first two decades of life. Becker's muscular dystrophy is a less severe variant and patients may not become symptomatic until later in life. Respiratory management of these muscular dystrophies is targeted toward the prevention and early treatment of respiratory infections via the use of pneumococcal and influenza vaccines and aggressive pulmonary toilet, which usually includes physiotherapy and incentive spirometry. Scoliosis is a common problem, and spinal fixation often improves patient comfort, although no conclusive data that this changes the clinical progression of respiratory failure exist [136]. Central respiratory drive is preserved in patients with muscular dystrophy, but as respiratory muscle weakness advances, they are unable to respond normally to hypoxemia or hypercarbia by increasing tidal volumes [137]. Instead, they are forced to increase minute ventilation by increasing respiratory rate, and tachypnea may be an early finding of impending respiratory compromise. When the FVC drops to below 30% of predicted value, acute decompensation may be precipitated by infection, pulmonary embolism, surgery, or the administration of respiratory depressants. Ideally, counseling regarding end-of-life decisions and mechanical ventilation will have been made well before this time.

Several different modes of ventilatory support have been advocated for advanced respiratory weakness in patients with muscular dystrophy. Noninvasive positive pressure systems such as bilevel positive airway pressure may be relatively well tolerated, although the risk of aspiration caused by associated bulbar dysfunction is not diminished. The use of intermittent positive pressure ventilation has met with marginal success in this population [138,139]. Nocturnal negative pressure ventilation may also forestall tracheostomy, although body ventilators may be cumbersome, uncomfortable, and associated with an increased risk of aspiration and intermittent upper airway obstruction [140]. These modes of nocturnal ventilatory support can reduce the incidence of complications such as cor pulmonale and pulmonary hypertension, as well as improve daytime respiratory function [138,141]. Ultimately, however, patients require tracheostomy for pulmonary toilet and continuous ventilatory support.

Myotonic Dystrophy

Myotonic dystrophy is the most common form of muscular dystrophy in adults, with an estimated incidence of 1 in 8,000 [142]. This condition is often associated with myotonia, cataracts, muscle weakness, and cardiac conduction abnormalities. Respiratory insufficiency commonly occurs and may be disproportionate to limb weakness. Alveolar hypoventilation is often caused by diaphragmatic dysfunction; both myotonia and weakness have been documented by EMG even in early disease, when symptomatic extremity involvement is minimal [143,144]. In addition to diaphragmatic involvement, respiratory function may be further compromised by myotonia of the chest wall. In patients with intercostal myotonia, respiratory function may improve after the administration of antimyotonic agents such as quinine or phenytoin [145]. Patients with advanced myotonic dystrophy may also have associated pharyngeal weakness and are particularly prone to aspiration [146]. Specific aspiration precautions, such as elevating the head of the bed, may help to reduce the incidence of pulmonary infections. Obstructive sleep apnea is also commonly seen in patients with myotonic dystrophy and should be considered in individuals who complain of excessive daytime somnolence. Definitive diagnosis of this condition can be made by polysomnography. Extreme sensitivity to anesthesia and depolarizing paralytic agents has also been described in myotonic dystrophy [147]. If general anesthesia is unavoidable, the respiratory status of these patients should be monitored closely after surgery.

Acid Maltase Deficiency

Acid maltase deficiency is a glycogen storage disease characterized by infiltration of affected organs with glycogen vacuoles. The infantile variant (Pompe's disease) is fulminant and is usually rapidly fatal. An adult variant of acid maltase deficiency also exists and may present as a subacute proximal myopathy, often in the third or fourth decade of life. A preferential involvement of the muscles of respiration exists, including the diaphragm, intercostals, and pectoralis muscles [148,149]. Early symptoms of respiratory compromise are common; acid maltase deficiency may present as isolated diaphragm weakness [150]. These patients may pose a diagnostic dilemma until the diagnosis is confirmed by muscle biopsy, which reveals a vacuolar myopathy with high glycogen content and acid phosphatase reactivity in vacuoles. No specific treatment other than supportive care exists for acid maltase deficiency at this time.

Inflammatory Myopathies

Three distinct disorders fall under the category of idiopathic inflammatory myopathy: dermatomyositis, polymyositis, and inclusion body myositis. Patients with inflammatory myopathy usually present with subacute proximal weakness. Respiratory weakness is uncommon, but may occur with fulminant cases of dermatomyositis or polymyositis. It has been advocated that a patient with known myositis and respiratory muscle involvement who presents with respiratory failure precipitated by infection receive a course of IVIG in addition to antibiotics [151]. Respiratory symptoms are more likely caused by interstitial lung disease, which is present in approximately 20–30% of patients with polymyositis or dermatomyositis [152]. Pneumonitis is usually associated with the clinical features of dry cough and dyspnea. The diagnosis is confirmed by a compatible chest radiograph and decreased diffusion coefficient on formal pulmonary function testing. Respiratory symptoms may also be secondary to pulmonary hypertension, which has been described with inflammatory myopathy [153]. Approximately 50% of patients with inflammatory myopathy and associated pneumonitis are steroid responsive. In patients who are unable to tolerate steroids or whose disease is refractory to these drugs, immunosuppressive agents may be of benefit.

Bulbar Weakness

Many of the same neuromuscular disease processes that cause respiratory weakness can also result in bulbar weakness. Weakness of the oropharyngeal musculature can lead to nasal regurgitation, dysphagia, and aspiration. These patients are particularly prone to recurrent pneumonia caused by aspiration of food and secretions. In the acute setting, endotracheal intubation is often justified for airway protection and to protect against aspiration of secretions. Patients with dysphagia caused by neuromuscular weakness often have particular difficulty with liquids, as opposed to patients with mechanical obstruction of the esophagus, who will have greater difficulty with solids. Pharyngeal weakness may be caused by disease that involves the bilateral upper motor neurons, lower motor neurons, neuromuscular junction, or muscle. As with respiratory insufficiency, a logical approach to pharyngeal weakness involves localization and identification of the disease process causing the deficit. Common causes of bulbar weakness are outlined in Table 1.1.

Bilateral interruption of the descending corticospinal tracts causes pseudobulbar palsy, an upper motor neuron weakness of the pharyngeal muscles. This condition is characterized by spastic paresis of the pharyngeal musculature and emotional lability. On examination, patients with pseudobulbar palsy have evidence of dysarthria and a hyperactive jaw jerk. This condition is particularly common in patients with diffuse intracranial small vessel disease and the lacunar state. Clinically, these patients may have evidence of gait apraxia and multi-infarct dementia as well. Pseudobulbar palsy is also common with the extrapyramidal syndromes such as Parkinson's disease and progressive supranuclear palsy. This diagnosis is aided by findings of bradykinesia, coarse tremor, rigidity, and postural instability on examination. Patients with progressive supranuclear palsy may have many of the same extrapyramidal features as patients with Parkinson's disease, but are resistant to Sinemet and may lose downgaze early in the course of their disease. Occasionally, demyelinating disease may also cause a pseudobulbar picture.

Intrinsic brain stem disease can also cause pharyngeal weakness. Because in this case lower motor neurons are injured, the jaw jerk and gag reflex is often diminished or absent. On clinical examination, patients with brain stem disease frequently have eye findings such as skew deviation or ipsipulsion. Common causes of brain stem impairment include (ischemic) vertebrobasilar disease, hemorrhage, demyelination, or neoplasm.

Pharyngeal function may also be affected by neuropathy or neuronopathy. GBS is an acute inflammatory polyradiculopathy frequently encountered in the ICU. Classically, GBS presents with ascending weakness, and bulbar function is affected relatively late in the course of disease. Variants of GBS have been described that preferentially affect brain stem function, and these patients may have early involvement of pharyngeal musculature. In either event, this disorder is usually self-limited. ALS may initially affect the lower or upper motor neurons that innervate the bulbar or extremity musculature. Regardless of the initial presentation, bulbar weakness is common, and patients are subject to repeated aspiration pneumonias and risk further ventilatory decompensation if gastrostomy is not performed. The lower motor neurons that innervate the palate (IX, X), tongue (XII), jaw (V), or face (VII) may also be compressed by skull base tumors or infiltrated in the subarachnoid space by infection or carcinomatous meningitis.

Myasthenia gravis is the most common disease of neuromuscular transmission encountered in the ICU. The muscles of mastication are commonly affected with disease exacerbation. These symptoms fluctuate, and usually respond to treatment with plasmapheresis, IVIG, corticosteroids, and anticholinesterase agents. Bulbar dysfunction may be exacerbated by the increased secretions associated with anticholinesterase treatment. This can be minimized by adding small doses of a peripherally acting anticholinergic drug, such as glycopyrrolate. Botulism is also associated with bulbar weakness secondary to impaired neuromuscular transmission. Again, symptoms may be prolonged but are usually self-limited.

Table 1.1 Common causes of bulbar dysfunction

Anatomic localization	Etiology	Associated history, signs, and symptoms	Diagnostic aids
Pseudobulbar palsy (bilateral disruption of cortico-bulbar tracts)	Vascular disease (lacunar state)	Vascular risk factors (diabetes, hypertension, smoking history) Dementia, gait apraxia	Neuroimaging study (computed tomography/magnetic resonance imaging [MRI]), neurosonology (carotid duplex, transcranial Doppler)
	Demyelinating disease (multiple sclerosis)	Previous history of optic neuritis, symptoms worse with heat; Lhermitte's phenomenon	Cerebrospinal fluid examination (pleocytosis, oligoclonal bands); MRI, visual and somatosensory evoked potentials
	Parkinson's and Parkinson's plus (PSP)	Rigidity, coarse tremor, postural instability, bradykinesia; ophthalmoparesis (PSP)	Response to levodopa (Parkinson's)
Brain stem (lower motor neuron)	Vascular disease (ischemic stroke or hemorrhage)	Vascular risk factors (diabetes mellitus, hypertension, smoking, cardiogenic emboli); skew deviation, ipsipulsion	MRI
Neuropathy or neuronopathy	Amyotrophic lateral sclerosis	Fasciculations, evidence of upper and lower motor neuron disease	Electrodiagnostic testing (electromyography [EMG]/nerve conduction studies)
	Guillain-Barré syndrome	Areflexia, ascending paresthesias and weakness	Lumbar puncture, electrodiagnostic studies
Neuromuscular junction	Myasthenia gravis	Jaw weakness, ptosis, fluctuates with fatigue	Edrophonium test, electrodiagnostic studies (single-fiber EMG), acetylcholine receptor antibody
	Botulism	Dilated, unreactive pupil, bradycardia, constipation; may be associated with gastrointestinal symptoms	Electrodiagnostic studies, serum bioassay
Muscle	Muscular dystrophy (earlier involvement in oculo-pharyngeal, myotonic, then Duchenne's)	Myotonia, frontal balding, cataracts (myotonic dystrophy); family history (Duchenne's)	Electrodiagnostic testing; muscle biopsy, genetic analysis, creatine phosphokinase (CPK)
	Inflammatory myopathy	Subacute onset of proximal muscle weakness; rash (dermatomyositis)	Electrodiagnostic testing; muscle biopsy, CPK
	Associated with steroids, paralytic agents	Recent steroids, nondepolarizing paralytics; failure to wean, may be fulminant	Electrodiagnostic studies, muscle biopsy

PSP = progressive supranuclear palsy.

Finally, pharyngeal weakness may be the result of an inherited or acquired muscle disorder. Pharyngeal weakness may be present with Duchenne's muscular dystrophy, but it is a much more prominent symptom early in the course of oropharyngeal dystrophy. In this setting, patients often require gastrostomy. Inflammatory myopathies may also affect bulbar function but are usually responsive to treatment with corticosteroids or immunosuppressive agents.

In many instances, such as after acute stroke or GBS, bulbar dysfunction is self-limited, and patients should be monitored closely at bedside for signs of aspiration. If any concern exists about the patient's ability to protect the airway from aspiration of food or secretions, a formal swallowing study is often helpful. Barium swallow with cine-esophagogram may help to define the coordination and function of the oral and pharyngeal muscles, as well as resolve the question of whether nasal regurgitation or aspiration of food is taking place. In borderline situations, aspiration precautions may be helpful. These include elevating the head of the bed, swallowing small volumes, and tucking the chin before swallowing. If the patient is at high risk for aspiration, or a prolonged period of pharyngeal weakness is anticipated, gastrostomy is indicated.

REFERENCES

1. Lumsden T. Observation on the respiratory centers in the cat. J Physiol (Lond) 1923;57:153.
2. Lumsden T. The regulation of respiration. J Physiol (Lond) 1923;58:81.
3. Bertrand F, Hugelin A, Vivert JF. A stereologic model of pneumotaxic oscillator based on spatial and temporal distributions of neuronal bursts. J Neurophysiol 1974;37:91.
4. Gautier H, Bertrand F. Respiratory effects of pneumotaxic center lesions and subsequent vagotomy in chronic cats. Respir Physiol 1975;23:71.
5. Berger AJ, Mitchell RA, Herbert DA. Properties of apneutic respiration. Fed Proc 1976;35:633.
6. Khan N, Wang SC. Electrophysiological basis for pontine apneustic center and its role in the integration of the Hering-Breuer reflex. J Neurophysiol 1967;30:301.
7. Cohen MI, Piercey MF, Gootman PM. Synaptic connections between medullary inspiratory neurons and phrenic motor neurons as revealed by cross-correlation. Brain Res 1974;81:319.
8. Merrill EG. Preliminary studies of nucleus retroambigualis—nucleus of the solitary tract interactions in cats. J Physiol (Lond) 1975;244:54.
9. Richter DW, Spyer KM. Cardiorespiratory Control. In A Loewy, KM Spyer (eds), Central Regulation of Autonomic Functions. New York: Oxford University Press, 1990;189.
10. Feldman JL. Neurophysiology of Breathing in Mammals. In FE Bloom (ed), Handbook of Physiology: The Nervous System (Vol 4). Bethesda, MD: American Physiology Society, 1987;463.
11. Merril EG. Finding Respiratory Function for Medullary Respiratory Neurons. In R Bellairs, EG Gray (eds), Essays on the Nervous System. Oxford, UK: Claredon, 1974;451.
12. Newsom DJ, Plum F. Separation of descending spinal pathways to respiratory motor neurons. Exp Neurol 1972;34:78.
13. Newsom DJ. An experimental study of hiccup. Brain 1970;93:851.
14. Weiner WJ, Bergen D. Prevention and Management of the Side Effects of Levodopa. In HL Klawans (ed), Clinical Neuropharmacology (Vol 2). New York: Raven, 1977;1.
15. Lahiri S, Delaney RG. Stimulus interaction in response to the carotid by the chemoreceptor single afferent fibers. Respir Physiol 1975;24:249.
16. Biscoe TJ, Purves MJ, Sampson SR. The frequency of nerve impulses in single carotid by the chemoreceptor afferent fibers recorded in vivo with intact circulation. J Physiol (Lond) 1970;28:121.
17. Berger AJ, Mitchell RA, Severinghaus JW. Regulation of respiration (first of 3 parts). N Engl J Med 1977;297:92.
18. Gelfand R, Lambertson CJ. Dynamic respiratory response to abrupt change if inspired CO_2 at normal and high Po_2. J Appl Physiol 1973;35:903.
19. Bruce EN, Cherniack NS. Central chemoreceptors. J Appl Physiol 1987;62:389.

20. Price WM, Batsel HL. Respiratory neurons participating in sneeze and in response to expiration. Exp Neurol 1970;29:554.
21. Batsel HL, Lanes AJ. Bulbar respiratory neurons participating in the sniff reflex in cats. Exp Neurol 1973;39:469.
22. Tomori Z, Widdicomb JG. Muscular and bronchomotor and cardiovascular reflexes elicited in mechanical stimulation of the respiratory tract. J Physiol (Lond) 1969;200:25.
23. von Euler C, Herrero F, Wexler I. Control mechanisms determining rate and depth of respiratory movements. Respir Physiol 1970;10:93.
24. Clark FJ, von Euler C. On the regulation and depth of breathing. J Physiol (Lond) 1972;222:267.
25. Sampson SR, Vidruk EH. Properties of irritant receptors in the canine lung. Respir Physiol 1975;25:9.
26. Nadel JA. Neurophysiological Aspects of Asthma. In KF Austen, LM Lichtenstein (eds), Asthma. New York: Academic, 1973;29.
27. Mines A. Anonymous Respiratory Physiology. New York: Raven, 1993;113.
28. Road JD. Phrenic afferents and ventilatory control. Lung 1990;168:137.
29. Duron B. Intercostal and Diaphragmatic Muscle Endings and Afferents. In TF Hornbein (ed), Regulation of Breathing. New York: Dekker, 1981;473.
30. Kao FF. An Experimental Study of the Pathway Involved in Exercise Hyperpnea Employing Cross-Circulation Technique. In DJ Cunningham, BB Loyd (eds), The Regulation of Human Respiration. Oxford, UK: Blackwell, 1963;461.
31. McCloskey DI, Mitchel JH. Reflex cardiovascular and respiratory responses originating in exercising muscle. J Physiol (Lond) 1975;250:431.
32. Senapti JM. Effect of stimulation of muscle afferents on ventilation in dogs. J Appl Physiol 1966;21:242.
33. Teitelbaum JS, Magder SA, Roussos C, et al. Effects of diaphragmatic ischemia on inspiratory muscle drive. J Appl Physiol 1966;21:242.
34. Banzett RB, Inbar GF, Brown R, et al. Diaphragm electrical activity during negative lower torso pressure in quadriplegic men. J Appl Physiol 1981;51:654.
35. Fryman DL, Frazier DT. Diaphragm afferent modulation of phrenic motor drive. J Appl Physiol 1987;62:2436.
36. Cheeseman M, Revelette WR. Phrenic afferent contribution to reflexes elicited by changes in diaphragm length. J Appl Physiol 1990;69:640.
37. Speck DF, Revelette WR. Attenuation of phrenic motor discharge by phrenic nerve afferents. J Appl Physiol 1987;62:941.
38. Teitelbaum M, Borel CO, Magder S, et al. Effect of selective diaphragmatic paralysis on the inspiratory motor drive. J Appl Physiol 1993;74:2261.
39. Plum F. Neurological Integration of Behavioural and Metabolic Control of Breathing. In R Porter (ed), Ciba Foundation Hering-Breuer Centenary Symposium: Breathing. London: J & A Churchill, 1970;159.
40. Simon RP. Breathing and the Nervous System. In JM Aminoff (ed), Neurology and General Medicine. New York: Churchill Livingstone, 1990;1.
41. Coulter DL. Partial seizures with apnea and bradycardia. Arch Neurol 1984;41:173.
42. Nelson DA, Ray CD. Respiratory arrest from seizure discharges in limbic system. Arch Neurol 1968;19:199.
43. Fluck DC. Chest movements in hemiplegia. Clin Sci 1966;31:383.
44. Heyman A, Birchfield RI, Sieker HO. Effects of bilateral cerebral infarction on respiratory center sensitivity. Neurology 1958;8:694.
45. Levin BE, Margolis G. Acute failure of autonomic respirations secondary to unilateral brainstem infarct. Ann Neurol 1977;1:583.
46. Atack EA, Suranyi L. Respiratory inhibitory apraxia. Can J Neurol Sci 1975;2:37.
47. Feldman MH. Physiological observations in a chronic case of "locked in" syndrome. Neurology 1971;21:459.
48. Devereaux MW, Keane JR, Davis RL. Automatic respiratory failure associated with infarction in the medulla. Arch Neurol 1973;29:46.
49. Bogousslavsky J, Khurana R, Deruaz JP, et al. Respiratory failure and unilateral caudal brain infarction. Ann Neurol 1990;28:668.
50. Khurana RK. Autonomic dysfunction in pontomedullary stroke [abstract]. Ann Neurol 1982;12:86.
51. Tranmer BI, Tucker WS, Bilbao JM, et al. Sleep apnea following percutaneous cervical cordotomy. Can J Neurol Sci 1987;14:262.
52. Plum F. Apneustic breathing in man. Arch Neurol 1964;10:115.

53. Steegman ET. Primary pontine hemorrhage. J Nerv Ment Dis 1951;114:35.
54. Plum F. Apneustic breathing in man. Arch Neurol 1964;10:101.
55. Sears TA. The respiratory motoneuron and apneusis. Fed Proc 1977;36:2412.
56. Posner JB, Plum F. Toxic effects of carbon dioxide and acetazolamide in hepatic encephalopathy. J Clin Invest 1980;39:1246.
57. Rout MW, Lanhe DJ, Wollner L. Prognosis in acute cerebrovascular accidents in relation to respiratory pattern and blood gas tensions. BMJ 1971;3:7.
58. Bateman DN, Cooper RG, Gibson GJ, et al. Levodopa dosage and ventilatory function in Parkinson's disease. BMJ 1981;190:181.
59. Langer H, Woolf CR. Changes in pulmonary function after treatment with L-dopa. Am Rev Respir Dis 1971;104:440.
60. Lilker ES, Woolf CR. Pulmonary function in Parkinson's syndrome: the effect of thalamotomy. Can Med Assoc J 1968;99:752.
61. Mehta AD, Wright WB, Kirby BJ. Ventilatory function in Parkinson's disease. BMJ 1978;1:1456.
62. Petit JM, Delhez L. Activité électrique du diaphragme dans la maladie de Parkinson. Arch Int Physiol Biochim 1961;69:413.
63. Schiffman PL. A "saw-tooth" pattern in Parkinson's disease. Chest 1985;87:124.
64. Vincken W, Gauthier SG, Dolfuss RE. Involvement of the upper airway muscles in extrapyramidal disorders: a cause of airflow limitation. N Engl J Med 1984;311:428.
65. Vincken WG, Darauay CM, Cosio MG. Reversibility of upper airway obstruction after levodopa therapy in Parkinson's disease. Chest 1989;96:210.
66. Apps MCP, Sheaff PC, Ingram DA, et al. Respiration and sleep in Parkinson's disease. J Neurol Neurosurg Psychiatry 1985;48:1240.
67. Neu HC, Connolly JJ, Schwertley FW. Obstructive respiratory dysfunction in parkinsonian patients. Am Rev Respir Dis 1967;95:33.
68. Granerus AK, Jagenburg R, Nilsson NJ, et al. Respiratory disturbance during L-dopa treatment of Parkinson's syndrome. Acta Med Scand 1974;195:39.
69. Weiner WJ, Goetz CG, Nausieda PA, et al. Respiratory dyskinesias: extrapyramidal function and dyspnea. Ann Intern Med 1978;88:327.
70. Zupnick HM, Brown LK, Miller A, et al. Respiratory dysfunction due to L-dopa therapy for parkinsonism: diagnosis using serial pulmonary function tests and respiratory inductive plethysmography. Am J Med 1990;89:109.
71. Sosin DM, Sacks JJ, Smith SM. Head injury–associated deaths in the United States from 1979 to 1986. JAMA 1989;262:2251.
72. Kraus JF, Franti CE, Riggins RS. Incidence of traumatic spinal cord lesions. J Chronic Dis 1975;28:471.
73. Huldtgren AC, Fugl-Meyer AR, Jonasson E, et al. Ventilatory dysfunction and respiratory rehabilitation in post-traumatic quadriplegia. Eur J Respir Dis 1980;61:347.
74. Goldmann AL, George J. Postural hypoxemia in quadriplegic patients. Neurology 1976;26:815.
75. Mackerssie RC, Karaoianes TG. Use of end-tidal carbon dioxide for monitoring induced hypocapnia in head-injured patients. Crit Care Med 1990;18:764.
76. Suderman VS, Crosby ET, Lui A, et al. Elective oral tracheal intubation in the cervical spine–injured patient. Can J Anaesth 1991;38:785.
77. Meschino A, Devitt JH, Kock JP, et al. The safety of awake tracheal intubation in cervical spine injury. Can J Anaesth 1992;39:114.
78. Twiner LM. Cervical spine immobilization with axial traction: a practice to be discouraged. J Emerg Med 1989;39:114.
79. Smith RB, Crenvik A. Cardiac arrest following succinylcholine administration in patients with central nervous system injuries. Anesthesiology 1970;33:558.
80. Bhaskar KR, Brown R, O'Sullivan DD, et al. Bronchial mucous hypersecretion in acute quadriplegia. Am Rev Respir Dis 1991;143:640.
81. Estenne M, De Troyer A. Cough in tetraplegic patients: an active process. Ann Intern Med 1990;112:22.
82. North JB, Jennett S. Abnormal breathing pattern associated with acute brain damage. Arch Neurol 1974;31:338.
83. Schumacker GR, Rhodes GR, Newell JC, et al. Ventilation-perfusion imbalance after head trauma. Am Rev Respir Dis 1979;119:33.
84. Eberhardt KE. Dose-dependent rate of nosocomial pulmonary infection in mechanically ventilated patients with brain oedema receiving barbiturates: a prospective case study. Infection 1992;20:12.

85. Rogers FB, Shackford SR, Trevisani GT, et al. Neurogenic pulmonary edema in fatal and nonfatal injuries. J Trauma Inj Infect Crit Care 1995;39:860.
86. Martin AM, Simmons RL, Heisterkamp CA. Respiratory insufficiency in combat casualties: I. Pathologic changes in the lungs of patients dying of wounds. Ann Surg 1969;170:30.
87. Ell SR. Neurogenic pulmonary edema: a review of the literature and a perspective. Invest Radiol 1991;26:499.
88. Darnell JC, Jay SJ. Recurrent postictal pulmonary edema: a case report and review of the literature. Epilepsia 1982;23:71.
89. Hardmann JM, Earle KM. Meningococcal infections: a review of 200 fatal cases. J Neuropathol Exp Neurol 1967;26:119.
90. Meyrignac C, Poirier J, Degos JD. Amyotrophic lateral sclerosis presenting with respiratory insufficiency as the primary complaint. Eur Neurol 1985;24:115.
91. Paul GR, Appenzeller O. Dyspnea as the presenting symptom in amyotrophic lateral sclerosis: case report. Dis Chest 1962;42:558.
92. Borel CO, Tilford C, Nichols DG, et al. Diaphragmatic performance during recovery from acute ventilatory failure in Guillain-Barré syndrome and myasthenia gravis. Chest 1991;99:444.
93. Black LF, Hyatt RE. Maximal static respiratory pressures in generalized neuromuscular disease. Am Rev Respir Dis 1971;103:641.
94. Schiffman PL, Belsh JM. Effect of inspiratory resistance and theophylline on respiratory muscle strength in patients with amyotrophic lateral sclerosis. Am Rev Respir Dis 1989;139:1418.
95. Collier CR, Offeldt JE. Ventilatory efficiency in the cuirass respirator in totally paralyzed chronic poliomyelitis patients. J Appl Physiol 1954;6:532.
96. Spalding JMK, Opie L. Artificial respiration with the Tunnicliffe breathing-jacket. Lancet 1958;1:613.
97. Braun SR, Sufit RL, Giovannoni R, et al. Intermittent negative pressure ventilation in the treatment of respiratory failure in progressive neuromuscular disorder. Neurology 1987;37:1874.
98. Braun NMT, Marino WD. Effect of daily intermittent rest of respiratory muscles in patients with severe chronic airflow limitation. Chest 1984;85:59S.
99. Alter M. The epidemiology of Guillain-Barré syndrome. Ann Neurol 1990;27(suppl):S7.
100. Schonberger LB, Hurwitz ES, Katona P. Guillain-Barré syndrome: its epidemiology and associations with influenza vaccination. Ann Neurol 1981;9(suppl):31.
101. Gracey DR, McMichan JC, Divertie MB, et al. Respiratory failure in Guillain-Barré syndrome: a six year experience. Mayo Clin Proc 1982;57:742.
102. Dowling PC, Menonna JP, Cook SD. Guillain-Barré syndrome in greater New York–New Jersey. JAMA 1977;238:317.
103. Ropper AH. *Campylobacter* diarrhea and Guillain-Barré syndrome. Arch Neurol 1988;45:655.
104. Kleyweg RP, Van der Meche FG, Banffer JR. *Campylobacter* infection in the Guillain-Barré syndrome (abstract). J Neurol 1988;235:23.
105. Loh L. Neurological and neuromuscular disease. Br J Anaesth 1986;58:190.
106. Ropper AH. The Guillain-Barré syndrome. N Engl J Med 1992;326:1130.
107. Ropper AH, Kehne SM. Guillain-Barré syndrome: management of respiratory failure. Neurology 1985;35:1662.
108. Newton-John H. Prevention of pulmonary complications in severe Guillain-Barré syndrome by early assisted ventilation. Med J Aust 1985;142:444.
109. Ropper AH. Acute Inflammatory Post-infectious Polyneuropathy. In AH Ropper, SF Kennedy (eds), Neurological and Neurosurgical Intensive Care. Gaithersburg, MD: Aspen, 1996;361.
110. Beach TP, Stone WA, Hamelberg W. Circulatory collapse following succinylcholine: report of a patient with diffuse lower motor neuron disease. Anesth Analg 1971;50:431.
111. Sunderrajan EV, Davenport J. The Guillain-Barré syndrome: pulmonary neurological complications. Medicine 1985;64:333.
112. Ropper A, Wijdicks EFM, Truax BT. Guillain-Barré Syndrome. Philadelphia: Davis, 1991.
113. Marsh MH, Gillespie DJ, Baumgartner AE. Timing of tracheostomy in critically ill patients. Chest 1989;96:190.
114. Dalos NP, Borel C, Hanley DF. Cardiovascular autonomic function in Guillain-Barré syndrome. Therapeutic implications of Swan Ganz monitoring. Arch Neurol 1988;45:115.
115. Greenland P, Griggs RC. Arrhythmic complications in the Guillain-Barré syndrome. Arch Intern Med 1980;140:1053.
116. Spitzer RA, Giancarlo T, Maher L, et al. Neuromuscular causes of prolonged ventilator dependency. Muscle Nerve 1992;15:682.

117. Zochodne DW, Bolton CF, Wells GA, et al. Critical illness polyneuropathy: a complication of sepsis and multiple organ failure. Brain 1987;110:819.
118. Wijdicks J, Fulgham J. Failure of high dose IVIG in critical care neuropathy. Muscle Nerve 1994;17:1494.
119. Donaldson DH, Ansher M, Horan SK. The relationship of age to outcome in myasthenia gravis. Neurology 1990;40:786.
120. Perlo VP, Poskanzer DC, Schwab RS, et al. Myasthenia gravis: evaluation of treatment in 1355 patients. Neurology 1966;16:431.
121. Cohen MS, Younger D. Aspects of the natural history of myasthenia gravis: crisis and death. Ann N Y Acad Sci 1981;377:670.
122. Mantegazza R, Beghi E, Pareyson D, et al. A multicentre follow-up study of 1152 patients with myasthenia gravis in Italy. J Neurol 1990;237:339.
123. Simpson JA. Myasthenia Gravis and Myasthenic Syndromes. In JN Walton (ed), Diseases of Voluntary Muscle (5th ed). Edinburgh: Churchill Livingstone, 1988;626.
124. Patel AM, Davila DG, Peters SG. Paraneoplastic syndromes associated with lung cancer. Mayo Clin Proc 1993;68:278.
125. Gracey DR, Southorn PA. Respiratory failure in Lambert-Eaton myasthenic syndrome. Chest 1987;91:716.
126. Laroche CM, et al. Respiratory weakness in the Lambert-Eaton myasthenic syndrome. Thorax 1989;44:913.
127. Hirano M, Ott BR, Raps EC, et al. Acute quadriplegic myopathy: a complication of treatment with steroids, nondepolarizing blocking agents, or both. Neurology 1992;42:2082.
128. Faragher MW, Day BJ, Dennet X. Critical care myopathy: an electrophysiological and histological study. Muscle Nerve 1995;19:516.
129. MacFarlane IA, Rosenthal FD. Severe myopathy after status asthmaticus. Lancet 1977;2:615.
130. Rouleau G, Karpati G, Carpenter S, et al. Glucocorticoid excess induces preferential depletion of myosin in denervated skeletal muscle fibers. Muscle Nerve 1987;10:428.
131. DuBois DC, Almon RR. A possible role for glucocorticoids in denervation atrophy. Muscle Nerve 1981;4:370.
132. Sher JH, Shafiq SA, Shutta HS. Acute myopathy with selective lysis of myosin filaments. Neurology 1979;29:100.
133. Danon MJ, Carpenter S. Myopathy with thick filament (myosin) loss following prolonged paralysis with vecuronium during steroid treatment. Muscle Nerve 1991;14:1131.
134. Knox AJ, Mascie-Taylor BH, Muers MF. Acute hydrocortisone myopathy in acute severe asthma. Thorax 1986;41:411.
135. Van Marle W, Woods KL. Acute hydrocortisone myopathy. BMJ 1980;281:271.
136. Miller RG, Chalmers AC, Dao H, et al. The effect of spine fusion on respiratory function in Duchenne muscular dystrophy. Neurology 1991;41:38.
137. Begin R, Bureau MA, Lupien L, et al. Control of breathing in Duchenne's muscular dystrophy. Am J Med 1980;69:227.
138. Mohr CH, Hill NS. Long-term follow-up of nocturnal ventilatory assistance in patients with respiratory failure due to Duchenne muscular dystrophy. Chest 1990;97:91.
139. McCool FD, Mayewski RF, Shayne DS, et al. Intermittent positive pressure breathing in patients with respiratory muscle weakness. Chest 1986;90:546.
140. Baydur A, Gilgoff I, Prentice W, et al. Decline in respiratory function and experience with long-term assisted ventilation in advanced Duchenne's muscular dystrophy. Chest 1990;97:884.
141. Curran FJ. Night ventilation by body respirators for patients in chronic respiratory failure due to late stage Duchenne muscular dystrophy. Arch Phys Med Rehabil 1981;62:270.
142. Harper PS. Myotonic Dystrophy. London: Saunders, 1989;21.
143. Caughey JE, Pachomov N. The diaphragm in dystrophia myotonica. J Neurol Neurosurg Psychiatry 1959;22:311.
144. Smorto MP, Vignieri MR, Firro B. The diaphragm in dystrophia myotonica. Rev Neurobiol 1972;18:48.
145. Fitting JW, Leuenberger P. Procainamide for dyspnea in myotonic dystrophy. Am Rev Respir Dis 1989;140:1442.
146. Swick HM, Werlin SL, Dodds WJ, et al. Pharyngoesophageal motor function in patients with myotonic dystrophy. Ann Neurol 1981;10:454.
147. Boheimer N, Harris JW, Ward S. Neuromuscular blockade in dystrophia myotonica with atracurium besylate. Anaesthesia 1985;40:872.

148. van der Walt JD, Swash M, Leake J, et al. The pattern of involvement of adult-onset acid maltase deficiency at autopsy. Muscle Nerve 1987;10:272.
149. Rosenow EC, Engel AG. Acid maltase deficiency in adults presenting as respiratory failure. Am J Med 1978;64:485.
150. Sivak ED, Salanga VD, Wilbourn AJ, et al. Adult onset acid maltase deficiency presenting as diaphragmatic paralysis. Ann Neurol 1981;9:613.
151. Frankel RJ, Bennett ED, Borland CD. Pulmonary edema in meningococcal meningitis. Postgrad Med J 1976;52:529.
152. Dickey BF, Myers AR. Pulmonary disease in polymyositis/dermatomyositis. Semin Arthritis Rheum 1984;14:60.
153. Herbert CA, Byrnes TJ, Baethge BA, et al. Exercise limitation in patients with polymyositis. Chest 1990;98:352.

2
Guillain-Barré Syndrome

John B. Winer

Guillain-Barré syndrome (GBS) is a clinical syndrome of acute neuromuscular paralysis caused by a neuropathy. It almost certainly encompasses a number of different pathologic entities, some of which have been identified. It is the major cause of acute neuromuscular paralysis in the Western world and is an important neurologic cause of respiratory failure. Patients with GBS frequently occupy intensive care beds for a considerable length of time, and the management of this disease is challenging and becoming increasingly complex. An attempt was made in 1981 to define the syndrome by specifying required and supportive criteria [1] (Table 2.1). The definition was later refined [2]. The diagnosis essentially is based on a progressive areflexic weakness of more than one limb with onset of less than 4 weeks, together with the exclusion of other recognized discrete causes of similar acute neuropathies, such as toxin exposure or porphyria (Table 2.2). The clinical syndrome includes an acute axonal motor neuropathy synonymous with the Chinese paralytic syndrome and an acute axonal motor and sensory neuropathy originally described by Feasby and associates [3] and defined mainly by its electrophysiology. The classic pathology with demyelination and inflammatory infiltrate is usually known as *acute inflammatory demyelinating polyradiculoneuropathy* [4].

CLINICAL FEATURES

The inflammatory neuropathies constitute a spectrum of disease in which GBS is at one end and chronic inflammatory demyelinating polyneuropathy (CIDP) is at the other (Table 2.3). By convention, disease that continues to progress for at least 8 weeks is termed *CIDP* [5], whereas disease that reaches its nadir within 4 weeks is labeled *GBS*. Disease that progresses for more than 4 weeks, but less than 8, has been termed *subacute inflammatory demyelinating polyneuropathy* [6], although debate exists about whether this group deserves a separate classi-

33

Table 2.1   Diagnostic criteria for Guillain-Barré syndrome

Required	Supportive
Progressive weakness of at least two limbs caused by neuropathy	Relatively symmetric weakness
Areflexia	Mild sensory signs
Progression less than 4 wks	Cranial nerve involvement, especially facial nerve
Neuropathy (e.g., porphyria, toxins, diphtheria)	Absence of other causes for autonomic dysfunction
	Absence of fever with neuropathic symptoms
	Cerebrospinal fluid protein increased
	Cell count normal
	Electrophysiologic evidence of demyelination

fication. Patients with chronic disease have been shown to respond well to steroids [7], which have been proven ineffective for the acute disorder [8,9]. Diagnosis of the classic presentation with very rapidly progressive paralysis associated with absent reflexes and distal numbness and tingling is not difficult (Table 2.4). A purely motor disorder may be confused with botulism and polymyositis. An acute neuropathy in the context of disturbed mental function should arouse suspicion of porphyria or toxin exposure, particularly with lead or hydrocarbons. Occasional patients with sudden-onset bulbar palsy and quadriplegia may be misdiagnosed as having experienced an acute brain stem stroke.

Approximately half of patients with GBS have pain at presentation, usually around the back and sides [10]. A completely sensory presentation has been described, but this is unusual [11,12]. The disease typically starts in the lower limbs, but occasionally begins in the arms and spreads downward. The cranial nerves are frequently involved, usually the facial nerve and the cranial nerves concerned with bulbar function.

Papilledema occasionally develops and can mimic a cerebral tumor. This rare complication of GBS was reviewed extensively by Morley and Reynolds [13]. No convincing correlation appeared to exist between the severity of the neuropathy and the occurrence of papilledema. One proposed mechanism to explain this physical finding was the development of communicating hydrocephalus secondary to the rise in cerebrospinal fluid (CSF) protein. However, no clear correlation with the extent of the CSF protein rise was noted by Morley and Reynolds. Attempts to monitor the absorption of radiolabeled albumin injected into the lumbar CSF have shown normal absorption [14]. Impaired absorption of technetium

Table 2.2   Differential diagnosis of Guillain-Barré syndrome

Toxins, especially lead and organophosphates
Vasculitis—polyarteritis, systemic lupus erythematosus, Churg-Strauss syndrome
Porphyria—acute intermittent and variegate
Polymyositis
Botulism
Acute transverse myelitis

Table 2.3 Inflammatory neuropathies

Guillain-Barré syndrome
   Acute inflammatory demyelinating polyradiculoneuropathy
   Acute motor axonal neuropathy
   Acute motor and sensory axonal neuropathy
Subacute demyelinating polyradiculoneuropathy
Chronic demyelinating polyradiculoneuropathy

pertechnetate from the CSF has been noted to support a degree of communicating hydrocephalus [15]. An alternative explanation of cerebral edema has been proposed [16] based on the histology of cortical tissue removed from a patient with intracellular edema.

Approximately 25% of patients have sufficient respiratory compromise to require assisted ventilation [17]. Recognition of respiratory difficulties in patients with GBS can be extremely difficult and incipient respiratory failure can remain undetected until an acute respiratory paralysis occurs. Careful observation of respiratory rate and tachycardia is important, and regular monitoring of vital capacity is essential. Peak flow, which is a measure of airway diameter, is inappropriate for this monitoring. Similarly, blood gases are very insensitive and do not predict impending respiratory catastrophe. A vital capacity approaching 1 liter, or 15 ml/kg, is usually a sign that assisted ventilation is required. The rate of decrease of vital capacity is important in predicting which patients may need respiratory support. Many patients with respiratory difficulties with GBS do not show the typical features of respiratory distress seen in patients with no neurologic disease. This may, in part, be caused by involvement of vagal receptors, which can mediate the psychological sensation of breathlessness.

Autonomic nerves are typically involved in the pathologic process of GBS, leading to a sinus tachycardia in at least 75% of patients with GBS. Abnormal sweating and variations in RR interval occur very frequently as well [18]. Patients who are being ventilated in intensive care units also often show swings in blood pressure and may show tachy- and bradyarrhythmias [19]. The bradyarrhythmias appear to be the most dangerous, and well-reported cases of sudden cardiac

Table 2.4 Major presenting features of Guillain-Barré syndrome

Feature	Percentage
Limb weakness	100
Numbness	79
Paresthesias	75
Pain	50
Difficulty in swallowing	46
Urinary disturbance	32

Source: J Winer. A clinical and immunological study of Guillain-Barré syndrome. MD Thesis, London University, 1986.

asystole are described. Such episodes often follow tracheal suction or some other form of vagal stimulation [18].

Approximately 34% of patients reach the worst severity of disease within 7 days, 70% within 2 weeks, and 84% within 3 weeks. The severity of the illness was found to be widely variable in one clinical survey [10], with 12% of patients retaining the ability to walk unaided throughout their illness, 7% requiring support to walk, 47% becoming bed bound, 33% requiring ventilation, and 3% dying without being ventilated.

INVESTIGATIONS

A number of investigations are helpful in confirming the diagnosis. Guillain-Barré and Strohl [20] described the striking rise in CSF protein that occurs in their original description. The CSF may contain a small increase in white cells but this is usually less than 50 µl. CSF protein measurements can reach several grams per liter. The rise in CSF usually takes a week to become apparent, causing some diagnostic confusion in the first few days of the illness. In occasional well-documented patients, a raised CSF protein never develops despite repeated CSF analysis throughout the course of the disease [13]. Nerve conduction studies are extremely valuable in confirming the diagnosis of GBS and excluding atypical presentations of cord and muscle disease. Early in the disease these may simply show evidence of conduction block with a decrement in the size of the muscle action potential when recorded proximally to distally [21]. Another early electrophysiologic abnormality is a prolongation of F waves [22]. Sometimes, distal motor latencies are prolonged, particularly in the feet but also in the upper limbs. This finding sometimes leads to the paradox of a totally paralyzed patient in whom the striking electrophysiologic abnormality is a carpal tunnel syndrome. Later in the course of the disease, conduction velocities begin to slow and muscle action potentials fall in size. In variants of the disease, specific electrophysiologic findings may be seen. In the acute motor neuropathy, the sensory action potentials remain normal [23], whereas in the acute motor and sensory axonal neuropathy, the sensory action potentials become unrecordable early in the course of the disease. In the latter variant of the illness, motor responses are frequently absent, leading to what has been described as "dead" nerves [3]. Electromyographic findings are usually relatively normal until several weeks into the illness, when denervation as indicated by fibrillation potentials and positive sharp waves emerge [24]. These signs indicate differing degrees of axonal damage and have been correlated with poor prognosis.

Hyponatremia is a well-recognized complication of GBS that rarely requires treatment other than fluid restriction [25]. Few studies have investigated its cause, which is presumed to be inappropriate antidiuretic hormone release. Abnormal liver enzymes are present in approximately 15% of patients [26]. In some individuals, this may reflect asymptomatic infection with agents such as hepatitis A or B, cytomegalovirus, and Epstein-Barr virus. In others, the abnormal liver function may be a nonspecific reflection of the severity of their illness, especially in an intensive care environment.

ANTECEDENT EVENTS

It has been known for many years that a number of antecedent events are associated with attacks of GBS, including infections, transfusions, operations, and vaccinations. A very large number of associated antecedent events have been described, but it is likely that the majority of these are simple coincidence. Good evidence exists that certain specific vaccinations are associated with GBS some weeks later. The best data are probably associated with the swine flu epidemic of the mid-1970s [27]. In this study, an increase above background of between four- and eightfold was seen for 6 weeks after immunization. This study has been criticized because of the limited clinical information and also because of the lack of an increase in the numbers of military personnel in whom the disease developed after vaccination [28]. Despite this, most observers have concluded that swine flu vaccination did confer an increased risk of development of GBS. Although occasional cases of GBS are still reported after current flu vaccines [29], no evidence has been found that this is any more than coincidence. Ascertainment for cases of GBS still relies on yellow card reporting, however, which almost certainly considerably underestimates the possible association. Reasonable evidence also exists that rabies vaccine can trigger GBS. The original Semple vaccine was associated with cases of encephalomyelitis and less commonly GBS [30]. Peripheral nervous system complications were probably approximately a tenth less common than central nervous system complications, with an incidence of approximately 1 in 4,000 [31]. No theoretical reason why human diploid cell culture–derived cell vaccine should precipitate GBS exists, but cases of GBS after the administration of these newer vaccines are still reported [32].

Upper respiratory tract infections are associated far more often than would be predicted by chance with GBS, as are gastrointestinal infections [10]. A history of triggering infection is found in at least 75% of patients with GBS. The most commonly identified infections are those of *Campylobacter jejuni* [33], cytomegalovirus [34], and Epstein-Barr virus [34]. Well-documented examples of GBS after human immunodeficiency virus infection [35] and *Mycoplasma* [36] are recorded in the literature. However, these associations have not been subjected to controlled studies. Reports of GBS occurring after operation also exist [17], and also transfusion [37], possibly by transmission of cytomegalovirus infection in transfused blood. Approximately 25% of cases of Guillain-Barré syndrome are associated with an identifiable infectious agent [10]. The incidence of *C. jejuni* infection as a precipitating agent varies according to the study and the serologic tests used but appears to account for at least 15% of all cases of the disease in the United Kingdom. Cytomegalovirus infection probably accounts for a further 10% and a variety of different infections for the remainder.

PATHOLOGY

Most histologic studies of GBS have found the pathologic basis of the disease to represent an acute inflammatory demyelinating lesion within the peripheral nerve associated with perivascular infiltration [4]. In the first few days of the lesion's appearance, lymphocytes seem to predominate but later in the disease they may be very scant [38]. Electron microscopic studies have found similar changes to the animal model of GBS—experimental allergic neuritis (EAN) [39]. Macrophages appear to be in close proximity to the Schwann cell myelin sheath invading the basal lamina and giving the impression that they are ingesting the myelin lamellas and leaving the axon bare. On the other hand, pathologic studies of patients with the acute motor and sensory axonal syndrome show wallerian degeneration in the absence of inflammation and only minimal demyelination. Periaxonal macrophages have been described, which has been interpreted as suggesting a primary immune attack against the axon [40]. In acute motor axonal neuropathy, pathologic studies have been similar, with minimal inflammation and predominantly wallerian degeneration without demyelination [41].

IMMUNOLOGY

The close association between GBS and a preceding infectious agent strongly argues for an immune basis to the syndrome in the majority of cases. Considerable evidence of an activated immune response with the presence of activation markers on lymphocytes in peripheral blood also exists [42] and the expression of adhesion markers in nerve biopsy and in postmortem material. The histology of the acute inflammatory demyelinating polyradiculoneuropathy form of the syndrome is very similar to an experimental model of the disease in rats, EAN [43]. EAN can be transferred between experimental animals using T cells alone, suggesting that it is primarily a T cell–mediated disease [44]. However, the degree of demyelination is influenced strongly by the presence of antibodies. A series of experiments on EAN during the 1990s [45] demonstrated that a breakdown in the blood-nerve barrier is T cell mediated and allows antibodies to penetrate the peripheral nerve, and that antibodies are largely responsible for mediating the demyelination. Whether the situation in the human disease is similar remains to be proved.

A large body of evidence has demonstrated the presence of a variety of different antibodies in patients with GBS. Initial experiments showed that only a small percentage of patients had complement-fixing antibodies in the acute stage of the disease [46]. More subtle measures of complement fixation, such as the C1 fixation technique, have demonstrated that this incidence may be as high as 80% or 90% [47]. These C1 fixation tests rapidly return to normal over a period of a few weeks, paralleling the clinical improvement. Antibodies against P0 and P2 proteins in peripheral blood are found only rarely in patients with GBS [48]. The most frequently occurring antibody is an antibody against gangliosides. Antiganglioside antibodies are seen in approximately 30% of patients with GBS [49]. They react with a number of different gangliosides, including GD_{1a} or GM_1 or asialo GM_1. Antibodies against the ganglioside GQ_{1b} are associated with Miller Fisher syndrome, which is discussed later in this chapter. It is tempting to speculate that plasma exchange (PE) mediates its beneficial effect in GBS by removing antiganglioside antibodies, although this has not been unequivocally demonstrated.

Attempts to transfer disease to animals have met with limited success. GQ_{1b} antiganglioside antibodies appear to reduce neuromuscular transmission in a mouse model of Miller Fisher syndrome, lending some support to a pathogenic role for these antibodies in that syndrome [50]. Only one case report has been published of mother-to-fetus transmission of ganglioside antibodies with neonatal GBS [51]. This case is of considerable interest because of the implications that it has to a pathogenic role for a humoral factor. A correlation seems to exist between the presence of an antiganglioside antibody and preceding infection with *Campylobacter* [52]. A number of reports have shown that the lipopolysaccharide of *Campylobacter* shares structural similarity with epitopes in ganglioside [53]. This raises the possibility that antiganglioside antibodies may be produced after *Campylobacter* infection, which leads to cross-reacting antibodies that combine with host ganglioside. This hypothetical mechanism is attractive and is the subject of intensive current research.

MANAGEMENT

The first and most important aspect of the management of GBS is the provision of supportive care during the acute and progressive phase. Recognition of imminent respiratory failure is of prime importance, as is the institution of ventilation. Prolonged intubation and ventilation can lead to trauma to the vocal cords and, although this can be helped with low-pressure and high-volume cuffed tubes, ventilation of a GBS patient for more than a few days almost inevitably means a tracheostomy will be required. This tracheostomy is conveniently carried out as a percutaneous dilation technique that leaves extremely minimal postoperative scars. Management of alert patients with neuromuscular respiratory disease is specialized and is probably best performed in units that are accustomed to dealing with these patients. Sedation and paralysis are frequently used in general intensive care units in which patients with multisystem disease are treated in an effort to reduce anxiety in an awake, ventilated patient. Such management is not appropriate as a matter of routine for neurologic patients, who do best with a minimum of sedation so that they can be weaned as soon as possible and so that adequate assessment of voluntary limb power is possible. Monitoring of voluntary vital capacity using Wright's spirometer or the equivalent is helpful in this regard, and the same data cannot be deduced from the settings of the respirator or the number of triggered breaths. Ventilation is frequently set up to allow patient-triggered breaths with a small amount of positive end-expiratory pressure to prevent accumulation of secretions and "elephant lung."

Patients should be turned at least every 2 hours to avoid pressure sores. Careful positioning of limbs is of vital importance in reducing pain and preventing compressive neuropathies or permanent contractures, which lead to persistent deficits, such as footdrop, that make active rehabilitation at a later stage far more difficult. Splinting of limbs can aid in this. Eye and mouth care is important in reducing infection and limiting the patient's distress. The two most common causes of death in patients managed in intensive care units are sudden cardiac asystole and focal collapse and consolidation of the lungs, leading to serious infection. Careful attention to respiratory care, frequent turning, and chest physiotherapy can reduce the frequency of chest infection. The incidence of infection is also reduced by careful hand-washing before procedures and by thorough hygiene before adjustment of urinary catheters; these should be removed if bacteriologic monitoring of catheter urine specimens suggests pyuria. Urinary tract infections should be treated early and assiduously if they develop. Patients should be monitored continuously for possible cardiac rhythm disturbances. We institute electrocardiographic (ECG) monitoring at the time of admission to the hospital and do not disconnect the patient from an ECG monitor until improvement has begun. Patients in the intensive care unit should have continuous ECG monitoring. Patients in whom significant bradyarrhythmias develop should have a temporary cardiac pacing wire inserted to prevent sudden asystole, which is reported to be associated with sudden death. Sinus tachycardia is not usually a significant clinical problem. The use of suxamethonium should be discouraged because this drug can precipitate rhythm disturbance in the presence of low serum potassium levels.

Gastrointestinal stasis occurs in GBS patients, and ileus is occasionally profound, with rare instances of cecal or colonic rupture reported. Nevertheless, management is usually relatively easy with regular stool softeners. Constipation may be worsened by intensive use of antacids, which are advocated by some to reduce the risk of stress ulcers. Hyponatremia is frequently observed but is seldom an important clinical problem. Fluid restriction is usually all that is required to correct the electrolyte imbalance.

Counseling is an extremely important part of the management of patients with GBS. The Guillain-Barré Support Group is very helpful in this aspect of care, and a local area network exists that allows patients and their relatives to be visited by recovered GBS patients. Intensive care units that deal regularly with GBS have their own methods of communication and communication charts that prevent frustration on the part of patients. Patients should be regularly reassured that the disease is a monophasic one, with recovery the norm.

Venous thrombosis and pulmonary embolism are other common problems among ventilated patients. Elastic stockings should be used routinely, and prophylactic subcutaneous heparin is helpful in reducing this complication. It may be more convenient to warfarinize some patients who require prolonged anticoagulation. As improvement begins, passive physiotherapy should be introduced initially, followed by active physiotherapy to maximize the use of limbs. Passive physiotherapy prevents the formation of contractures and provides optimum preparation for recovery. Physiotherapy may need to continue for many months in patients with extensive axonal damage. Later in the recovery phase, occupational therapists can provide appropriate aids to maximize function and independence.

Pain is a common problem in GBS patients in intensive care. Careful positioning and frequent turning do much to reduce the extent of limb pain in many patients. Massage and local application of heat and cold can also help. Some authorities have reported small doses of methylprednisolone to be useful [54]. Codeine may be effective but exacerbates any constipation that may be present, and occasionally pain is so severe as to require morphine. Careful use of antidepressants may be required and reassurance and counseling are often helpful. Combinations of sedation (propofol) and analgesics (morphine/fentanyl) may be required for severe, intractable pain. These patients frequently experience sleep deprivation, and care should be taken to reduce its occurrence.

ACTIVE MANAGEMENT

In the 1950s, steroids began to be used in patients with GBS, and their use gradually increased despite the conflicting anecdotal reports and series that documented their possible effect. The first controlled trials were published in the 1970s. The earliest of these consisted of 18 patients, of whom 10 received adrenocorticotropic hormone, 100 units, and the remaining 8 received placebo [55]. No striking immediate improvement was seen in the disease, but the time taken to recover was 4.4 months in the adrenocorticotropic hormone group compared to 9.0 months in the placebo group. This difference was considered significant, although the numbers were very small and the analysis was not carried out on an intention-to-treat basis.

The largest available randomized control trial of oral prednisolone was published in 1978 [8] and included 40 GBS patients, of whom 21 received a tapering dose of 60 mg prednisolone. This trial was the first to use a six-point disability scale in the assessment of the severity of the neuropathy. This scale has been subsequently used in a number of other trials (Table 2.5). The two treatment groups were very similar at randomization in terms of their duration of disease, disability grade, and CSF parameters. The improvement in the average disability grade was slightly greater in the control group, although this was not significant, thus giving no support to the potential benefit of steroid medication in hastening recovery from the disease. Of note was the fact that three relapses occurred among the steroid-treated group and none among the controls, raising the possibility that steroids might increase the chance of converting a monophasic disease into CIDP. This trial, though small, was in keeping with the trial methodology that was common at the time. It subsequently became clear that study of a much larger number of patients would be required to be certain that steroids did not convey a useful benefit that would not have been detected by this trial in view of the large variation in recovery time of GBS patients.

Modern multicenter trials include at least 200 patients to reduce this chance of error. A subsequent large-scale clinical trial of methylprednisolone was carried out in 1990–1993 that involved 242 patients [9]. Disability was assessed using the same slightly modified disability scale, and 4 weeks after treatment the difference in average disability grade was only 0.06 (confidence intervals +0.36, –0.23). The sample size gave a 91% chance of detecting a 0.5 grade difference between the two groups at the 5% probability level with a two-tailed test. Forty-eight weeks

Table 2.5   Disability grades in Guillain-Barré syndrome for clinical trials

Grade	Signs and symptoms
0	Healthy: no signs or symptoms of Guillain-Barré syndrome
1	Minor symptoms or signs; able to run
2	Able to walk 5 m across an open space without assistance
3	Able to walk 5 m across an open space with the help of one person and waist level walking frame, stick, or sticks
4	Chair bound/bed bound; unable to walk as in 3
5	Requires assisted ventilation (for at least part of day or night)
6	Dead

after randomization the mean disability grades were 1.33 (1.56) in the IVMP group and 1.13 (1.15) in the placebo group. Five deaths and seven relapses occurred in the IVMP group and two deaths and four relapses in the placebo group during the 48-week follow-up. This negative study was influential in reducing the use of steroids for the acute patient with GBS and contrasted with the results for trials of PE. The only other controlled trial of steroids in GBS was reported in 1985; in this study, 13 patients received 100 mg prednisolone daily for 10 days together with PE, and a further 12 patients received neither treatment. No difference was seen in outcome, which was perhaps not surprising in view of the small numbers studied [56].

A single report of a beneficial benefit of PE to a patient with GBS was published in 1978 [57]. Over the next 6 years, a number of anecdotal reports of GBS patients responding favorably to PE were published, leading up to the first published controlled trial in 1984 [58]. This small British trial involved 14 patients randomized to receive PE compared with 15 who did not receive it. The time from onset of the disease to receiving PE was quite long, at almost 14 days. The benefit of PE was not significant, although a trend was seen toward greater improvement in the PE group; 0.67 functional grade (0.37) compared with 0.18 (0.30) in the control group. The sample sizes were chosen with the intention of detecting a 1.0 grade change in disability, which is greater than that used for the subsequent large-scale multicenter studies, which used a 0.5 grade change as clinically significant. A Swedish study of 38 patients was published in 1982 [59]. In this study, significant benefits were found in the patients receiving PE, who stopped progressing earlier than the other group and had less severe disability at 2 months. The trial had an unusual alternate rather than truly random allocation arrangement for treatment and was not blinded.

Two large-scale multicenter trials have provided the clearest evidence in favor of PE [60,61]. In the North American trial, 122 patients were randomly allocated to PE and 123 to conventional treatment. Exchange consisted of approximately 250 ml/kg body weight over up to 14 days with 5% albumin as replacement fluid. Twelve patients were excluded from analysis because they did not complete their PE, and therefore the analysis was not strictly by intention to treat. Despite this, the findings were clear-cut. At 4 weeks, 59% of patients treated with PE had improved compared with only 39% of the control subjects ($p < .01$). Although sham exchange was not considered ethical, a blinded assessor was used for the 4-week assessment in an attempt to reduce bias. Similar highly significant changes were seen in the difference in mean functional grades at 4 weeks, the proportion of patients who failed to improve one grade at 6 months, and in the time spent on a ventilator. The study used a one-tailed *t* test for these analyses, and this has been controversial; even if more conventional two-tailed *t* tests had been used, however, the results would have still been significant. Patients who were randomized early in the course of their disease appeared to respond much more than did those who were randomized later, which is consistent with the hypothesis that PE is removing a serum factor that contributes to the nerve damage. PEs performed by machines using a continuous process appeared to be more effective than those with an intermittent process. At 4 weeks, 64% of patients who had been treated with continuous exchange had improved one disability grade compared with 51% treated with intermittent flow machines.

A French multicenter trial with 220 patients reached very similar results 2 years later [61]. Four exchanges were used on alternate days of two plasma volumes. A different neurologic scoring system was used in this trial and only half of the patients had replacement with 5% albumin; the rest received fresh frozen plasma. Of the PE group, 67% had improved at 4 weeks, compared with only 44% of the control subjects who received conventional supportive care. Significant advantages to PE were also seen in the time to start weaning from the ventilator, time to walk unaided, and time to walk with assistance. Patients who received fresh frozen plasma had a higher incidence of complications, such as rashes and hepatitis, without any additional benefit. In this study, the GBS patients were allocated to PE earlier than in the North American study (mean, 6.6 days), and this has been cited as a reason why the French results were slightly more impressive than those of the North American study, in which patients did not receive PE until, on average, 11.1 days after their first neuropathic symptom. The only other controlled trial of PE was a small Finnish study [62], which only involved 26 patients and found no significant differences in time of hospital stay or time to recover with the PE group, although some improvement in hand strength was noted.

In 1992, a Dutch group published a trial suggesting that intravenous immunoglobulin (IVIG) was at least as effective as PE in improving the time required for patients to recover from the syndrome [63]. This trial was criticized for the relatively poor response to PE seen in the control patients. A 1997 multicenter trial compared PE, IVIG, and the combination of the two treatments [26]. This confirmed that IVIG and PE are roughly equivalent in their efficacy in shortening the time taken for patients to recover from the syndrome. A small but insignificant advantage was found in giving both treatments together. The mean change after 4 weeks on a seven-point disability scale was 0.9 for PE, 0.8 for IVIG, and 1.1 for the combination group. In the combination group, PE was given over 8 to 13 days and was followed by 5 days of IVIG, 0.4 g/kg per day. A theoretical advantage exists in giving IVIG at a time when B cells that produce antinerve antibodies can be stimulated by the PE and the lack of negative feedback. The difference between PE alone and IVIG alone was so small that a difference between the treatments of 0.5 grades was excluded at the 95% confidence level. Secondary variables, such as the time to walk unaided and the time to discontinue ventilation, were similarly not significantly different between PE and IVIG. This result confirmed the Dutch uncontrolled study and was consistent with a small pilot trial that compared PE with IVIG [64].

As a result of this trial, it seems likely that IVIG will become the treatment of choice for patients with GBS. It is easier to deliver and requires less specialized care than does PE. PE is associated with a number of complications, including hemorrhage, central line and other infections, and exacerbation of autonomic disturbance. It is not always possible to achieve adequate plasmapheresis through a large peripheral line, and attempts at central line insertion can add to morbidity through pneumothorax and increased risk of infection. The frequency of such complications is low in clinical trials but likely to be greater in widespread clinical practice. PE is still a useful treatment in circumstances in which IVIG cannot be used or in patients who relapse on IVIG. The Dutch group has published a small uncontrolled study suggesting that patients who receive both methylprednisolone and IVIG do better than those given IVIG alone [65]. A larger randomized multicenter trial is in progress and should be reported soon.

PROGNOSIS

The prognosis of GBS is extremely variable, with some patients making a rapid recovery over a few weeks and others remaining ventilated for many months and either dying or making only a minimal recovery. A review of the available large-scale clinical studies in 1984 containing almost 1,000 patients suggested that only 24% are back to all normal activities at 3 months and that 77% eventually make a full recovery by this criterion [66]. In a study of 100 patients with GBS followed for a year, 3 were still bed bound, 4 required aid to walk, and 14 were unable to work [17]. These data were obtained before the use of PE or IVIG became widespread. Although both PE and IVIGs shorten the time that patients spend in the hospital and the time required to regain the ability to walk unaided, little evidence that they improve the disability that is present at the end of 2 or 3 years exists. A survey carried out in 1985 showed that approximately 25% of patients were left with persistent disability at the end of 1 year after the onset of GBS [17]. This survey was repeated in 1995 [67] and showed very similar results. In the initial study, no patients were treated with IVIG and only a handful were given PE. In the repeated study 10 years later, almost all the patients received some form of specific therapy. The eventual number of patients left with disability at the end of the year was virtually identical in the two studies, suggesting that treatment does not really influence the number of disabled individuals. It seems likely that it is this group of patients who will be the subject of ongoing clinical trials. Some preliminary work has been done looking at growth factors within this group, and a multicenter trial may follow.

Mortality for the syndrome varies from 1.25% [68] to 13% [17]. It is much higher in unselected surveys of patients across many centers than in the trial situation or in specialized centers of excellence.

A number of authors have sought factors that might predict prognosis more accurately. This would have considerable clinical usefulness in planning care and in deciding which patients should be subjected to future clinical trials aimed at reducing long-term deficit. A small motor compound action potential recorded distally, a rapid deterioration over a few days, a history of *Campylobacter* infection, and a requirement for ventilation all appear to be adverse prognostic factors [17,69]. The development of denervation is accompanied by appreciable axonal damage and has been associated with poor prognosis in several studies [24]. However, denervation is less useful clinically because this information is only available late in the course of the illness.

MILLER FISHER SYNDROME

In 1956, C. Miller Fisher described a new clinical syndrome that consisted of ophthalmoplegia associated with areflexia and absent reflexes [70]. Patients with Miller Fisher syndrome differed from individuals with GBS in that they had no demonstrable weakness. For some time, this disorder has been considered to be a variant of GBS (and clinical overlap features often exist), although there has been debate about whether the clinical syndrome of Miller Fisher could be mimicked by a brain stem encephalitis. Electrophysiologic examination of patients with Miller Fisher syndrome suggests that it is predominantly a disease of the sensory neurons with small sensory action potentials. The prognosis seems to be slightly better than that of traditional GBS, and anecdotal reports suggest a response to both PE and IVIG. Patients with Miller Fisher syndrome almost always have antibodies against the ganglioside GQ_{1b}. These have been reported in approximately 90% of patients in several studies [71,72]. One report indicates that the serum from these patients produces neuromuscular block in a mouse diaphragm preparation. It has been suggested that anti-GQ_{1b} in these patients may actually be the pathogenic serum factor [50].

CHRONIC INFLAMMATORY DEMYELINATING POLYNEUROPATHY

Patients who have a chronic course of disease with progression of motor deficit for longer than 8 weeks are considered separately from those with acute GBS, and this condition is given the diagnostic label of *CIDP*. Included within this label are the small number of GBS patients who are identified at an early stage and continue to progress and those individuals with a relapsing demyelinating polyneuropathy. The distinction of this group of patients seems justified in view of their clear response to steroid therapy that is ineffective in GBS [7]. The name is a misnomer because only a small minority of patients have a significant inflammatory infiltrate on nerve biopsy. CIDP seldom represents a clinical problem in the intensive care unit because the occurrence of respiratory failure is unusual. For this reason, it is discussed only briefly here.

Clinical Features

Like GBS, CIDP occurs more commonly in men than in women, and evidence has been found of an HLA association with DR3 and B8 [73]. It presents with weakness and sensory symptoms, aching pain in the muscles, and tendon areflexia. Cranial nerve involvement is seen less frequently than with GBS, with facial weakness occurring in approximately 15% and bulbar symptoms in only 6% of patients. Tremor occurs in occasional patients. Approximately 11% of patients exhibit thickening of peripheral nerves. A small number of patients have some associated upper motor neuron signs, and magnetic resonance imaging has shown cerebral white matter abnormalities in rare patients who appear to have both central and peripheral nerve demyelination [74].

Electrophysiology shows evidence of conduction block or severely slowed velocities, and the electrophysiologic criteria for demyelination have been defined [5]. Nerve biopsy reveals demyelination with typically little if any inflammatory infiltrate. Onion bulb formation from chronic demyelination and remyelination is frequently seen.

Treatment

Controlled trials have demonstrated the efficacy of steroids [7], PE [75,76], and IVIG [77] in improving muscle strength in CIDP. Steroids at a dose of approximately 60 mg prednisolone daily have been the mainstay of treatment, and some authors advocate a gradual increase in dose to prevent occasional worsening of the weakness with the start of therapy. IVIG represents an alternative initial treatment that has fewer side effects but is more difficult to deliver and more expensive. Maintenance of remission sometimes requires the use of azathioprine, but other immunosuppressants, such as cyclosporin and cyclophosphamide, have been used successfully.

The prognosis with treatment is good, with an average 80% response and only a small percentage of patients severely disabled at 10 years [78].

Etiology

Occasional patients with CIDP have antibodies against gangliosides, but the possible relevance of these to the demyelination is unknown. The efficacy of PE in the treatment of CIDP argues for a role for circulating factors in the etiology of the disease, but studies so far have shown conflicting results, and the relative role of cell-mediated and humoral immunity remains to be determined.

ACUTE PANDYSAUTONOMIA

GBS is frequently accompanied by an autonomic neuropathy, but autonomic disturbance in the absence of weakness, although exceptionally rare, has been described as a presumed postinfectious phenomenon. This syndrome is termed *acute pandysautonomia*. In one well-documented example, postural hypotension, blurred vision, dry eyes, and sphincter disturbance evolved over a few weeks [79]. The pathology of this rare syndrome is unknown. In one case, evidence of improvement with IVIG treatment was found [80].

REFERENCES

1. Asbury AK. Diagnostic considerations in Guillain-Barré syndrome. Ann Neurol 1981;9(suppl):1.
2. Asbury AK, Cornblath DR. Assessment of current diagnostic criteria for Guillain-Barré syndrome. Ann Neurol 1990;27(suppl):S21.
3. Feasby TE, Gilbert JJ, Brown WF, et al. An acute axonal form of Guillain-Barré polyneuropathy. Brain 1986;109(pt 6):1115.
4. Asbury AK, Arnason AB, Adams RD. The inflammatory lesion in idiopathic polyneuritis. Its role in pathogenesis. Medicine 1969;48:173.
5. Ad Hoc Committee of the American Academy of Neurology AIDS Task Force. Research criteria for the diagnosis of chronic demyelinating polyradiculoneuropathy (CIDP). Neurology 1991;41:617.
6. Hughes RA. The spectrum of acquired demyelinating polyradiculoneuropathy. Acta Neurol Belg 1994;94:128.
7. Dyck PJ, O'Brien PC, Oviatt KF, et al. Prednisone improves chronic inflammatory demyelinating polyradiculoneuropathy more than no treatment. Ann Neurol 1982;11:136.
8. Hughes RA, Newsom-Davis JM, et al. Controlled trial prednisolone in acute polyneuropathy. Lancet 1978;2:750.
9. Guillain-Barré Syndrome Steroid Trial Group. Double-blind trial of intravenous methylprednisolone in Guillain-Barré syndrome. Lancet 1993;341:586.

10. Winer JB, Hughes RA, Anderson MJ, et al. A prospective study of acute idiopathic neuropathy. II. Antecedent events. J Neurol Neurosurg Psychiatry 1988;51:613.
11. Dawson DM, Samuels MA, Morris J. Sensory form of acute polyneuritis. Neurology 1988;38:1728.
12. Miralles F, Montero J, Rene R, et al. Pure sensory Guillain-Barré syndrome [letter]. J Neurol Neurosurg Psychiatry 1992;55:411.
13. Morley JB, Reynolds EH. Papilloedema and the Guillain-Barré syndrome. Brain 1966;89:205.
14. Davidson DLW, Jellinek EH. Hypertension and papilloedema in the Guillain-Barré syndrome. J Neurol Neurosurg Psychiatry 1977;40:144.
15. Farrell K, Hill A, Chuang S. Papilledema in Guillain-Barré syndrome. A case report. Arch Neurol 1981;38:55.
16. Joynt R. Mechanisms of production of papilloedema in the Guillain-Barré syndrome. Neurology 1958;8:8.
17. Winer JB, Hughes RA, Osmond C. A prospective study of acute idiopathic neuropathy. I. Clinical features and their prognostic value. J Neurol Neurosurg Psychiatry 1988;51:605.
18. Winer JB, Hughes RA. Identification of patients at risk of arrhythmia in the Guillain-Barré syndrome. QJM 1988;68:735.
19. Lichtenfeld P. Autonomic dysfunction in Guillain-Barré syndrome. Am J Med 1971;50:772–780.
20. Guillain G, Barré JA, Strohl A. Sur un syndrome de radiculo-nevrite avec hyperalbuminose du liquide cephalorachidien sans reaction cellulaire. Remarques sur les caracteres cliniques et graphique des reflexes tendineux. Bull Soc Med Hop Paris 1916;40:1462.
21. Feasby TE, Brown WF, Gilbert JJ, Hahn AF. The pathological basis of conduction block in human neuropathies. J Neurol Neurosurg Psychiatry 1985;48:239.
22. Kimura J, Butzer JF. F wave conduction velocity in Guillain-Barré syndrome. Arch Neurol 1975;32:524.
23. McKhann GM, Cornblath DR, Ho T. Clinical and electrophysiological aspects of acute paralytic disease of children and young adults in northern China [see comments]. Lancet 1991;338:593.
24. McLeod JG. Electrophysiological studies in the Guillain-Barré syndrome. Ann Neurol 1981;9(suppl):20.
25. Posner JB, Ertel NH, Kossman RJ, Scheinberg LC. Hyponatraemia in acute polyneuropathy. Arch Neurol 1967;17:530.
26. Anonymous. Randomised trial of plasma exchange, intravenous immunoglobulin, and combined treatments in Guillain-Barré syndrome. Lancet 1997;349:225.
27. Schonberger LB, Hurwitz ES, Katona P, et al. Guillain-Barré syndrome: its epidemiology and associations with influenza vaccination. Ann Neurol 1981;9(suppl):31.
28. Kurland LT, Wiederholt WC, Kirkpatrick JW, et al. Swine influenza vaccine and Guillain-Barré syndrome. Epidemic or artifact? Arch Neurol 1985;42:1089.
29. Hughes R, Rees J, Smeeton N, Winer J. Vaccines and Guillain-Barré syndrome [letter]. BMJ 1996;312:1475.
30. Hemachudha T, Phanuphalc P, Johnson RT, et al. Neurologic complications of Semple-type rabies vaccine: clinical and immunological studies. Neurology 1987;37:550.
31. Hughes RA. Guillain-Barré Syndrome. London: Springer-Verlag, 1990.
32. Boe E, Nyland H. Guillain-Barré syndrome after vaccination with human diploid cell rabies vaccine. Scand J Infect Dis 1980;12:231.
33. Vriesendorp FJ, Mishu B, Blaser MJ, Koski CL. Serum antibodies to GMT, GDlb, peripheral nerve myelin, and *Campylobacter jejuni* in patients with Guillain-Barré syndrome and controls: correlation and prognosis. Ann Neurol 1993;34:130.
34. Dowling PC, Cook SD. Role of infection in Guillain-Barré syndrome: laboratory confirmation of herpesviruses in 41 cases. Ann Neurol 1981;9(suppl):44.
35. Hagberg L, Malmvall BE, Svennerholm L, et al. Guillain-Barré syndrome as an early manifestation of HIV central nervous system infection. Scand J Infect Dis 1986;18:591.
36. Goldschmidt B, Menonna J, Fortunato J, et al. *Mycoplasma* antibody in Guillain-Barré syndrome and other neurological disorders. Ann Neurol 1980;7:108.
37. Merelli E, Sola P, La Spina I, et al. Guillain-Barré polyradiculoneuritis after blood transfusion. Ital J Neurol Sci 1991;12:313.
38. Honavar M, Tharakan JK, Hughes RA, et al. A clinicopathological study of the Guillain-Barré syndrome. Nine cases and literature review. Brain 1991;114(pt 3):1245.
39. Prineas J. Acute idiopathic polyneuritis. An electron microscope study. Lab Invest 1972;26:133.
40. Griffin JW, Li CY, Ho TW, et al. Pathology of the motor-sensory axonal Guillain-Barré syndrome. Ann Neurol 1996;39:17.
41. Griffin JW, Li CY, Ho TW, et al. Guillain-Barré syndrome in northern China. The spectrum of neuropathological changes in clinically defined cases. Brain 1995;118(pt 3):577.

42. Hartung HP, Hughes RA, Taylor WA, et al. T cell activation in Guillain-Barré syndrome and in MS: elevated serum levels of soluble IL-2 receptors. Neurology 1990;40:215.
43. Prineas JW. Pathology of the Guillain-Barré syndrome. Ann Neurol 1981;9(suppl):6.
44. Linington C, Mann A, Izumo S, et al. Induction of experimental allergic neuritis in the BN rat: P2 protein-specific T cells overcome resistance to actively induced disease. J Immunol 1986;137:3826.
45. Spies JM, Westland KW, Bonner JG, Pollard JD. Intraneural activated T cells cause focal breakdown of the blood-nerve barrier. Brain 1995;118(pt 4):857.
46. Winer JB, Gray IA, Gregson, NA, et al. A prospective study of acute idiopathic neuropathy. III. Immunological studies. J Neurol Neurosurg Psychiatry 1988;51:619.
47. Koski CL, Humphrey R, Shin ML. Anti-peripheral myelin antibody in patients with demyelinating neuropathy: quantitative and kinetic determination of serum antibody by complement component 1 fixation. Proc Natl Acad Sci U S A 1985;82:905.
48. Hughes RA, Gray IA, Gregson NA, et al. Immune responses to myelin antigens in Guillain-Barré syndrome. J Neuroimmunol 1984;6:303.
49. Gregson NA, Koblar S, Hughes RA. Antibodies to gangliosides in Guillain-Barré syndrome: specificity and relationship to clinical features [see comments]. QJM 1993;86:111.
50. Roberts M, Willison H, Vincent A, Newsom-Davis J. Serum factor in Miller-Fisher variant of Guillain-Barré syndrome and neurotransmitter release. Lancet 1994;343:454.
51. Luijckx GJ, de Baets M, Buchwald B, Troost J. Guillain-Barré syndrome in mother and newborn child. Lancet 1997;349:27.
52. Yuki N, Yoshino H, Sato S, Miyatake T. Acute axonal polyneuropathy associated with anti-GMI antibodies following *Campylobacter* enteritis. Neurology 1990;40:1900.
53. Yuki N, Taki T, Inagaki F, et al. A bacterium lipopolysaccharide that elicits Guillain-Barré syndrome has a GM_1 ganglioside-like structure. J Exp Med 1993;178:1771.
54. Ropper AH, Shahani BT. Pain in Guillain-Barré syndrome. Arch Neurol 1984;41:511.
55. Swick HM, McQuillen MP. The use of steroids in the treatment of idiopathic polyneuritis. Neurology 1976;26:205–212.
56. Mendell JR, Kissel JT, Kennedy MS, et al. Plasma exchange and prednisone in acute inflammatory polyradiculoneuropathy: a controlled randomized trial. J Clin Apheresis 1985;2:332.
57. Brettle RP, Gross M, Legg NJ, et al. Treatment of acute polyneuropathy by plasma exchange [letter]. Lancet 1978;2:1100.
58. Greenwood R, Newsom-Davis J, Hughes RA, et al. British multicentre trial of plasma exchange in acute inflammatory polyradiculoneuropathy (AIP). Prog Clin Biol Res 1982;106:189.
59. Osterman PO, Fagius J, Safwenberg J, et al. Treatment of the Guillain-Barré syndrome by plasmapheresis. Arch Neurol 1982;39:148.
60. Anonymous. Plasmapheresis for acute Guillain-Barré syndrome. Neurology 1985;35:1096.
61. French Cooperative Group on Plasma Exchange in Guillain-Barré Syndrome. Efficiency of plasma exchange in Guillain-Barré syndrome: role of replacement fluids. Ann Neurol 1987;22:753.
62. Farkkila M, Kinnunen E, Haapanen E, Iivanainen M. Guillain-Barré syndrome: quantitative measurement of plasma exchange therapy. Neurology 1987;37:837.
63. van der Meché FG, Schmitz PI. A randomized trial comparing intravenous immune globulin and plasma exchange in Guillain-Barré syndrome. Dutch Guillain-Barré Study Group. N Engl J Med 1992;326:1123.
64. Bril V, Ilse WK, Pearce R, et al. Pilot trial of immunoglobulin versus plasma exchange in patients with Guillain-Barré syndrome. Neurology 1996;46:100.
65. The Dutch Guillain-Barré Study Group. Treatment of Guillain-Barré syndrome with high-dose immune globulins combined with methylprednisolone: a pilot study [see comments]. Ann Neurol 1994;35:749–752. [Published erratum appears in Ann Neurol 1994;36:457.]
66. Hughes R, Winer JB. Guillain-Barré Syndrome. In GH Glaser, WB Matthews (eds), Recent Advances in Clinical Neurology. Edinburgh: Churchill Livingstone, 1984;19–49.
67. Rees JH, Soudain SE, Gregson NA, Hughes RA. *Campylobacter jejuni* infection and Guillain-Barré syndrome. N Engl J Med 1995;333:1374.
68. Ropper AH, Shahani BT. Diagnosis and Management of Acute Areflexic Paralysis with Emphasis on Guillain-Barré Syndrome. In RW Gilliatt, AK Asbury (eds), Peripheral Nerve Disorders. A Practical Approach. London: Butterworth, 1984;21–45.
69. Cornblath DR, Mellits ED, Griffin JW, et al. Motor conduction studies in Guillain-Barré syndrome: description and prognostic value. Ann Neurol 1988;23:354.
70. Fisher M. Syndrome of ophthalmoplegia, ataxia and areflexia. N Engl J Med 1956;255:57.
71. Chiba A, Kusunoki S, Shimizu T, Kanazawa I. Serum IgG antibody to ganglioside GQ_{1b} is a possible marker of Miller Fisher syndrome. Ann Neurol 1992;31:677.

72. Willison HJ, Veitch J, Paterson G, Kennedy PG. Miller Fisher syndrome is associated with serum antibodies to GQ_{1b} ganglioside. J Neurol Neurosurg Psychiatry 1993;56:204.
73. Feeney DJ, Pollard JD, McLeod JG, et al. HLA antigens in chronic inflammatory demyelinating polyneuropathy. J Neurol Neurosurg Psychiatry 1990;53:170.
74. Thomas PK, Walker RW, Rudge P, et al. Chronic demyelinating peripheral neuropathy associated with multifocal CNS demyelination. Brain 1987;110:53.
75. Dyck PJ, Daube J, O'Brien P, et al. Plasma exchange in chronic inflammatory demyelinating polyradiculoneuropathy. N Engl J Med 1986;314:461.
76. Hahn AF, Bolton CF, Pillay N, et al. Plasma exchange in chronic inflammatory demyelinating polyneuropathy. A double-blind sham-controlled cross-over study. Brain 1996;119:1055.
77. Hahn AF, Bolton CF, Zochodne D, Feasby TE. Intravenous immunoglobulin treatment in chronic inflammatory demyelinating polyneuropathy. A double-blind placebo-controlled cross-over study. Brain 1996;119(pt 4):1067.
78. McCombe PA, Pollard JD, McLeod JG. Chronic inflammatory demyelinating polyradiculoneuropathy. A clinical and electrophysiological study of 92 cases. Brain 1987;110(pt 6):1617.
79. Young RR, Asbury AK, Corbett JL, Adams RD. Pure pan-dysautonomia with recovery. Description and discussion of diagnostic criteria. Brain 1975;98:613.
80. Heafield MT, Gammage MD, Nightingale S, Williams AC. Idiopathic dysautonomia treated with intravenous gamma-globulin. Lancet 1996;347:28.

3
Myasthenia Gravis

Laurence Loh

Myasthenia gravis is a disorder of neuromuscular transmission characterized by fatigable muscle weakness. It is an autoimmune disease brought about through the action of a circulating antibody that dramatically reduces the density of acetylcholine receptors on the postjunctional membrane of the neuromuscular junction [1]. To understand the clinical features of the disease and its management, it is necessary to be aware of the underlying pathophysiology. In this chapter, I first discuss the normal anatomy of the neuromuscular junction, the safety margin, and the effects of the antiacetylcholine receptor antibody; then the epidemiology and clinical features are described. The clinical management, particularly with reference to intensive care management, follows.

PATHOPHYSIOLOGY

Safety Margin

Figure 3.1 shows a schematic diagram of the structure of the neuromuscular junction [2]. Vesicles containing quanta of acetylcholine molecules are generated and stored in the presynaptic nerve terminal and released from active zones in the presynaptic membrane. The active zones are sited opposite the synaptic folds of the postsynaptic muscle membrane where the acetylcholine receptors are most densely concentrated. The architectural arrangement ensures efficient neurochemical transmission by acetylcholine. When the nerve terminal is at rest, quanta of acetylcholine molecules are occasionally randomly liberated from vesicles. Some of the released acetylcholine molecules are destroyed by the enzyme cholinesterase in the synaptic cleft, but some molecules attach to acetylcholine receptors on the postjunctional membrane and cause a small change in membrane potential called the *miniature end-plate potential*. This change of approximately 0.8 mV is small compared to the resting membrane potential of

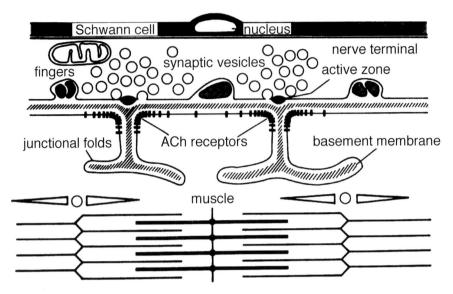

Figure 3.1   Diagram of the neuromuscular junction. (ACh = acetylcholine.) (Adapted from F Dreyer. Acetylcholine receptor. Br J Anaesth 1982;54:4168.)

–70 mV and is not sufficient to stimulate a muscle contraction. When a nerve impulse arrives at the nerve terminal, however, a large number of quanta of acetylcholine are released. Sufficient acetylcholine receptors are stimulated at one time to change the membrane potential so that it exceeds a critical firing threshold, and a muscle action potential is propagated. The depolarization opens calcium channels in the sarcolemmal reticulum of the muscle and muscle contraction takes place. The safety factor for neuromuscular transmission is the margin by which the change in membrane potential exceeds the critical firing threshold [3]. Although the safety margin in humans is not large compared to that of other mammals, such as the rat, it is large enough to make neurotransmission very certain under normal circumstances. In myasthenia gravis, structural changes in the architecture of the neuromuscular junction as well as dynamic alterations in the turnover of acetylcholine receptors erode the safety margin and efficiency of neuromuscular transmission.

Effects of the Antiacetylcholine Receptor Antibody

Of patients with myasthenia gravis, 80–85% have an identifiable and quantifiable antibody found in the immunoglobulin G (IgG) fraction of plasma, which is responsible for the changes that take place at the neuromuscular junction [4]. This is called the *antiacetylcholine receptor antibody*; it has the following effects:

1. The antibody attaches to the acetylcholine receptor and increases the rate of breakdown and internalization of the receptor.

2. The antibody may also block the receptor to the action of acetylcholine.
3. The antibody causes destruction of the postjunctional folds through complement-mediated lysis. This hinders the insertion of new acetylcholine receptor into postjunctional membrane.
4. The result is a marked reduction in the density of acetylcholine receptor at the neuromuscular junction.
5. The synaptic cleft is widened, and the receptor area is also increased. This increases the destruction of acetylcholine by cholinesterase and decreases the efficiency of acetylcholine targeting a receptor.
6. The result of all the preceding is a progressive erosion of the safety margin. By the time clinical weakness is present, acetylcholine receptor density is severely reduced (approximately 30% of normal). Successful neuromuscular transmission is therefore markedly affected by small and subtle changes in the amount of acetylcholine release. A small decrement in acetylcholine release occurs during repetitive stimulation, giving rise to the failure in transmission of some motor units and the characteristic fatigable muscle weakness.

Anticholinesterase Therapy

Anticholinesterase drugs inhibit the action of cholinesterase and increase the survival of acetylcholine molecules in the synaptic cleft. In patients with myasthenia gravis, this improves the probability of successful neuromuscular transmission. Therefore, some anticholinesterase drugs are clinically useful in improving muscle power in myasthenia gravis. If too much anticholinesterase is present, however, persistent depolarization of the muscle end plate occurs and this cholinergic state causes failure of neuromuscular transmission.

Role of the Thymus Gland

It has been observed for many years that the removal of the thymus gland frequently improves the clinical state of patients with myasthenia gravis [5,6]. The precise reason for this is not clear. Cells in the thymus gland have been shown to produce antiacetylcholine receptor antibody. However, the amount of antibody produced is small, because most antiacetylcholine receptor antibody is manufactured in the periphery, outside the thymus gland. Acetylcholine receptor–like protein has been identified in thymic tissue and may act as an antigenic stimulus for antibody production [7]. It may be that thymectomy removes this antigenic stimulus, allowing a decrease in antibody production. Most likely, the thymus gland is a source of thymic lymphocytes that stimulate antibody production elsewhere in the body. In the younger age group of patients with myasthenia gravis, the medulla of the thymus gland shows striking hyperplasia of the lymphoid tissue in the germinal centers. Total removal of the thymus gland is usually followed by a decrease in antiacetylcholine receptor antibody level in those patients with a histologically active-looking thymus gland. The precise trigger for the onset of myasthenia gravis is not known, but it is thought that the thymus gland is the primary site of autosensitization [8].

ASSESSMENT

Epidemiology

The incidence of myasthenia gravis in the general population is 1 per 20,000. The disease occurs in all countries. No familial tendency exists, but some HLA associations exist. Frequently, other members of the family have other autoimmune diseases such as rheumatoid arthritis, thyrotoxicosis, and pernicious anemia. The female-to-male ratio is 3 to 2. The onset of the disease tends to be earlier in women than in men, with a peak incidence in the second decade in women and in the fourth decade in men, although the spread is wide, with the disease occurring in all age groups. Ten percent of patients with myasthenia gravis have an associated thymoma. This tumor is usually benign (two-thirds), but one-third become locally invasive. Thymomas should generally be excised to prevent local damage to important structures such as the phrenic nerves and the great vessels in the mediastinum.

Presentation

The characteristic of myasthenia gravis is fatigable muscle weakness, which is improved by rest and usually improved with the administration of an anticholinesterase drug. The muscle weakness can affect all voluntary muscle groups, but often one muscle group is more affected than others and, as the disease progresses, additional muscle groups become involved.

Ocular Muscles

Frequently, the presenting symptoms in myasthenia gravis are diplopia and ptosis. Sometimes these are the only symptoms and, if the disease does not progress to affect other muscles within 2 years of onset, it is likely that it will remain confined to the extraocular muscles.

Generalized Muscle Weakness

The proximal limb muscles tend to be more affected than distal muscles, although exceptions occur (e.g., isolated finger drop). Weakness of the shoulders and hips impairs mobility and normal activity. Neck muscle weakness is common: The patient may have difficulty in supporting his or her head upright.

Bulbar Weakness

Some patients complain of difficulty with chewing and speech (poor phonation caused by vocal cord weakness and impaired articulation caused by weakness of the tongue and lips). In more severe cases, difficulty with swallowing and poor protection of the airway occur and can result in choking and aspiration of oral secretions. A characteristic nasal speech and inability to smile properly often allow easy recognition of this condition. A typical stance of a patient with severe generalized myasthenia is arms folded across the chest, one fist held below the chin keeping the jaw closed, and the head tilted up to enable the patient to see ahead despite partial ptosis.

Respiratory Muscle Weakness

The inability to take a deep breath and to cough efficiently is often associated with bulbar weakness, and this is a particularly dangerous combination. The inability to swallow oral secretions and to clear secretions aspirated into the trachea is a crisis situation that can lead to acute respiratory failure, with or without superadded chest infection caused by aspiration or collapse/consolidation.

Clinical Grading of Disability

Several methods of staging disability in myasthenia gravis have been used in the past. The best known is that of Osserman and Genkins [9], which divides myasthenic patients into four classes (Table 3.1). However, more useful clinical scoring systems have been devised based on the patient's ability to perform a few simple tasks. One system is shown in Table 3.2 [10]. The clinical scoring systems are preferred, as they can chart the course of the disease and reflect the response to treatment.

DIAGNOSIS

History

The diagnosis is usually made from the history of fluctuating, fatigable muscle weakness, made worse by exercise of the muscle group involved and improved by rest, and tending to be worse toward the end of the day. Examination should confirm fatigable motor weakness with no sensory or reflex changes.

Table 3.1   Classification of myasthenia gravis

Class	Signs and Symptoms
I	Ocular signs and symptoms only
IIA	Mild, generalized muscle weakness with slow progression; no crises; drug-responsive
IIB	Moderate, generalized muscle weakness; skeletal and bulbar muscle involvement but no crises; drug response less than satisfactory
III	Acute fulminating presentation; rapid progression of severe symptoms with respiratory crises and poor drug response; high incidence of thymoma
IV	Late, severe myasthenia; respiratory crises and poor drug response as in III but with slower progression over 2 years or more from class I or II

Source: Adapted from KE Osserman, G Genkins. Studies in myasthenia gravis: review of a twenty-year experience in over 1200 patients. Mt Sinai J Med 1971;38:497–537.

Table 3.2　Example of scheme of clinical scoring for patients with myasthenia gravis

Weakness grades	None (0)	Mild (1)	Moderate (2)	Severe (3)	Score*
Muscles of limbs and trunk					
Arms outstretched (90 degrees, standing), secs	>240	90–240	10–90	<10	
Leg outstretched (45 degrees, supine), secs	>100	30–100	0–30	0	
Head lifted (45 degrees, supine), secs	>120	30–120	0–30	0	
Grip strength (dynamometer; percent decrement after 10 maximal closures)	<15	15–30	30–75	>75	
Vital capacity, liters					
Men	3.5	2.5–3.5	1.5–2.5	<1.5	
Women	2.5	1.2–2.5	1.2–1.8	<1.2	
Oropharyngeal muscles					
Facial muscles	Normal	Mild weakness on lid closure, snarl	Incomplete lid closure	No mimic expressions	
Chewing	Normal	Fatigue on chewing solid foods	Only soft foods	Gastric tube	
Swallowing	Normal	Fatigue on normal foods	Incomplete palatal closure, nasal speech		

*For calculation of score, weakness grades of each item are added and divided by the number of items tested. The upper test limit was taken from patients and healthy control subjects without neuromuscular weakness.

Source: Adapted from UA Besinger, KV Toyka, M Homberg, et al. Myasthenia gravis: long-term correlation of binding and bungarotoxin blocking antibodies against acetylcholine receptors with changes in disease severity. Neurology 1983;33:1316–1321.

Response to Edrophonium

Edrophonium (Tensilon) is a short-acting anticholinesterase that can be administered intravenously. In myasthenia gravis, a transient improvement in muscle strength occurs within 30 seconds of the administration of 4–8 mg edrophonium and lasts only a minute or two. Useful signs to look for are improvements in ptosis and diplopia, vital capacity, and arm outstretch time. The test is positive in approximately 90% of newly presenting, untreated patients. A positive response may not be seen in a myasthenic patient treated with anticholinesterase drugs if he or she is in a cholinergic state. In fact, such an individual can be made considerably worse by the test. A patient who is receiving anticholinesterase therapy should be pretreated with intravenous atropine first to prevent bradycardia and excessive salivation, and resuscitation facilities should always be available when the test is performed.

Repetitive Nerve Conduction and Electromyography

Abnormal decrement in the compound action potential is seen on repetitive stimulation at approximately 3 Hz in myasthenia gravis, and post-tetanic facilitation followed by decrement is seen after tetanic stimulation [11]. Jitter is often seen on single-fiber electromyography because of variable conduction at the nerve terminal. Neurophysiologic abnormalities are not present in all cases.

Antiacetylcholine Receptor Antibody

An immunoprecipitation assay is available for the antiacetylcholine receptor antibody. An assay value greater than 2×10^{-10} mmol/liter is virtually diagnostic of myasthenia gravis. No close relationship exists between antibody level and severity of illness in a population of individuals. In a single individual, however, a direct relationship exists between antibody level and clinical weakness. Of patients with myasthenia gravis, 15–20% have no detectable antiacetylcholine receptor antibody and yet respond to treatments designed to lower antibody levels [12]. In these individuals, it is assumed that an antibody is present that has not yet been detected.

Radiologic Investigation of the Mediastinum

Posteroanterior and lateral chest x-rays may reveal a thymic mass in the anterior mediastinum. Currently, computed tomography or magnetic resonance imaging of the mediastinum provides better evidence of thymoma, although it is not always possible to distinguish thymic hyperplasia from thymoma or benign from malignant thymoma. The presence and appearance of a tumor may determine the surgical approach to thymectomy and pre- and postoperative management.

OTHER MYASTHENIC CONDITIONS

Congenital Myasthenic Syndromes

Some patients have a congenital abnormality in the type of acetylcholine receptor on the postjunctional membrane or a presynaptic defect in acetylcholine release, giving rise to fatigable muscle weakness. Several variants of these uncommon disorders manifest at an early age [13]. Some are thought to be a form of slow-channel syndrome [14]. The weakness may be responsive to anticholinesterase drugs and 3,4-diaminopyrimidine but does not respond to thymectomy or immunosuppression. Life-threatening bulbar and respiratory weakness rarely occurs.

Neonatal Myasthenia Gravis

Neonatal myasthenia gravis is seen in 10–15% of babies born of myasthenic mothers. The weakness responds to anticholinesterase drugs and the babies recover completely in approximately 6 weeks. The disorder is likely to be caused by transplacental passage of the maternal antibody into the baby.

Lambert-Eaton Myasthenic Syndrome

Lambert-Eaton myasthenic syndrome is a disorder of neuromuscular transmission in which the primary defect is an autoimmune interference of presynaptic voltage-gated calcium channels that control acetylcholine release from the nerve terminal [15]. A deficiency of acetylcholine release gives rise to muscular weakness, and although fatigue occurs (with decrement on repetitive stimulation), the muscle power temporarily improves with activity (seen as an increment in the compound muscle action potential after a short period of muscle contraction). Approximately 90% of patients with Lambert-Eaton myasthenic syndrome have antibodies to voltage-gated calcium channels. Proximal limb muscles are most often involved. Respiratory failure is much less common than in myasthenia gravis, but can occur. Symptomatic treatment with 3,4-diaminopyrimidine (a potassium-channel blocker that prolongs the nerve action potential arriving at the motor end plate, thus enhancing calcium uptake) is often gratifyingly successful. The condition is also improved with plasma exchange and immunosuppression. Approximately 50% of patients with this condition have an associated neoplasm, usually an oat-cell carcinoma of the lung, which sometimes does not manifest until several years after onset of the neurologic syndrome.

TREATMENT

Several forms of treatment are available for myasthenia gravis. It is through the clarification of the immunopathogenesis of this disease that management has improved and mortality and morbidity have been dramatically reduced.

Anticholinesterase Drugs

Pyridostigmine (Mestinon) is probably the anticholinesterase drug of choice in the majority of patients with myasthenia gravis. The half-life of the drug is reasonably long (90 minutes), but the drug does not accumulate easily. It can be given orally as a tablet or elixir and has relatively mild cholinergic side effects. It is frequently used to improve muscle strength, but it should be appreciated that the drug only produces symptomatic improvement and does not tackle the underlying immunopathogenic mechanisms. Neostigmine is the other anticholinesterase drug used in myasthenia gravis. It has the advantage of being able to be administered intravenously but is shorter acting than pyridostigmine and generally the muscarinic side effects are more prominent. Given in too large a dosage, anticholinesterase drugs produce a cholinergic neuromuscular blockade and increase muscle weakness. In the longer term, these drugs in high dosage can probably damage the neuromuscular junction itself and cause muscle weakness. Anticholinesterase drugs can produce cholinergic (muscarinic) side effects such as excessive salivation, abdominal cramps and diarrhea, sweating, and bradycardia. An average dosage of pyridostigmine is 30–60 mg four to five times a day. Only a minority of myasthenic patients have their symptoms controlled satisfactorily by anticholinesterases alone.

Thymectomy

Removal of the thymus gland in the younger age group (<50 years old) with generalized myasthenia gravis is likely to produce remission (return to normal activity without medication) in 25% of cases and partial remission (return to normal activity with the addition of medication) in a further 50%, although the remission may take 6 months or more to be achieved. Thymectomy is the treatment of first choice in young women of childbearing age because the operation alone may prevent the need for immunosuppressant drugs. Patients older than the age of 50 years are helped less by thymectomy because the gland is more atrophic in middle age. Patients who have a thymoma should have a thymectomy to decrease local complications from the tumor. In patients with thymoma, however, the myasthenic symptoms are less likely to benefit from thymectomy alone.

Thymectomy is usually performed through a transsternal incision. This approach exposes the thymus gland well and makes total removal more certain. It is currently the most favored method and the safest approach when large thymomas are excised. A supraclavicular, transcervical incision has been used if no thymoma is present, but total thymectomy may not be achieved. Nevertheless, good results have been recorded from the transcervical approach [16]. More recently, minimally invasive, video-assisted, thoracoscopic thymectomies have been performed with success and with little in the way of complications and postoperative morbidity [17,18]. Further studies of this novel technique are required, however. Thymomas are relatively radiosensitive, and radiotherapy after surgery is often used in locally invasive tumors.

Steroids

Immunosuppression with steroids, such as prednisolone, is effective in decreasing antiacetylcholine receptor antibody levels and improving the clinical state in the majority of patients with myasthenia gravis. Ocular myasthenia is frequently controlled with prednisolone alone. An alternate-day steroid regimen typically starts with a low dose of prednisolone, for example, 5–10 mg, and then increases weekly by 5–10 mg until a maintenance dosage of 1 mg/kg on alternate days is reached. This gradual introduction reduces the chances of an initial steroid-induced worsening of the myasthenia. The dosage is then maintained until the patient has been in remission for several months. Next, the steroids are reduced slowly over months (but not more than 5 mg/month) until a minimum effective dose is achieved. Starting with a high dose of steroid or increasing the dose too fast can cause a deterioration of muscle power before improvement begins. However, remission is achieved more rapidly. If a high-dose regimen is contemplated, the patient is best managed in a hospital or even an intensive care environment where respiratory support is rapidly available.

Azathioprine

Azathioprine immunosuppression is also successful in producing remission in myasthenia gravis. A dosage of 2.5 mg/kg per day is used. However, remission can take 6 months or more to be achieved. The side effects of this drug are less pronounced than those of steroids. Liver function should be checked regularly. Some patients cannot tolerate the drug because of gastrointestinal disturbance or rash.

Because of the lengthy period required to achieve remission with azathioprine, a combined regimen of steroids and azathioprine is commonly used in patients with generalized myasthenia gravis. This strategy has the benefit of a more rapid steroid-induced remission, better long-term maintenance control, and an overall higher success rate than either steroids or azathioprine alone [19].

Plasma Exchange

The antiacetylcholine receptor antibody is in the IgG fraction of the plasma. The level of the antibody can be rapidly reduced by plasma exchange. A typical course of plasma exchange is five daily sessions when 2–3 liters of plasma is removed at each exchange and replaced by a plasma substitute. Improvement in clinical state may be seen within 3 days of the start of plasma exchange, and improvement is optimal by approximately the tenth day. The benefit may be maintained for a month or more but is not sustained. Repeated courses are often needed to maintain the clinical improvement while waiting for other forms of immunosuppression to have an effect. Plasma exchange is often useful to achieve an optimal clinical state before thymectomy.

Immunoglobulin G Immunoadsorption

It is now possible to pass the plasma separated during plasma exchange through a gel column of tryptophan-linked polyvinyl alcohol resin. The IgG fraction is absorbed onto the surface of the gel, but a substantial amount of albumin can be returned to the patient, and protein replacement is therefore unnecessary. The clinical benefits are otherwise similar to those of plasma exchange [20].

Intravenous Immunoglobulin

Several studies have shown a temporary clinical improvement in myasthenia gravis after the administration of intravenous immunoglobulin [21]. The results are comparable to those of plasma exchange, but administration of the immunoglobulin is considerably easier than plasma exchange. The precise mechanism of action of immunoglobulin in myasthenia gravis has yet to be determined.

CRISIS IN MYASTHENIA GRAVIS

Before adequate immunosuppressive treatment for myasthenia gravis was available, the disease tended to pursue a fluctuating but downward course in which anticholinesterase therapy became less effective and the eventual mortality was high (30%). The terminal event was usually respiratory failure. As with several other neuromuscular disorders, the inability to swallow and deal with normal oral secretions, when combined with weak respiratory muscles (manifested as an inability to take a deep breath or to generate an effective cough), leads to aspiration of oral secretions into the lungs and acute respiratory failure. With more effective treatment for myasthenia gravis, the mortality from the disease is now very low, and most patients can be brought into remission. Nevertheless, some individuals still develop bulbar weakness and life-threatening respiratory failure requiring control of the airway and artificial ventilation. This situation is known as a *crisis*. The three main causes of a crisis in myasthenia gravis are (1) myasthenic crisis (most common), (2) cholinergic crisis (rare), and (3) steroid crisis (not uncommon when treatment is started in patients with generalized myasthenic weakness).

Myasthenic Crisis

Several situations can precipitate a myasthenic crisis:

1. A sudden worsening of the myasthenic weakness may be the result of an inability to take or absorb the prescribed anticholinesterase therapy (e.g., persistent vomiting, coma, surgery).
2. Infection appears to worsen the myasthenic state. The weakness could be the result of a sudden general rise in antibody production, including the anti-acetylcholine receptor antibody.
3. Mental or physical stress also seems to influence and exacerbate myasthenic weakness, although the cause is not understood.
4. The natural progression of the disease untreated can lead to bulbar and respiratory weakness and a crisis state.
5. The marked erosion of the safety margin in myasthenia gravis means that small changes in the efficiency of neurotransmission occurring on either side of the neuromuscular junction (which, with a normal safety margin, would not be revealed) can have a profound effect on muscle power. The effects of drugs

on neuromuscular transmission in myasthenia gravis has been reviewed by Wittbrodt [22]. Several types of drugs can have a deleterious effect on muscle power in myasthenia gravis. A neuromuscular blocking agent that occupies the acetylcholine receptor, making it unavailable to acetylcholine, dramatically alters neuromuscular transmission. Thus, myasthenic patients are exquisitely sensitive to the nondepolarizing muscle relaxants used in anesthesia, even in low dosage. The situation may be further complicated by anticholinesterase medication. The aminoglycoside group of antibiotics, ciprofloxacin [23], ampicillin, and erythromycin can worsen myasthenic weakness. Quinine, quinidine, procainamide, chloroquine, beta blockers, verapamil, phenytoin [24], and lithium carbonate have all been noted to exacerbate myasthenic weakness. Penicillamine can produce a myasthenic state itself and also exacerbate myasthenia gravis [25].

Cholinergic Crisis

The most common cause of a cholinergic crisis is anticholinesterase overdose in a self-medicating patient. Initially the patient, already marginally cholinergic and experiencing substantial myasthenic weakness, may increase the dose of anticholinesterase to achieve optimal strength. On finding that the medication is less effective and not appreciating the symptoms and dangers of the cholinergic state, the patient increases the dose even further. If the bulbar and respiratory muscles become weak, the excessive salivation of the cholinergic state can precipitate acute respiratory failure.

Medically prescribed overdose of anticholinesterase therapy can occur. Not infrequently, some muscle groups are more cholinergic than others. If a Tensilon test is performed and it is observed that one muscle group improves with Tensilon, the patient may be thought to be myasthenically weak and the anticholinesterase is increased. Failure to examine or take note of the lack of improvement or worsening in power in other important muscle groups, such as the bulbar and respiratory muscles, may lead the physician to misinterpret the Tensilon test and precipitate the patient into a cholinergic crisis.

Pure cholinergic weakness is very rare: The usual scenario of cholinergic crisis is in fact a combination of serious myasthenic weakness with superimposed cholinergic overdose and neuromuscular blockade. In such a setting, the patient is best admitted to the intensive care unit and managed as described in Management of a Crisis.

Steroid Crisis

Steroid crisis is not an uncommon occurrence when a rapid increase in steroid dosage occurs at the start of steroid therapy in a patient with pre-existing generalized myasthenic weakness [26]. The patient can become rapidly weak and unresponsive to anticholinesterase therapy. The safe procedure is to manage such an individual in the intensive care unit and to intubate and ventilate the patient until the situation improves. Usually, within 7–10 days the crisis has resolved and remission begins.

Management of a Crisis

If a myasthenic patient presents in a distressed state with breathing difficulties, it may not be an appropriate time to investigate the situation with a Tensilon test. If the patient is anxious, breathless, and unwilling to lie supine and if the accessory muscles of respiration are being used and swallowing is a problem, it is essential that the airway is controlled first and that satisfactory ventilation and oxygenation are provided. This means rapid and efficient intubation either orally or nasally. Often, nasal intubation is preferable because it is more comfortable and patients may not require much in the way of sedation and analgesia, which makes the neurologic assessment easier.

Whether the patient is myasthenically weak or cholinergic (or both) can be gleaned from the history. The cholinergic patient may complain of muscarinic symptoms. Once the respiratory distress is under control and the patient is more comfortable and cooperative, a Tensilon test can be performed cautiously, bearing in mind that cholinergic patients can be made acutely worse with Tensilon. Although the result may clarify the situation, not uncommonly the response to Tensilon at the time of crisis is equivocal. In this case, it is best to stop all anticholinesterase treatment, support ventilation, and wait until the patient is definitely myasthenic before introducing anticholinesterase medication again.

It is useful to pass a nasogastric tube to administer nutrition and medication. Intravenous access is essential and an indwelling arterial cannula is advisable to monitor blood gases.

If an obvious precipitating factor for the crisis is found, such as an infection, this should be treated. However, very often the damage sustained by the neuromuscular junction is such that anticholinesterase drugs cannot improve the situation and only lowering of the antiacetylcholine receptor antibody level can allow recovery to occur.

Plasma exchange is probably the most efficient method of reducing antibody levels quickly. Usually within 4 days of the start of treatment, an improvement in neuromuscular function occurs, and by 10 days the crisis is over. Other short-term methods of improving the myasthenic state, such as intravenous immunoglobulin, can be used as well to achieve a rapid improvement.

This is also a good time to review long-term therapy and consider the introduction of immunosuppression or to optimize the dosage in those who are already receiving immunosuppression. In the case of crisis that occurs after the start of high-dose steroid therapy, it is perfectly reasonable, having run into problems requiring intubation and ventilation, to continue with high-dose therapy to try to achieve an early remission. It is not known whether plasma exchange before the administration of high-dose steroids reduces the incidence of steroid crisis. If a patient in myasthenic crisis is already ventilated, and a decision is made to start steroids, a daily high-dose regimen is appropriate (prednisolone, 60–80 mg/day) to achieve a more rapid improvement.

If recovery is slow and bulbar and respiratory weakness is likely to persist for some time, tracheostomy should be considered. It provides more comfortable security of the airway, protection of and easy access to the lower respiratory tract, and an unhurried, safe weaning period. With the advent of percutaneous tracheostomy techniques and their lower morbidity and good cosmetic result, tracheostomy is a small price to pay for the benefits it affords.

PERIOPERATIVE MANAGEMENT OF THYMECTOMY

Whereas today thymectomy is the treatment of choice in the younger age group with generalized myasthenia, 25 or more years ago it was a treatment of last resort and usually was performed on patients in a poor clinical state when conservative medical management had already failed. Thymectomy in those days was a hazardous undertaking, and postoperative complications frequently occurred. It used to be routine to perform a tracheostomy before thymectomy, and the operation had a poor reputation, with a high morbidity and mortality.

With the development of immunosuppression therapy and techniques such as plasma exchange, it became possible to electively perform thymectomy when the patient was in an optimal clinical state. This has made the operation and postoperative management a much less hazardous procedure. Improvements in anesthesia, postoperative pain control, ventilation techniques, and intensive care management have also contributed to the safety of thymectomy.

Preoperative Assessment and Management

To a certain degree, the precise management of thymectomy depends on the surgical approach proposed. Transcervical supraclavicular and video-assisted thoracoscopic thymectomy require different anesthetic approaches from those for transsternal thymectomy. An ongoing debate exists as to whether the decreased morbidity and length of hospitalization of the less invasive surgical techniques can produce as good an end result as the more complete removal of all thymic tissue achieved by the extensive exposure of the mediastinal anatomy through a transsternal operation. In this chapter, the discussion relates to the transsternal surgical operation but is also relevant to other approaches.

History

The general medical history of previous illness, drug therapy, surgery, allergies, and so forth may affect subsequent management and is important. However, particular attention must be directed to the severity and course of the myasthenic illness. The duration of the illness, the muscle groups affected, the drug requirements, previous episodes of crisis, and the response to previous anesthesia all give a flavor of the severity of the disease and the likely postoperative problems. Perhaps the most important predictor of postoperative complications, however, is the presence of bulbar or respiratory muscle weakness. Should this be a feature preoperatively, further medical treatment to improve respiratory and bulbar function is advisable.

Examination and Investigations

General physical examination should confirm the history. Simple bedside measurements of muscle power and degree of muscle fatigue are useful as a baseline for subsequent comparison, and measurement of vital capacity (VC) is a useful rough index of respiratory muscle power. A VC of less than 1.5 liters in an adult in the upright posture should give rise to concern, and a fall in VC of more than 50% on assuming the supine position is indicative of severe diaphragm weakness. Respiratory distress in the supine posture and the use of accessory muscles of respiration at rest are also signs of significant respiratory muscle weakness.

The diagnosis of myasthenia gravis should have been confirmed by previous investigations, but posteroanterior and lateral chest x-rays and computed tomography or magnetic resonance imaging of the mediastinum should be available to demonstrate whether a thymoma is present. The possibility of phrenic nerve involvement should always be borne in mind if the patient has a thymoma and radiologic evidence of unilateral diaphragm weakness is seen. Full blood count, urea, electrolytes, blood group, cross-match, and so forth should be checked routinely.

Preanesthetic Management

If the patient's medical condition can be improved by adjustment of medication, antibiotics, or procedures such as plasma exchange or intravenous immunoglobulin, it would be advisable to provide such treatment preoperatively to give the patient the best chance of a trouble-free postoperative recovery [27]. A full account of the likely procedures and outcome of the anesthesia, surgery, postoperative pain relief, and recovery or intensive care management should be given at the preoperative visit and consent for the procedures obtained.

Commonly, the normal dose of anticholinesterase medication is omitted on the morning of the operation because the majority of patients do not appear to require this treatment for the first 2 days or so postoperatively. If given their normal medication postoperatively, these patients may show cholinergic signs. The reasons for this are not clear but may possibly be related to the decrease in mobility in the postoperative period, a slight preoperative tendency to anticholinesterase overdose, or perhaps to some unrealized immune response to surgery and anesthesia. Should the patient predict that uncomfortable weakness would occur by omitting the anticholinesterase on the day of the operation, however, it would be best to give the drug. Preoperative anticholinesterases promote salivation and can interfere with the actions of muscle-relaxant drugs, but as muscle relaxants are seldom administered during a thymectomy, this is rarely a major problem.

Premedication before operation may be a kindness, and the use of opioid drugs is not contraindicated. Steroid cover should follow usual practice if the patient is having steroid medication. Preoperative starvation and preparation should proceed as with any other thoracic surgical operation, and a preoperative chest shave should be given if necessary. Prophylactic antibiotic cover should be considered and prescribed at this stage.

Induction of Anesthesia and Intraoperative Management

As many ways exist of conducting anesthesia thymectomy as there are anesthetists. Baraka [28] and Eisenkraft [29] have reviewed anesthesia for myasthenia gravis and thymic surgery. The following is an outline of my practice when anesthetizing for a transsternal thymectomy. However, other drugs and techniques have been used equally successfully.

Anesthesia is induced with an intravenous bolus of fentanyl followed by propofol, and intubation with an oral endotracheal tube is performed without the use of any muscle relaxant; anesthesia is maintained with artificial ventilation using nitrous oxide, oxygen, and isoflurane. If intubation is predicted to be difficult, no contraindication to the use of suxamethonium exists, as resistance to this relaxant is hardly noticeable with normal dosage [30,31]. However, the normal fasciculations after suxamethonium may not be seen. Should it be predicted that the patient might require assisted ventilation postoperatively in intensive care, a nasotracheal tube can be used for greater comfort during recovery.

Use of nondepolarizing muscle relaxants in patients with myasthenia gravis is best avoided, as the sensitivity of the patient to such drugs is unpredictable and prolonged paralysis can occur. Atracurium is the nondepolarizing relaxant of choice if such a drug is required, as its rate of elimination is more predictable [32]. However, it should be administered in approximately one-fourth of the normal dose, and monitoring of neuromuscular blockade both before and after administration of the drug is advisable. Muscle relaxation is not required by the surgeon for transsternal thymectomy, and adequate anesthesia and mild hyperventilation are all that are needed to suppress respiratory movement.

Technically, thymectomy is a straightforward operation. Care must be taken not to damage the phrenic nerves during dissection of the thymus gland. Opening of the pleural cavity should not cause a problem unless the visceral pleura has been breached, giving rise to an alveolar leak. The operation can be considerably more difficult if an associated thymoma is present, especially if local invasion of important mediastinal structures, such as the phrenic nerves, aorta, or superior vena cava, has occurred. In this situation, it may be advisable to debulk the tumor but leave a remnant behind to be dealt with by radiotherapy rather than to attempt a hazardous clearance of the thymoma. It is possible for a patient to manage with a unilateral phrenic nerve palsy, but a bilateral palsy is a disaster.

After careful hemostasis, the two halves of the sternum should be firmly wired together to reduce postoperative pain. Mediastinal or chest drains are inserted as necessary, and the wound is closed while a positive pressure is maintained in the airway to expel air out of the pleural cavity and mediastinum. Local anesthetic infiltration of the wound is also a help in reducing postoperative pain.

Postoperative Management

The majority of patients who are in good condition preoperatively can be extubated at the end of surgery and can be observed in a high-dependency unit for a time postoperatively. The main requirement is adequate postoperative analgesia. A combination of nonsteroidal anti-inflammatory analgesic and intravenous opioid infusion (usually patient-controlled) is adequate.

A postoperative chest x-ray is advisable to exclude a pneumothorax. Some widening of the mediastinum is to be expected after operation. Output from the drains should be observed. Measurements of VC and arm strength are unreliable owing to wound pain in the first 3 days postoperatively. Facial, bulbar, and lower limb strength can be assessed, however, and the patient's own assessment of weakness is a good guide to the need for anticholinesterase medication. It is usually wise to restart anticholinesterase drugs at a lower dose and increase the dose as the patient becomes more mobile.

In patients with significant bulbar and respiratory weakness preoperatively, airway complications may develop postoperatively as a result of the inability to clear oral secretions. This can precipitate acute respiratory failure. Should this be a possibility, it is advisable to provide postoperative care in an intensive care environment with elective intubation until respiratory and bulbar function can be properly assessed, with the patient recovered adequately from the anesthetic and in a stable, comfortable state. Postoperative respiratory failure should be managed in much the same way as outlined in the section on crisis.

REFERENCES

1. Drachman DB. Myasthenia gravis. N Engl J Med 1994;330:1797.
2. Dreyer F. Acetylcholine receptor. Br J Anaesth 1982;54:4168.
3. Paton WDM, Waud DR. The margin of safety of neurotransmission. J Physiol 1967;191:59.
4. Vincent A, Newsom-Davis J. Acetylcholine receptor antibody as a diagnostic test for myasthenia gravis: results in 153 validated cases and 2967 diagnostic assays. J Neurol Neurosurg Psychiatry 1985;48:1246.
5. Detterbeck FC, Scott WW, Howard JF Jr, et al. One hundred consecutive thymectomies for myasthenia gravis. Ann Thorac Surg 1996;62:242.
6. Masaoka A, Yamakawa Y, Niwa H, et al. Extended thymectomy for myasthenia gravis patients: a 20-year review. Ann Thorac Surg 1996;62:853.
7. Kao I, Drachman DB. Thymic muscle cells bear acetylcholine receptors: possible relation to myasthenia gravis. Science 1997;195:74.
8. Truffault F, Cohen-Kaminsky S, Khali I, et al. Altered intrathymic T-cell repertoire in human myasthenia gravis. Ann Neurol 1997;41:732.
9. Osserman KE, Genkins G. Studies in myasthenia gravis: review of a twenty-year experience in over 1200 patients. Mt Sinai J Med 1971;38:497.
10. Besinger UA, Toyka KV, Homberg M, et al. Myasthenia gravis: long-term correlation of binding and bungarotoxin blocking antibodies against acetylcholine receptors with changes in disease severity. Neurology 1983;33:1316.
11. Stalberg E. Clinical electrophysiology in myasthenia gravis. J Neurol Neurosurg Psychiatry 1980;43:622.
12. Soliven BC, Lange DJ, Penn AS, et al. Seronegative myasthenia gravis. Neurology 1988;38:514.
13. Vincent A, Newland C, Croxen R, Beeson D. Genes at the junction—candidates for congenital myasthenic syndromes. Trends Neurosci 1997;20:15.
14. Engel AG, Lambert EH, Mulder DM, et al. A newly recognized congenital myasthenic syndrome attributed to a prolonged open time of the acetylcholine-induced ion channel. Ann Neurol 1982;11:553.
15. Lennon VA, Kryzer TJ, Griesmann, GE, et al. Calcium-channel antibodies in the Lambert-Eaton syndrome and other paraneoplastic syndromes. N Engl J Med 1995;332:1467.
16. DeFilippi VJ, Richman DP, Ferguson MK. Transcervical thymectomy for myasthenia gravis. Ann Thorac Surg 1994;57:194.
17. Yim APC, Kay RLC, Ho JKS. Video-assisted thoracoscopic thymectomy for myasthenia gravis. Minimally invasive techniques. Chest 1995;108:1440.
18. Mack MJ, Landreneau RJ, Yim AP, et al. Results of video-assisted thymectomy in patients with myasthenia gravis. J Thorac Cardiovasc Surg 1996;112:1352.
19. Myasthenia Gravis Clinical Study Group: Gajdos P, Elkharrat D, Chevret S, et al. A randomised clinical trial comparing prednisone and azathioprine in myasthenia gravis. Results of the second interim analysis. J Neurol Neurosurg Psychiatry 1993;56:1157.
20. Grob D, Simpson D, Mitsumoto H, et al. Treatment of myasthenia gravis by immunoadsorption of plasma. Neurology 1995;45:338.

21. Gajdos PH. Intravenous immune globulin in myasthenia gravis. Clin Exp Immunol 1994;97(suppl 1):49.
22. Wittbrodt ET. Drugs and myasthenia gravis. Arch Intern Med 1997;157:399.
23. Roquer J, Cano A, Seoane JL, Pou Serredell A. Myasthenia gravis and ciprofloxacin. Acta Neurol Scand 1996;94:419.
24. So EL, Penry JK. Adverse effects of phenytoin on peripheral nerves and neuromuscular junction: a review. Epilepsia 1981;22:467.
25. Kuncl RW, Pestronk A, Drachman DB, Rechtland E. The pathophysiology of penicillamine-induced myasthenia gravis. Ann Neurol 1986;20:740.
26. Miller RG, Milner-Brown HS, Mirka A. Prednisone-induced worsening of neuromuscular function in myasthenia gravis. Neurology 1986;36:729.
27. d'Empaire G, Hoaglin DC, Perlo VP, Pontoppidan H. Effect of prethymectomy plasma exchange on postoperative respiratory function in myasthenia gravis. J Thorac Cardiovasc Surg 1985;89:592.
28. Baraka A. Review article. Anaesthesia and myasthenia gravis. Can J Anaesth 1992;39;476.
29. Eisenkraft JB. Myasthenia Gravis and Thymic Surgery—Anaesthetic Considerations. In JWW Gothard (ed), Bailliere's Clinical Anaesthesiology (Vol 1, No. 1). Thoracic Anaesthesia. London: Bailliere Tindall, 1987;133–162.
30. Eisenkraft JB, Book WJ, Mann SM, et al. Resistance to succinylcholine in myasthenia gravis: a dose-response study. Anesthesiology 1988;69:760.
31. Baraka A. Suxamethonium block in the myasthenic patient: correlation with plasma cholinesterase. Anaesthesia 1992;47:217.
32. Vacanti CA, Ali HH, Schweiss JF, Scott RP. The response of myasthenia gravis to atracurium. Anesthesiology 1985;62:692.

4
Other Causes of Acute Weakness in the Intensive Care Unit

James W. Teener, Mark M. Rich, and Shawn J. Bird

Since the 1970s, neuromuscular disorders have been recognized as common causes of prolonged weakness and ventilator dependence in the setting of critical illness [1,2]. The list of neuromuscular disorders encountered in the intensive care unit (ICU) is extensive (Table 4.1). One useful way to organize the differential diagnosis of generalized weakness is to divide the list between conditions that themselves produce weakness severe enough to warrant ICU care, and those that develop as a consequence of another disorder or treatment in the ICU. Myasthenia gravis and Guillain-Barré syndrome (GBS) are examples of the former and are discussed elsewhere in this book. This chapter focuses on less common causes of generalized weakness, as well as on the neuromuscular complications of critical illness: critical illness polyneuropathy, acute quadriplegic myopathy, and prolonged neuromuscular blockade.

A generalized neuropathy that develops in the setting of sepsis and multiorgan failure, critical illness polyneuropathy (CIP), was first described and then characterized by Bolton and colleagues [3]. More recently, numerous authors have reported a myopathy that develops in the same setting of critical illness, often associated with the use of nondepolarizing neuromuscular blocking agents (NMBAs), corticosteroids, or both. It has been increasingly identified as a cause of prolonged weakness [4,5]. This myopathy has been termed *acute quadriplegic myopathy* (AQM), *thick filament myopathy*, *acute myopathy of critical illness*, and *critical illness myopathy*, among others.

Other neuromuscular diseases may develop de novo in the ICU. GBS may rarely develop in this setting. Transient muscle weakness may develop as a result of metabolic abnormalities, such as hypokalemia or hypermagnesemia. Preexisting, but unsuspected, disorders may become symptomatic. Myasthenia gravis or motor neuron disease may first be identified in the ICU, often in the setting of infection that precipitates respiratory failure.

Table 4.1   Differential diagnosis of generalized weakness in the intensive care unit

Brain
  Encephalopathy
  Multiple infarcts
  Brain stem lesion
Spinal cord
  Cord infarct
  Transverse myelitis
  Tetanus
  Many acute causes such as epidural compression, infection
Anterior horn cell
  Amyotrophic lateral sclerosis
  Poliomyelitis or poliomyelitis-like syndrome
  Paralytic rabies
  Paraneoplastic effect of lymphoma
Multiple radiculopathy
  Carcinomatous meningitis
  Lymphomatous meningitis
  Acquired immunodeficiency syndrome–related
  Polyradiculitis (Lyme and others)
Peripheral nerve
  Critical illness polyneuropathy
  Guillain-Barré syndrome
  Porphyria
  Vasculitis
  Acute massive intoxication
Neuromuscular junction
  Persistent neuromuscular blockade
  Myasthenia gravis
  Hypermagnesemia
  Botulism
  Marine toxins
Muscle
  Acute quadriplegic myopathy
  Hypokalemia
  Periodic paralysis
  Metabolic/inflammatory myopathy (acid maltase deficiency, polymyositis, etc.)
  Disuse atrophy
  Rhabdomyolysis

CLINICAL EVALUATION OF ACUTE QUADRIPARESIS

Close attention to historical clues and examination findings is the first step in elucidating the cause of generalized weakness in the ICU. Evidence of subtle preexisting sensory and motor dysfunction should be sought. Although some neuromuscular disorders, particularly myasthenia gravis and amyotrophic lateral sclerosis, may initially present with respiratory failure, often subtle hints of weakness become apparent on careful questioning of the patient or the patient's family. A history of exposure to medications or other toxins also should be thoroughly sought. A history of travel or exposure to unusual foods or animals may be important, as discussed later.

Examination is often complicated by the presence of encephalopathy, which itself can cause weakness and mask other causes of weakness. Attention to the pattern of weakness, facial and ocular motor involvement, muscle tendon reflexes, and sensory examination often allows localization of the disorder and guides further evaluation. Table 4.2 presents the typical characteristics of the most common causes of generalized weakness in the ICU.

Imaging studies, particularly computed tomography and magnetic resonance imaging, are most useful in identifying lesions of the brain and spinal cord. Electrodiagnostic studies are used to evaluate the peripheral nervous system. These studies may confirm neuromuscular abnormalities as well as demonstrate subtle abnormalities that are not apparent on clinical evaluation. They are often difficult to perform in the ICU, however, and their usefulness may be limited by a variety of factors. Electrical equipment in the ICU produces electrical noise, making recording of small potentials, particularly sensory potentials, difficult. Recording and stimulating sites are often obscured by bandages and other monitoring equipment, making optimal studies difficult. Finally, encephalopathic patients are often unable to cooperate with the voluntary portions of the electrodiagnostic examination.

Electrodiagnostic evaluations performed in the ICU may be so limited as to preclude positive identification of the cause of weakness, or even determination of the definite location of the lesion. For example, both CIP and AQM produce reduced motor amplitudes on nerve conduction studies. These disorders can be distinguished in the ideal setting through differences in voluntary motor unit recruitment and the sensory involvement typically present in CIP. If the sensory potentials cannot be reliably recorded and the recruitment patterns cannot be evaluated, it may be impossible to make an electrodiagnostic distinction between these two disorders.

Table 4.2   Clinical features of common causes of generalized weakness in the intensive care unit

Cause of weakness	Limb weakness	Cranial nerve involvement	Reflexes	Sensory deficits
Brain stem lesion	Asymmetric quadriparesis	Common, ocular motility	Increased	Common
Spinal cord lesion	Paraparesis	None	Reduced early, increases later	Below lesion
Guillain-Barré syndrome	Distal	Common, facial diplegia	Absent	Common
Myasthenia gravis	Proximal	Common, ptosis, oculomotor, and facial	Normal	None
Critical illness polyneuropathy	Distal	Rare	Absent	Present
Acute quadriplegic myopathy	Diffuse	Rare	Normal or reduced	None

Nerve conduction studies nevertheless play the primary role in identifying disorders of peripheral nerve. Features of demyelination (prolonged distal motor latencies, conduction slowing, and conduction block) are typically identified in the demyelinating form of GBS. The absence of features of demyelination in combination with reduced sensory and motor nerve conduction response amplitudes suggest that the process primarily involves axonal loss. Axonal neuropathies are relatively common, and definitive identification of the etiology of the axonal neuropathy may not be possible. For example, it can be difficult to determine with certainty whether the patient has axonal GBS or CIP.

Nerve conduction studies with repetitive nerve stimulation allow identification of defects in neuromuscular transmission. Such defects can be further classified as presynaptic, as seen in the Lambert-Eaton syndrome and botulism, or postsynaptic, as seen in myasthenia gravis or persistent paralysis caused by NMBAs.

Needle electromyography (EMG) typically allows separation of neuropathic from myopathic processes but requires the cooperation of the patient, which is often lacking in encephalopathic, critically ill patients. Additional studies, such as nerve and muscle biopsy, may be required to make a more definite diagnosis.

NEUROMUSCULAR COMPLICATIONS OF CRITICAL ILLNESS

Three distinct syndromes, persistent neuromuscular blockade, CIP, and AQM, develop in critically ill patients as a consequence of the illness or its treatment. Interest in these disorders has grown since the description of CIP by Bolton and others in the 1980s. It has become apparent that nerve and muscle dysfunction is common in the ICU and substantially contributes to slow weaning from mechanical ventilation, prolonging the ICU stay.

Persistent Neuromuscular Blockade

NMBAs are being used increasingly often in the ICU to improve lung compliance and allow more efficient mechanical ventilation. These medications have been strongly linked to the development of AQM and perhaps to CIP as well. In addition, the recovery of neuromuscular transmission after either short- or long-term blockade with nondepolarizing agents may be prolonged in patients with impaired hepatic or renal function [6–11]. Return of muscle strength after acute discontinuation of atracurium or pancuronium for anesthesia was studied and, despite neostigmine reversal, grip strength ranged from 44% to 60% for at least 1 hour [12]. Prolonged neuromuscular blockade requiring mechanical ventilation has been reported after short-term use of atracurium as well [6].

Prolonged neuromuscular blockade after long-term vecuronium administration has been reported in patients with renal or hepatic failure [10,13,14]. Because vecuronium is metabolized primarily by the liver, the association with renal insufficiency is surprising but can result from delayed excretion of active metabolites. A 3-desacetyl metabolite of vecuronium, elevated magnesium levels, and female gender have all been associated with prolonged neuromuscular blockade in patients with renal failure [10]. Prolonged blockade should be considered in any patient who remains weak after discontinuation of NMBAs. It is easily detected through nerve conduction studies with repetitive stimulation in which a decrement in the compound muscle potential amplitude is seen. Weakness should not persist beyond 2 weeks after stopping the blocking agent and typically lasts for only a few days. One method of decreasing the incidence of prolonged neuromuscular blockade is to titrate dosage by using a peripheral nerve stimulator and monitoring twitch response to train-of-four stimulation [15].

Critical Illness Polyneuropathy

CIP was first described by Bolton and colleagues [3] in five patients in whom a severe sensorimotor polyneuropathy developed during a period of critical illness (sepsis and multiorgan failure). With detailed nerve conduction studies and EMG, they were able to identify a distal axonal sensory and motor neuropathy. This entity was convincingly shown to differ from the GBS on electrophysiologic and morphologic, as well as clinical, grounds [16]. Subsequently the clinical, electrophysiologic, and pathologic features were well characterized [17–21]. In their prototypic form, these features define a distinctive type of acute polyneuropathy (Table 4.3).

In patients with CIP, peripheral nerve degeneration develops in the setting of the systemic inflammatory response syndrome (SIRS). SIRS is a severe systemic response that occurs in up to 50% of those in a critical care setting in response to infection or other insults, such as burns or trauma [22]. In the setting of infection, the term *sepsis* is appropriate [23]. In addition to the inciting insult, the clinical features of this syndrome are two or more of the following: temperature higher than 38°C or lower than 36°C, heart rate greater than 90, respiratory rate greater than 20 or $Paco_2$ less than 32 mm Hg, and white blood cell count greater than 12,000 or less than 4,000 cells/μl. The major risk factor for the development of CIP in the ICU is SIRS, usually sepsis. A prospective study demonstrated that as many as 70% of patients with sepsis and multiple organ failure develop abnormalities on nerve conduction studies [19]. Subsequent prospective studies have reported on the incidence of this disorder, with a wide range of results [24–27]. The variability in incidence between these studies is likely owing to the definition used for identifying neuropathy and the difficulty in separating CIP from the myopathy that can occur in the same setting. With careful attention to this issue, Lacomis and coworkers [2] prospectively evaluated 92 patients in the ICU over a 4.5-year period. Of those in whom acute weakness developed in the ICU, the most common cause was myopathy (42%). An acute neuropathy, CIP, was seen in 13%.

The pathophysiology of CIP is uncertain. Evidence is lacking to support drugs, toxins, nutritional deficiencies, autoimmune disorders, or specific infectious agents as causative. One hypothesis is that in the setting of SIRS, humoral and cellular mechanisms are initiated that disturb microcirculation, including that of brain and nerve [28].

On clinical examination, those with CIP have distally predominant limb weakness, atrophy, and reduced reflexes. Sensory loss can be demonstrated in patients who are able to cooperate with the examination. However, many patients in the critical care setting are not easily examined owing to sedation or coexistent encephalopathy, an even more common complication of SIRS. Quadriparesis

Table 4.3   Features of critical illness polyneuropathy, acute quadriplegic myopathy, and indeterminate forms

Feature	Critical illness polyneuropathy	Acute quadri- plegic myopathy	Indeterminate
Risk factors	SIRS	NMBA and/or steroids	SIRS, NMBA, and/or steroids
Clinical findings	Sensory and motor deficits	Purely motor	Predominantly motor
Creatine phospho- kinase	Normal	Normal to slightly elevated	Normal to elevated
Pathology	Nerve: axonal loss	Nerve: normal	Nerve: ?
	Muscle: denervation	Muscle: patchy myosin loss; min- imal necrosis	Muscle: ?
Clinical course	Slow recovery	Often rapid recovery	Variable
Nerve conduction studies	Decreased SNAPs and CMAPs	Normal SNAPs Very decreased CMAPs	Normal to decreased SNAPs Decreased CMAPs
Spontaneous activity	Yes, often prominent	None to prominent	None to prominent
MUP morphology	Normal to long/large	Decreased amplitude and decreased duration	No voluntary units or indeterminate due to poor effort
MUP recruitment	Increased recruitment ratio (neurogenic)	Early full (myopathic)	No or few voluntary units
Direct muscle CMAP amplitude	Normal	Absent or minimal	Often reduced

SIRS = systemic inflammatory response syndrome; NMBA = neuromuscular blocking agent; CMAP = compound muscle action potential; MUP = motor unit potential; SNAP = sensory nerve action potential.

should be suspected when little movement is provoked by painful stimulation of the distal limb, despite vigorous facial grimacing. Failure to wean from the ventilator, a feature common to other neuromuscular disorders in this setting, may be the first recognized manifestation. In an early prospective clinical and electrophysiologic study of 21 patients who had difficulty in being weaned from the ventilator, Spitzer and colleagues [1] identified a neuromuscular cause in 62%. Although most may have acute myopathy [2], CIP has developed as the underlying cause in a significant percentage.

Witt and coworkers [19] prospectively followed 43 patients with sepsis and multiorgan failure. The mean age of patients was 64 (21–78 years) with a mean of 28 days (5–89) in the ICU. Thirty patients (70%) had abnormal nerve conduction studies or spontaneous activity on needle examination, or both. Half of these (35%) had clinical evidence of neuropathy defined as distal weakness and hyporeflexia or otherwise unexplained inability to wean from the respirator. The severity of the neuropathy correlated with the total time in the ICU. All patients had evidence of encephalopathy. Nearly half of the patients affected by CIP died of their critical illness. Of those who survived, recovery mirrored that seen in most axonal neuropathies. Those who survived with mild to moderate neuropathy recovered fully over months, likely as a result of collateral sprouting from remaining motor neurons. Those with severe neuropathy, requiring axonal regeneration for recovery, either had no recovery or had a significant persistent deficit.

Electrophysiologic studies have characterized CIP as an axonal sensorimotor polyneuropathy [1,3,16,17,19,21]. Nerve conduction studies typically demonstrate reduced motor and sensory response amplitudes, without evidence of demyelination. Those patients who have reduced motor responses, with preserved sensory responses, may have a motor variant of CIP (discussed in Does a "Pure Motor" Form of Critical Illness Polyneuropathy Exist?), or more likely have myopathy [2]. Repetitive nerve stimulation studies are normal. Needle EMG examination of limb muscle shows fibrillation potentials and positive sharp waves in many patients. With voluntary recruitment, an excess of polyphasic motor unit potentials is seen. Motor unit recruitment is typically reduced. These EMG features are consistent with acute denervation.

Phrenic nerve conduction studies are notable for reduced responses bilaterally. In those with severe neuropathy, the phrenic nerve motor responses are absent [17,21]. Denervation on needle EMG examination of the chest wall muscles or the diaphragm also has been demonstrated [29,30]. This can confirm the presumed neuromuscular cause of the failure to wean from the respirator in many patients with this disorder. Nerve biopsy and autopsy studies show axonal degeneration of both sensory and motor fibers without evidence of significant inflammation or primary demyelination [3,21].

ACUTE QUADRIPLEGIC MYOPATHY

AQM was first reported in 1977 in a woman with asthma treated with both corticosteroids and NMBAs [31]. In a subsequent report, Sher and colleagues [32] presented a critically ill patient with multiorgan failure and pneumonia who received corticosteroids and developed a myopathy. These and a number of subsequent reports gave rise to the hypothesis that a distinct myopathy develops in critically ill patients [33–41]. A 1998 report indicates that AQM is the most common cause of generalized weakness in the ICU [2]. In addition to AQM, other names given to this syndrome have included acute illness myopathy, acute myopathy of intensive care, rapidly evolving myopathy with myosin-deficient fibers, and critical illness myopathy.

The classic clinical picture of AQM is that of an asthmatic patient who is intubated for an exacerbation and treated with corticosteroids and NMBAs [31,33,34,36–39,41–53]. As the asthmatic crisis resolves, it becomes apparent that the patient is quadriparetic. Some patients have only mild weakness, but many are severely affected and weaning from the ventilator is often delayed secondary to the myopathy. Extraocular movements are often spared, but have occasionally been involved [37,51,53]. Sensation is spared and reflexes are decreased in parallel with the decrease in strength. After patients recover from the acute illness, improvement in strength usually occurs within 1–3 months to the point at which they are able to ambulate [5,31,33,34,36,37,39,40,42,43,45–49,52].

Nerve conduction studies in AQM reveal diminished compound muscle action potential (CMAP) amplitudes in the setting of normal sensory response amplitudes [5,34,37,42,46,49,50,52–59]. Conduction velocities and repetitive stimulation are normal [5,34,35,37,42,43,46,47,49–51,53,54,56–61]. Needle EMG often reveals scattered spontaneous activity with small, short-duration motor unit potentials that recruit in a myopathic manner [5,34,37,42–44,46,47,49–54,56–59,62]. However, many patients are unable to cooperate with voluntary portions of the needle examination owing to encephalopathy. Furthermore, some patients are so severely affected that they are unable to generate any voluntary activity.

Muscle biopsy may reveal loss of myosin adenosine triphosphatase staining, and electron microscopy confirms loss of myosin thick filament [5,32,42, 43,46,47,49,50,52,55,57,59,63]. In a few patients, necrosis is the predominant feature [5,41,42,44,45,51,53,55,57,61,64]. In these cases, serum creatine phosphokinase (CPK) levels are elevated, particularly early on, but in most instances the CPK is normal or minimally elevated [5,34,35,38,40,43,46–50,55,56,60]. In some biopsies, the only major abnormality is muscle fiber atrophy [5,33,34,44, 49,50,60]. Increased calpain expression has been demonstrated in muscle in AQM and may play a role in pathogenesis of the disorder [59]. It is likely that these pathologic patterns represent a spectrum of severity owing to the same pathophysiologic mechanism.

Muscle is electrically inexcitable in AQM [49,50]. Paralyzed muscle in AQM patients cannot be made to fire action potentials, even when directly stimulated. Clinical recovery of patients parallels recovery of muscle membrane excitability, indicating that weakness in AQM is primarily the result of muscle membrane inexcitability, although myosin loss and atrophy also contribute. The loss of muscle electrical excitability explains why CMAP amplitudes can be markedly reduced despite relatively normal muscle morphology. This mechanism of weakness is analogous to that of periodic paralysis in which profound weakness, markedly decreased CMAP amplitudes, and relatively normal muscle morphology are present. We have performed direct muscle stimulation on a patient during an attack of periodic paralysis and found the CMAP amplitudes to be markedly reduced during the attack, just as they are in severe AQM [50]. The CMAP amplitudes returned to normal when the patient with periodic paralysis regained strength, just as the CMAP amplitudes rise during recovery from AQM. The analogy between AQM and periodic paralysis is also instructive when trying to understand the presence of spontaneous activity in AQM. Fibrillations are common in hyperkalemic periodic paralysis and may increase during attacks when most muscle fibers are inexcitable [65,66]. Although the mechanism of electrical inexcitability in AQM remains unknown, it is possible that severely affected individual muscle fibers exist in a state of inexcitability, whereas less severely affected fibers might have poorly regulated excitability and fibrillate (Figure 4.1).

In an animal model of AQM, intracellular recording demonstrated loss of excitability in individual muscle fibers [67]. This loss could not be explained solely by changes in resting membrane potential or decreases in specific membrane resistance. Although most fibers lacked action potentials, in some mildly affected fibers small action potentials were present. The decreased rate of rise and reduced amplitude of action potentials in these mildly affected fibers are consistent with a severe reduction in sodium current (Figure 4.2).

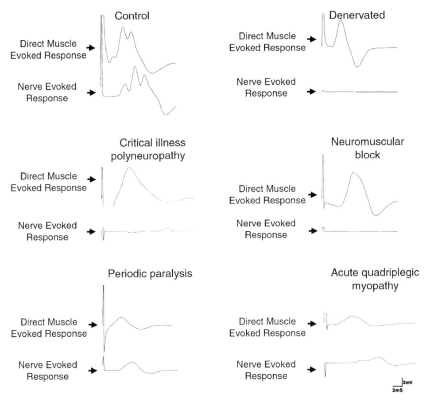

Figure 4.1 Compound muscle action potentials (CMAPs) from the tibialis anterior muscle in six patients. In each panel, the upper trace is the maximal amplitude CMAP recorded after direct muscle stimulation, and the lower trace is the CMAP recorded from the same electrode array after supramaximal peroneal nerve stimulation. In control muscle, large CMAPs are obtained after both direct muscle stimulation and nerve stimulation. In denervated muscle, a small or absent response is obtained after nerve stimulation, but a large response occurs when the muscle is directly stimulated. In critical illness polyneuropathy (CIP), the pattern obtained is the same as that seen in denervated muscle. In patients receiving neuromuscular blocking agents, a large response can be obtained after direct stimulation despite no response obtained after nerve stimulation. During an attack of periodic paralysis, in which weakness is caused by muscle fiber inexcitability, markedly reduced CMAPs are obtained after both nerve and muscle stimulation. Similarly, in acute quadriplegic myopathy (AQM), markedly low CMAPs are obtained after both nerve and direct muscle stimulation. The difference in response to direct muscle stimulation can be used to distinguish between CIP and AQM in critically ill patients.

The relationship between muscle fiber inexcitability and the muscle pathology findings in AQM is uncertain. We believe that muscle fiber inexcitability is an early event that can occur in the presence of only muscle fiber atrophy. More severely affected patients may have muscle fiber inexcitability and myosin loss. Ultimately, muscle fiber necrosis can result.

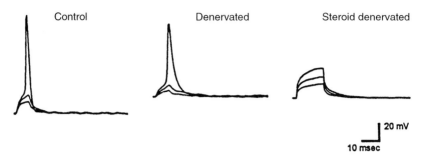

Figure 4.2   Intracellular action potentials from muscle fibers in an animal model of acute quadriplegic myopathy. In each panel, three superimposed traces are shown. Two subthreshold stimuli are shown in control and denervated muscle that do not elicit action potentials. In both control and denervated muscle, the third trace is suprathreshold and an action potential is seen. In steroid-treated denervated muscle (a model for acute quadriplegic myopathy) no action potential can be elicited despite strong depolarizing stimuli. This loss of excitability appears to be caused by a decrease in sodium currents in affected fibers.

DIFFERENTIATING ACUTE QUADRIPLEGIC MYOPATHY FROM CRITICAL ILLNESS POLYNEUROPATHY

When CIP and AQM present within the confines of their expected clinical, electrodiagnostic, and epidemiologic patterns, little difficulty in making an accurate diagnosis exists. However, most patients encountered in the ICU are not so easy to classify. A large heterogeneous group of patients has clinical and electrodiagnostic features common to both disorders. This group of indeterminate patients may include individuals with AQM, CIP, both, or other disorders (see Table 4.3).

Most patients who require care in the ICU for more than a few days are affected by sepsis and SIRS. Some of these patients have also received NMBA, corticosteroids, or both. Although CIP has been most closely linked to SIRS [30], there have been several reports in the 1990s of AQM developing in patients affected by SIRS who did not receive either NMBA or corticosteroids [50,59,60]. Furthermore, many patients thought to have CIP have received NMBA and corticosteroids. Given this overlap of risk factors, it is not possible to determine the cause of generalized weakness in the ICU based on clinical history alone.

Physical and electrodiagnostic examination may allow identification of a specific disorder in critically ill, weak patients. However, both examinations are limited in the ICU setting. Evaluation of strength and sensation is limited by sedation, encephalopathy, and mechanical ventilation. Ideally, CIP and AQM can be distinguished electrodiagnostically. However, the primary studies that allow differentiation of these disorders, sensory nerve conduction studies and evaluation of motor unit potential morphology and recruitment, are often limited in the ICU. Recording of sensory responses is limited by electrical noise in the ICU and by edema at recording sites. In addition, some reports suggest that CIP can exclusively involve motor fibers (see the following section). Needle EMG examination is limited by poor patient cooperation or the lack of voluntary motor unit potential recruitment in patients with severe weakness. Recruitment patterns often appear neurogenic when AQM is very severe. Only with recovery is myopathic recruitment apparent [62,68]. The two studies that are reliably performed in the ICU, motor nerve conduction studies and evaluation of spontaneous activity during needle EMG examination, cannot distinguish between AQM and CIP. The presence of spontaneous activity and reduced CMAP amplitudes are electrophysiologic findings common to both disorders. Even muscle biopsy may not allow differentiation of AQM from CIP. If the classic finding of loss of myosin is identified, AQM can be diagnosed. However, the biopsy findings can be limited to muscle fiber atrophy in both AQM and CIP.

Direct muscle stimulation may overcome some of the previously mentioned limitations and allow identification of patients with AQM in this heterogeneous group. Direct muscle stimulation can be performed even in encephalopathic, uncooperative patients. We have used direct muscle stimulation to study severe generalized weakness in 14 patients in the ICU [50]. In our study, 11 of 14 patients had reduced excitability of muscle as seen in AQM. Further prospective studies using direct muscle stimulation, serial nerve conduction studies, and muscle biopsy may allow better definition of this heterogeneous group of patients.

DOES A "PURE MOTOR" FORM OF CRITICAL ILLNESS POLYNEUROPATHY EXIST?

A "pure motor" form of CIP has been proposed in reports of patients with severe weakness, reduced CMAP amplitudes, and relatively preserved sensory function [69,70]. Identification of reduced CMAP amplitudes and spontaneous activity has been used as evidence of denervation. AQM also produces reduced CMAP amplitudes and spontaneous activity, however, and these two features are insufficient to distinguish reliably between AQM and motor neuropathy. Direct muscle stimulation was not performed in studies that have reported pure motor CIP. Using direct muscle stimulation, we have yet to find a patient with pure motor CIP and believe no direct evidence exists supporting distal axonopathy as the mechanism of weakness in most critically ill, weak patients. We believe that patients reported to have pure motor CIP have had AQM.

ARE SOME NEURONS ELECTRICALLY INEXCITABLE IN CRITICALLY ILL PATIENTS?

Electrical inexcitability of muscle is the major cause of weakness in AQM. It is possible that electrical inexcitability of neurons explains some of the observed clinical and electrophysiologic features of the heterogeneous group of patients who have neither classic AQM nor CIP. Although the predominant electrodiagnostic feature of most patients in this group is markedly reduced CMAP amplitudes, some patients also have decreased sensory nerve action potential (SNAP) amplitudes. This has been interpreted as being indicative of neuropathy. As some patients recover, however, we and others have noted a rapid increase in SNAP amplitudes, which is difficult to explain on a structural basis [53]. In such patients, several possible explanations exist for the initial decrease and subsequent rapid recovery of SNAP amplitudes. Technical factors, such as edema, might account for the loss of SNAP amplitude. However, often no edema or technical difficulty is present to account for the decrease in SNAP amplitude. A second potential explanation is rapid reversal of conduction block owing to demyelination. However, no pathologic or electrodiagnostic evidence has been found of demyelination in critically ill patients. Another appealing explanation is a temporary loss of nerve electrical excitability similar to the loss of excitability found in muscle in AQM. This may explain the observation in two reports in which sural nerve SNAP amplitude was markedly decreased, but sural nerve biopsy revealed no substantial pathology [60,61]. The results reported by Latronico and colleagues [60] are particularly interesting. In 19 of 24 patients, SNAP amplitudes were reduced, yet 14 of 22 sural nerve biopsies were normal.

If muscle and peripheral nerve are inexcitable in critically ill patients, could neurons in the central nervous system (CNS) become electrically inexcitable as well? We speculate that the encephalopathy seen during critical illness, so-called septic encephalopathy, might result in part from decreased excitability of CNS neurons and offer the hypothesis that acquired electrical inexcitability may potentially serve as a common theme in critically ill patients with neurologic abnormalities, both central and peripheral.

UNUSUAL NEUROMUSCULAR DISORDERS ENCOUNTERED IN THE INTENSIVE CARE UNIT

Tetanus

Tetanus is characterized by increased muscle tone and spasms. These typically begin in the masseter muscle, resulting in the classic finding of trismus, or "lockjaw." Pain and stiffness in the neck, shoulder, and back muscles often follow. Dysphagia may develop. Respiratory compromise, caused by spasm of respiratory muscles or laryngospasm, is the most serious development. The spasms may be episodic, provoked by the slightest movement or occurring spontaneously. Mentation is unaffected. Autonomic dysfunction is common in severe cases, resulting in heart rate and blood pressure lability, arrhythmia, fever, profuse sweating, peripheral vasoconstriction, ileus, and increased serum and urine catecholamine levels. Muscle rupture and rhabdomyolysis can complicate extreme cases. Neonatal tetanus develops in children born to inadequately immunized mothers. It results in poor feeding, rigidity, and spasms, but may be even more difficult to recognize in the neonate than in adults. Tetanus may occasionally remain restricted to areas around the portal of entry, resulting in local tetanus. Cephalic tetanus is a variant of local tetanus in which cranial nerve–innervated muscles are exclusively affected [71].

The neurologic manifestations of tetanus are caused by tetanospasmin, a protein toxin elaborated by the gram-positive, spore-forming bacilli *Clostridium tetani*, which is found worldwide in soil. Spores can persist for years in some environments and can withstand mild disinfectants. Wound contamination with *C. tetani* spores may be relatively common, but germination and toxin production require the specialized conditions found in devitalized tissue, around foreign bodies, or in wounds with another active infection. Toxin is produced in the wound and binds to peripheral motor nerve terminals. It is transported via retrograde axonal transport into the spinal cord or brain stem, or both. The toxin ultimately migrates to the presynaptic terminals where it has its pathophysiologic effect. It inhibits release of gamma-aminobutyric acid (GABA) and glycine, important inhibitory neurotransmitters. In the absence of the inhibitory influence of GABA and glycine, alpha motor neurons fire rapidly, producing rigidity. Preganglionic sympathetic neurons are also affected, resulting in increased catecholamine levels and sympathetic overactivity. Tetanospasmin also can produce weakness through blockade of acetylcholine release in a manner analogous to that of botulinum toxin. Tetanus remains localized if only the nerves near the wound are affected. If the toxin spreads via the lymphatics and bloodstream, generalized tetanus results.

Tetanus is a clinical diagnosis with few absolute confirmatory studies. It is unlikely to occur in a person who has had documented immunization with timely booster doses. In a patient with increased tone in the face, trunk, and proximal limb muscles with relative sparing of distal muscles, tetanus must be suspected. Tetanus can be cultured from wounds of clinically unaffected individuals but often cannot be cultured from patients who clearly are affected. Cerebrospinal fluid is normal. EMG may reveal involuntary discharges of motor units.

Treatment of tetanus begins with removal of the source of the toxin, usually through wound cleaning and débridement. Antibiotic therapy with metronidazole is recommended by most experts to eradicate vegetative cells. Human tetanus immunoglobulin neutralizes circulating toxin but has no effect once the toxin is neural-bound. Thus, early administration of tetanus immunoglobulin is desirable. It should be administered before wound manipulation if possible. Supportive care consists of treatment in a quiet ICU setting to allow cardiorespiratory monitoring with minimal stimulation. Benzodiazepines are most commonly used to control muscle spasm. Large doses may be required. Therapeutic paralysis with NMBAs may be necessary in severe cases. This treatment, of course, requires mechanical ventilation. Intubation may be required owing to hypoventilation caused by muscular rigidity or laryngospasm and should be performed in a controlled, elective manner if possible. The profound muscle rigidity increases energy needs, and insensible fluid losses and increased hydration and nutritional supplementation should be considered. Finally, patients should be vaccinated because immunity is not produced by the small toxin exposure.

Treatment in the ICU has resulted in a marked improvement in prognosis for patients with tetanus. Modern mortality is near 10%. Severe muscular rigidity may last for weeks, with mechanical ventilation required for up to 3–4 weeks. A complete recovery is typical, although mild painful spasms can persist for months [72].

Botulism

Botulism is caused by a toxin produced by another clostridium, *Clostridium botulinum*. Although eight immunologically distinct toxins have been identified, only three—A, B, and E—are associated with disease in humans. Four distinct clinical classifications of botulism have been identified. The classic form occurs after ingestion of food that contains toxin. A second form, infantile botulism, results when spores of *C. botulinum* germinate in the intestinal tract and produce botulinum toxin. A third form is wound botulism in which spores germinate in a wound leading to toxin production. The fourth form is one in which the source of toxin is never identified.

In the classic form, symptoms begin 12–36 hours after ingestion of contaminated food. Patients develop cranial nerve deficits, including blurred vision, diplopia, ptosis, dysarthria, and dysphagia. The weakness often affects the arms first and then progresses to the legs. In many patients, the weakness progresses until mechanical ventilation is required. Autonomic symptoms, including dry mouth, unreactive pupils, and ileus, often are present. Similar symptoms are seen in infantile and wound botulism. Botulism can be mistaken for myasthenia gravis or Guillain-Barré syndrome. Prominent gastrointestinal and autonomic symptoms in addition to weakness are indicative of botulism.

Definitive diagnosis requires detection of toxin in the patient's serum, stool, or food. In many individuals, however, detection of toxin is not possible and the diagnosis must be inferred from the clinical picture and electrophysiologic findings. Nerve conduction studies reveal normal sensory responses and decreased CMAP amplitudes. With repetitive stimulation, a decrement in amplitude is seen at low rates of stimulation, as occurs with any defect in neuromuscular transmission. A larger-amplitude muscle action potential is often seen with rapid rates of stimulation or immediately after exercise, indicating that a presynaptic defect in neuromuscular transmission is present. In severely affected patients, however, no increment may be seen. Needle EMG reveals small polyphasic motor units. Single-fiber EMG shows jitter and block, which improve after exercise or rapid repetitive stimulation.

Treatment consists primarily of supportive care. If patients survive the acute phase of illness, recovery is usually complete. Mortality in the era of the ICU is less than 10%. Antitoxin may be helpful, particularly in type E botulism, but in most adult patients treatment with antitoxin does not lead to significant improvement. Most experts recommend its use, although the problems of serum sickness and other reactions to the equine antiserum must be considered. In infant botulism, a new treatment with human-derived botulism antitoxin (botulism immunoglobulin) has been developed. In a study that is unpublished at this time, botulism immunoglobulin was very effective in treating infant botulism. Antitoxin was administered within 72 hours of the onset of symptoms and shortened the mean hospital stay from 5.5 to 2.5 weeks [73]. Length of stay in the ICU was also dramatically shortened, and the cost of hospital stays was greatly reduced.

Rabies

One form of rabies, paralytic rabies, produces neuromuscular weakness that can be difficult to differentiate from other causes of weakness such as GBS. The more common form of rabies, "furious rabies," is predominantly a CNS disorder, with prominent encephalopathy, intermittent muscle spasms, and bizarre neuropsychiatric symptoms.

Rabies is present in many countries throughout the world, although it is absent in some countries (e.g., Australia). Nearly 50,000 cases occur each year in India but fewer than 5 per year in the United States and central Europe [74].

Rabies is caused by a single-stranded RNA virus that is transmitted via secretions, typically saliva, through the bite of an animal or on to mucosa or broken skin. The virus spreads to the nervous system via axoplasmic flow from the site of infection; hematogenous spread is not important. The virus replicates in the dorsal root ganglion and then rapidly spreads throughout the CNS and ultimately to other organs via efferent nerves.

Rabies may begin with local pain and paresthesias followed by fasciculations near the site of inoculation. Flu-like symptoms and early manifestations of encephalopathy follow. The early symptoms may be indistinguishable from those of any number of viral encephalitides. Furious rabies begins with worsening encephalopathy, often with the classically described hydrophobia and aerophobia. Muscle spasms may be severe and can produce respiratory failure if diaphragm, sternocleidomastoid, or accessory muscles of inspiration become involved. Both upper and lower motor neuron signs may become apparent. Limbic disinhibition can be present as can autonomic instability. Death typically occurs within a week of onset of symptoms of furious rabies. Survival has been prolonged by ICU treatment, but little evidence exists that death is preventable in most cases even with the most sophisticated care.

Paralytic rabies is less common, perhaps because it is most frequently acquired from Latin American bat bites. After the flu-like prodrome, weakness, paresthesias, and pain develop first in the infected limb, followed by progression to quadriparesis and respiratory failure. Death follows in days, but again can be delayed, if not prevented, by ICU care.

Early treatment reliably prevents the onset of rabies. Thorough wound cleaning and disinfection should be followed by active and passive immunization if rabies exposure is possible. Active immunization is achieved by intramuscular injection of human diploid cell vaccine on days 0, 3, 7,14, and 30 of exposure. Passive immunization by injection of human rabies immunoglobulin as soon as possible after exposure is also recommended. Ten units per kilogram should be infiltrated around the wound and another 10 units/kg given intramuscularly. If immunization is not performed or is delayed beyond 7 days, clinical rabies will develop in more than 15% of individuals exposed to rabies virus. Despite aggressive ICU care, survival of patients with rabies who did not receive timely postexposure vaccination has not been reported [75].

Acute Hepatic Porphyrias

The acute hepatic porphyrias are a group of inherited disorders of heme biosynthesis that have prominent involvement of the nervous system. They may also have profound effects on the liver and less prominently on the skin. The acute hepatic forms of porphyria include acute intermittent porphyria, variegate porphyria, and hereditary coproporphyria. The main neurologic manifestation of the acute hepatic porphyrias is a polyneuropathy that can produce acute to subacute severe generalized weakness. The pathophysiology of this neuropathy is poorly understood. One interesting feature of the neuropathy is the tendency for shorter nerve fibers to be more involved than longer ones. This produces a rather distinctive phenomenon in which the ankle jerks may be preserved despite the quite severe weakness. Although the precise pathophysiology of the neuropathy is uncertain, it is clear that most attacks are precipitated either by certain medications or changes in hormonal levels. The medications most often implicated in initiating an attack of porphyria include barbiturates, most antiepileptics, sulfa antibiotics, many nondepolarizing NMBAs, anesthetic agents, theophylline, metoclopramide, and estrogens [76]. Just as the administration of estrogen can precipitate an attack, conditions such as pregnancy, menstruation, and puerperium can result in an exacerbation. Infection, starvation, and dieting also can result in an attack.

Porphyric neuropathy often begins with abdominal and low back pain followed by limb weakness. The combination of back pain and limb weakness may suggest GBS, but the porphyrias often cause greater proximal than distal weakness, which is unusual for GBS. The weakness is typically symmetric. Flaccid quadriplegia and respiratory failure may result. Sensory disturbance may be minimal and again is often more pronounced proximally than distally. The proximal distribution creates the so-called bathing trunk distribution of sensory loss. Autonomic disturbances, including fever, tachycardia, labile blood pressure, urinary retention, vomiting, constipation, and abdominal pain, are frequently seen. The CNS also can be involved. A wide variety of mental disturbances, including confusion, irritability, psychosis, depression, and coma, have been reported. Seizures occur in as many as 10% of patients.

Diagnosis of porphyria can be confirmed through the quantitative analysis of porphyrins and their precursors in the urine and stool. Both the urine and the stool should be studied because urine excretion of porphobilinogen is highly variable and may be low even during the acute attack in variegate porphyria. Direct enzyme analysis is also possible, typically through measurement of erythrocyte enzyme levels. No neuroradiographic hallmarks assist in establishing the diagnosis of porphyria, although brain magnetic resonance imaging abnormalities may occur. Electroencephalography may be abnormal but typically shows only nonspecific diffuse slowing. Nerve conduction studies are consistent with an axonal sensory motor neuropathy, but this is a relatively nonspecific finding.

Porphyria is most commonly mistaken either for GBS or lead or other heavy-metal poisoning. Preservation of ankle reflexes in the presence of severe weakness and evidence of neuropathy on electrodiagnostic studies suggests the presence of porphyria. Evidence of demyelination on electrodiagnostic studies suggests classic GBS. The axonal variant of GBS can be more troublesome to distinguish from porphyria, but axonal GBS does tend to involve more distal than proximal muscles. Lead poisoning can be particularly difficult to distinguish from porphyria because one of the main pathologic mechanisms of lead intoxication is through its interference with heme synthesis. Anemia with basophilic stippling is often present in lead in intoxication but not in porphyria. The serum and urine heavy-metal screening confirms the diagnosis.

The mainstay of therapy of porphyria is discontinuation of medications or correction of conditions that may have led to the exacerbation. Administration of a high carbohydrate load is thought to suppress porphyrin synthesis. Supportive care is of critical importance. Respiratory status should be closely monitored and respiratory failure should be supported through mechanical ventilation. In a life-threatening crisis, infusion of hematin may be useful. Treatment with these agents is complicated by peripheral thrombophlebitis and other disturbances of hemostasis. Treatment of seizures is extremely difficult because many antiepileptic medications worsen porphyria. Any treatable causes of the seizure, such as electrolyte disturbances, should be sought and treated first. Hyponatremia commonly occurs and should be corrected immediately. Clonazepam and valproate are among the safest medications, particularly when used in low doses. Bromides are the main alternative if seizures remain refractory.

The rate of recovery from the attack varies with the extent of axonal damage. With prompt treatment, rapid recovery can occur [77]. If axonal loss is severe, motor recovery can occur over many months and will likely be incomplete.

Animal Toxins

A variety of animals, from microscopic dinoflagellates to snakes and spiders, produce toxins that can result in neuromuscular weakness. A history of exposure should be sought in any patient with unexplained generalized weakness.

Approximately 20 species of venomous snakes are found in North America with neurotoxins potent enough to produce profound, rapid neuromuscular paralysis and respiratory distress. Only one spider species with such capability is found in North America, the female black widow spider. Black widow spider venom produces increased release of acetylcholine from motor nerve terminals. Treatment of snake or spider envenomization is largely supportive. Antivenom is available for some species in severe cases. Zoos often maintain a supply of antivenom for the species they handle and may be the local source of such antivenom.

Tick paralysis is an ascending weakness associated with the active feeding of several species of tick found in North America. Paralysis is thought to be caused by a toxin in the saliva of the tick and typically begins a few days after the tick begins feeding. Sensory and CNS functions are preserved. The paralysis can be severe and respiratory failure may result. The tick must be removed by firm traction at the point of attachment, and rupture of the tick body should be avoided if possible. Removal of the tick typically leads to recovery over hours to days. Supportive care may be needed for a brief time.

Several neuromuscular toxins may be present in fish and other seafood. Most toxins are produced by microscopic dinoflagellates or diatoms consumed by larger animals that may be subsequently consumed by humans. Table 4.4 summarizes the most common marine toxins. It should be noted that puffer fish poisoning is unique in that the toxin, tetrodotoxin, is produced by the fish itself.

CONCLUSIONS

Neuromuscular weakness is commonly seen in the ICU. AQM and CIP account for much of this weakness, but other relatively common disorders, such as GBS or myasthenia gravis, should be considered. Rare disorders, such as those discussed in this chapter, should be considered if other explanations seem unlikely. Combined careful review of recent medical history, the examination, and electrodiagnostic studies usually allow a definite diagnosis to be made. Specific treatments may be available, but supportive care is the mainstay of treatment of most of these disorders.

Table 4.4   Common marine neuromuscular toxins

Syndrome	Toxin	Source of toxin	Action of toxin	Symptoms	Treatment
Ciguatera	Ciguatoxin	Dinoflagellate *Gambierdiscus toxicus*	Prolonged depolarization caused by Na^+ channel opening	Nausea/vomiting, paresthesias, hot/cold reversal	Supportive
Paralytic shellfish poisoning	Saxitoxin	Dinoflagellate spp. *Alexandrium*	Blocks Na^+ channel	Oral paresthesias, jaw/facial weakness, respiratory failure	Supportive
Neurotoxic shellfish poisoning	Brevitoxin B	Dinoflagellate *Ptychodiscus brevis*	Prolonged depolarization caused by Na^+ channel opening	Nausea/vomiting, paresthesias, hot/cold reversal	Supportive
Puffer fish (fugu) poisoning	Tetrodotoxin	Puffer fish	Blocks Na^+ channel	Oral paresthesias, weakness, respiratory failure	Supportive; gastric lavage and charcoal for recent ingestion

REFERENCES

1. Spitzer AR, Giancarlo T, Maher L, et al. Neuromuscular causes of prolonged ventilator dependency. Muscle Nerve 1992;15:682.
2. Lacomis D, Petrella JT, Giuliani MJ. Causes of neuromuscular weakness in the intensive care unit: a study of ninety-two patients. Muscle Nerve 1998;21:610.
3. Bolton CF, Gilbert JJ, Hahn AF, Sibbald WJ. Polyneuropathy in critically ill patients. J Neurol Neurosurg Psychiatry 1984;47:1223.
4. Raps EC, Bird SJ, Hansen-Flaschen J. Prolonged muscle weakness after neuromuscular blockade in the intensive care unit. Crit Care Clin 1994;10:799.
5. Lacomis D, Giuliani MJ, Van Cott A, Kramer DJ. Acute myopathy of intensive care: clinical, electromyographic, and pathological aspects. Ann Neurol 1996;40:645.
6. Bizzari-Schmid MD, Desai SP. Prolonged neuromuscular blockade with atracurium. Can Anaesth Soc J 1986;33:209.
7. Gooch JL, Suchyta MR, Balbierz JM, et al. Prolonged paralysis after treatment with neuromuscular junction blocking agents. Crit Care Med 1991;19:1125.
8. Goudsouzian NG, Crone RK, Todres JD. Recovery from pancuronium blockade in the neonatal intensive care unit. Br J Anaesth 1981;53:1303.
9. Schindler MB. Prolonged neuromuscular blockade following the use of vecuronium for mediastinoscopy. Anaesth Intensive Care 1989;17:372.
10. Segredo V, Caldwell JE, Matthay MA, et al. Persistent paralysis in critically ill patients after long-term administration of vecuronium. N Engl J Med 1992;327:524.
11. Vandenbrom RHG, Wierda JMKH. Pancuronium bromide in the intensive care unit: a case of overdose. Anesthesiology 1988;69:996.
12. O'Conner M, Russel WJ. Muscle strength following anaesthesia with atracurium and pancuronium. Anaesth Intensive Care 1988;16:255.
13. Segredo V, Matthay MA, Sharma ML, et al. Prolonged neuromuscular blockade after long-term administration of vecuronium in two critically ill patients. Anesthesiology 1990;72:566.
14. Vanderheyden BA, Reynolds HN, Gerold KB, et al. Prolonged paralysis after long-term vecuronium infusion. Crit Care Med 1992;20:304.
15. Frankel H, Jeng J, Tilly E, et al. The impact of implementation of neuromuscular blockade monitoring standards in a surgical intensive care unit. Am Surg 1996;62:503.
16. Bolton CF, Laverty DA, Brown JD, et al. Critically ill polyneuropathy: electrophysiological studies and differentiation from Guillain-Barré syndrome. J Neurol Neurosurg Psychiatry 1986;49:563.
17. Bolton CF. Electrophysiologic studies of critically ill patients. Muscle Nerve 1987;10:129.
18. Williams AC, Sturman S, Kelsey S, et al. The neuropathy of the critically ill. BMJ 1986;293:790.
19. Witt NJ, Zochodne DW, Bolton CF, et al. Peripheral nerve function in sepsis and multiple organ failure. Chest 1991;99:176.
20. Zochodne DW, Bolton CF, Gilbert JJ. Polyneuropathy in critical illness: pathologic features. Ann Neurol 1985;18:160.
21. Zochodne DW, Bolton CF, Wells GA, et al. Critical illness polyneuropathy. Brain 1987;110:819.
22. Tran DD, Groeneveld ABJ, Van Der Meuien J. Age, chronic disease, sepsis, organ system failure, and mortality in a medical intensive care unit. Crit Care Med 1990;18:474.
23. American College of Chest Physicians Consensus Conference. Definition for sepsis and organ failure and guidelines for the use of innovative therapies in sepsis. Crit Care Med 1992;20:864.
24. Bleck TP, Smith MC, Pierre-Louis SJ, et al. Neurologic complications of critical medical illness. Crit Care Med 1993;21:98.
25. Kelly BJ, Mathay MA. Prevalence and severity of neurologic dysfunction in critically ill patients: influence on need for continued mechanical ventilation. Chest 1993;104:1818.
26. Leijten FSS, Harinck-De Weerd JE, Poortvliet DCJ, De Weerd AW. Critical illness polyneuropathy in multiple organ dysfunction syndrome and weaning from the ventilator. Intensive Care Med 1996;22:856.
27. Berek K, Margreiter J, Willeit J. Polyneuropathies in critically ill patients: a prospective evaluation. Intensive Care Med 1993;22:849.
28. Glauser MP, Zanetti G, Baumgartner JD, Cohen J. Septic shock: pathogenesis. Lancet 1991;338:732.
29. Bolton CF. Clinical neurophysiology of the respiratory system. AAEM Minimonograph #40. Muscle Nerve 1993;16:809.
30. Bolton CF. Sepsis and the systemic inflammatory response syndrome: neuromuscular manifestations. Crit Care Med 1996;24:1408.

31. MacFarlane IA, Rosenthal FD. Severe myopathy after status asthmaticus. Lancet 1977;2:615.
32. Sher JH, Shafiq SA, Schutta HS. Acute myopathy with selective lysis of myosin filaments. Neurology 1979;29:100.
33. Bachmann P, Gaussorgues P, Piperno D, et al. Acute myopathy after status asthmaticus. Presse Med 1987;16:1486.
34. Kaplan PW, Rocha W, Sanders DB, et al. Acute steroid-induced tetraplegia following status asthmaticus. Pediatrics 1986;78:121.
35. Knox AJ, Mascie-Taylor BH, Muers MF. Acute hydrocortisone myopathy in acute severe asthma. Thorax 1986;41:411.
36. Kupfer Y, Okrent DG, Twersky R, Tessler S. Disuse atrophy in a ventilated patient with status asthmaticus receiving neuromuscular blockade. Crit Care Med 1987;15:795.
37. Op de Coul AAW, Lambregts PCLA, Koeman J, et al. Neuromuscular complications in patients given Pavulon (pancuronium bromide) during artificial ventilation. Clin Neurol Neurosurg 1985;87:17.
38. Picado C, Montserrat J, Agusti-Vidal A. Muscle atrophy in severe exacerbation of asthma requiring mechanical ventilation. Respiration 1988;53:201.
39. Shee CD. Risk factors for hydrocortisone myopathy in acute severe asthma. Resp Med 1990; 84:229.
40. Van Marle W, Woods KL. Acute hydrocortisone myopathy. BMJ 1980;281:271.
41. Williams TJ, O'Hehir RE, Czarny D, et al. Acute myopathy in severe acute asthma treated with intravenously administered corticosteroids. Am Rev Respir Dis 1988;137:460.
42. Barohn RJ, Jackson CE, Rogers SJ, et al. Prolonged paralysis due to nondepolarizing neuromuscular blocking agents and corticosteroids. Muscle Nerve 1994;17:647.
43. Danon MJ, Carpenter S. Myopathy with thick filament (myosin) loss following prolonged paralysis with vecuronium during steroid treatment. Muscle Nerve 1991;14:1131.
44. Douglas OA, Tuxen DV, Horne M, et al. Myopathy in severe asthma. Am Rev Respir Dis 1992;146:517.
45. Griffin D, Fairman N, Coursin D, et al. Acute myopathy during treatment of status asthmaticus with corticosteroids and steroidal muscle relaxants. Chest 1992;102:510.
46. Hirano M, Ott BR, Raps EC, et al. Acute quadriplegic myopathy: a complication of treatment with steroids, nondepolarizing blocking agents, or both. Neurology 1992;42:2082.
47. Lacomis D, Smith TW, Chad DA. Acute myopathy and neuropathy in status asthmaticus: case report and literature review. Muscle Nerve 1993;16:84.
48. Margolis BD, Khachikian D, Friedman Y, Garrard C. Prolonged reversible quadriparesis in mechanically ventilated patients who received long-term infusions of vecuronium. Chest 1991;100:877.
49. Rich MM, Teener JW, Raps EC, et al. Muscle is electrically inexcitable in acute quadriplegic myopathy. Neurology 1996;46:731.
50. Rich MM, Bird SJ, Raps EC, et al. Direct muscle stimulation in acute quadriplegic myopathy. Muscle Nerve 1997;20:665.
51. Sitwell LD, Weinshenker BG, Monpetit V, Reid D. Complete ophthalmoplegia as a complication of acute corticosteroid- and pancuronium-associated myopathy. Neurology 1991;41:921.
52. Waclawik AJ, Sufit RL, Beinlicj BR, Schutta HS. Acute myopathy with selective degeneration of myosin filaments following status asthmaticus treated with methylprednisolone and vecuronium. Neuromusc Dis 1992;2:19.
53. Zochodne DW, Ramsay DA, Saly V, et al. Acute necrotizing myopathy of intensive care: electrophysiological studies. Muscle Nerve 1994;17:285.
54. Bird SJ, Mackin GA, Schotland DL, Raps EC. Acute myopathic quadriplegia: a unique syndrome associated with vecuronium and steroid treatment. Muscle Nerve 1992;15:1208.
55. Faragher MW, Day BJ, Dennett X. Critical care myopathy: an electrophysiological and histological study. Muscle Nerve 1996;19:516.
56. Gooch JL. AAEM Case report #29: prolonged paralysis after neuromuscular blockade. Muscle Nerve 1995;18:937.
57. Hanson P, Dive A, Brucher J-M, et al. Acute corticosteroid myopathy in intensive care patients. Muscle Nerve 1997;20:1371.
58. Kupfer Y, Namba T, Kaldawi E, Tessler S. Prolonged weakness after long-term infusion of vecuronium bromide. Ann Intern Med 1992;117:484.
59. Showalter CJ, Engel AG. Acute quadriplegic myopathy: analysis of myosin isoforms and evidence for calpain-mediated proteolysis. Muscle Nerve 1997;20:316.
60. Latronico N, Fenzi F, Recupero D, et al. Critical illness myopathy and neuropathy. Lancet 1996;347:1570.

61. Ramsay DA, Zochodne DW, Robertson DM, et al. A syndrome of acute severe muscle necrosis in intensive care unit patients. J Neuropathol Exp Neurol 1993;52:387.
62. Road J, Mackie G, Jiang T, et al. Reversible paralysis with status asthmaticus, steroids, and pancuronium: clinical electrophysiological correlates. Muscle Nerve 1997;20:1587.
63. Campellone J, Lacomis D, Kramer D, et al. Acute myopathy after liver transplantation. Neurology 1998;50:46.
64. Helliwell TR, Coakley JH, Wagenmakers AJM, et al. Necrotizing myopathy in critically-ill patients. J Pathol 1991;164:307.
65. Buchthal F, Engbaek L, Gamstorp I. Paresis and hyperexcitability in adynamia episodica hereditaria. Neurology 1958;8:347.
66. Layzer RB, Lovelace RE, Rowland LP. Hyperkalemic periodic paralysis. Arch Neurol 1967;16:457.
67. Rich MM, Pinter MJ, Kraner SD, Barchi RL. Loss of electrical excitability in an animal model of acute quadriplegic myopathy. Ann Neurol 1998;43:171.
68. Rich MM, Teener JW, Raps E, Bird S. Muscle inexcitability in patients with reversible paralysis following steroids and neuromuscular blockade. Muscle Nerve 1998;21:1231.
69. Hund E, Genzwurker H, Bohrer H, et al. Predominant involvement of motor fibres in patients with critical illness polyneuropathy. Br J Anaesth 1997;78:274.
70. Schwarz J, Planck J, Briegel J, Straube A. Single-fiber electromyography, nerve conduction studies, and conventional electromyography in patients with critical-illness polyneuropathy: evidence for a lesion of terminal motor axons. Muscle Nerve 1997;20:696.
71. Orowitz JI, Galetta SL, Teener JW. Bilateral trochlear nerve palsy and downbeat nystagmus in a patient with cephalic tetanus. Neurology 1997;49:894.
72. Bleck TP. Tetanus. In WM Scheld, RJ Whitley, DT Durack (eds), Infections of the Central Nervous System. New York: Raven, 1991;603.
73. Arnon SS. Infant Botulism. In RD Feigin, JD Cherry (eds), Textbook of Pediatric Infectious Diseases. Philadelphia: Saunders, 1998;359.
74. Steele JH. Rabies in the Americas and remarks on global aspects. Rev Infect Dis 1988;10:585.
75. Anderson LJ, Nicholson KG, Tauxe RV, Winkler WG. Human rabies in the United States 1960 to 1979: epidemiology, diagnosis and prevention. Ann Intern Med 1984;100:728.
76. Moore MR. International review of drugs in acute porphyria. Int J Biochem 1980;12:1089.
77. Kauppinen R, Mustajoki P. Prognosis of acute porphyria: occurrence of acute attacks, precipitating factors and associated diseases. Medicine 1992;71:1.

5
Coma, Vegetative State, and Locked-In Syndrome

Robin S. Howard and Nicholas P. Hirsch

Consciousness can be defined as a state of awareness of self and environment that gives significance to stimuli from the internal and external environment. It can be thought of as depending on two critical components: cognitive content and arousal. The content of consciousness is the sum of mental functions, leading to awareness of self and environment and the expression of psychological functions of sensation, emotion, and thought. The content of consciousness can be impaired independently by focal or generalized cortical damage, leading to a focal cognitive deficit or global impairment such as the akinetic or vegetative state. Impairment of arousal leads to obtundation, stupor, or coma with a secondary impairment of content that may be temporary or permanent, depending on the etiology [1–3].

Coma or impaired consciousness is therefore associated with either bilateral hemispheric damage or suppression, or a focal brain stem lesion or metabolic derangement that damages or suppresses the reticular activating system. In general, unilateral dysfunction of the cerebral hemispheres does not, by itself, cause stupor or coma, although large dominant hemispheric lesions can cause drowsiness or obtundation in the absence of brain stem compression [1].

STATES OF IMPAIRED CONSCIOUSNESS

A number of terms have been applied to different states of altered consciousness. *Clouding of consciousness* is a term applied to states of reduced wakefulness characterized by impaired attention and memory. The patient may be distractible, hyperexcitable, and irritable, and thought processes are slow.

Acute confusional state refers to more severe impairment of consciousness in which stimuli are misinterpreted, and patients are drowsy, bewildered, and disoriented for time and have poor short-term memory and comprehension. They also have difficulty in undertaking complex tasks and day-night reversal.

Delirium is characterized by the rapid onset of a floridly abnormal mental state with disturbed consciousness, disorientation, severe motor restlessness, fear, irritability, misperception of sensory stimuli, and visual hallucinations. Lucid periods can alternate with delirious episodes. The patient is commonly loud, talkative, irritable, suspicious, and agitated.

Obtundation refers to mental blunting and torpidity. The patient is drowsy and hypersomnolent with mild to moderate reduction of alertness accompanied by a lessened interest in the environment. Responses are slow, but the patient can be aroused to respond to verbal or tactile stimulation. *Stupor* is a condition of deep sleep or behaviorally similar unresponsiveness from which the patient can be aroused only by vigorous and repeated stimuli. As soon as the stimulus ceases, the stuporous subject lapses back into the unresponsive state. He or she communicates using only monosyllabic sounds and simple behaviors.

The term *locked-in syndrome* (see Locked-In Syndrome) describes a de-efferented state in which consciousness and cognition are preserved but the patient has lost motor function, making movement and speech impossible. The syndrome is caused by bilateral lesions of the ventral pons that disrupt corticospinal, corticopontine, and corticobulbar tracts. The patient remains able to breathe but often has total paralysis of voluntary motor activity below the level of the third nerve nuclei. The subject is usually able to communicate by opening and voluntarily moving his or her eyes in the vertical plane, but horizontal and other eye movements are lost.

Akinetic mutism is a rare syndrome characterized by pathologically slowed or virtually absent bodily movements and loss of speech. Patients are flaccid with no response to pain, and they lie immobile, mute, and unresponsive to commands, questions, and greetings. They display no emotion, agreeable or disagreeable, and ideation is minimal. Patients appear awake and their eyes may follow the movement of people around the bed or turn toward a sound in the environment. The ability to blink, both spontaneously and to visual threat, is preserved. Grasping and sucking reflexes may be prominent. The patient may have no evidence of paralysis or sensory deficit. Incontinence of bowel and bladder exists. Wakefulness, alertness, and self-awareness appear to be preserved, but cognitive function is reduced. Sleep-wake cycles are present and electroencephalography shows reactive alpha and theta rhythms. The condition characteristically accompanies gradually developing or subacute bilateral damage to the inferior frontal lobes, extensive bilateral hemispheric disease, or lesions of the paramedian mesencephalic reticular formation or posterior diencephalon.

Coma can be defined as a state of unarousable psychological unresponsiveness in which the subject lies with his or her eyes closed. No psychologically understandable response to external stimuli or inner need exists. The patient neither utters understandable responses nor accurately localizes noxious stimuli. Thus, the subject has a total absence of awareness of self and environment even when externally stimulated. No spontaneous eye opening, no response to voice, no localization to painful stimuli, and no verbal output exists. Coma is rarely a permanent state and most patients who survive the initial causative insult regain identifiable sleep-wake cycles after a few days or weeks, although the outcome may vary from complete recovery to a vegetative state [1].

CAUSES OF COMA

Several schemes have been proposed to classify the differential diagnosis of the causes of coma. None is entirely satisfactory, as many of the underlying conditions are either multifactorial (e.g., mass lesions with secondary herniation) or may affect the brain at different levels (e.g., meningitis) [4]. Nonetheless, the most important considerations in the initial assessment are (1) the presence of lateralizing signs, (2) the presence of meningism, and (3) the pattern of brain stem reflexes (Table 5.1). In most cases, the cause of coma is associated with a clear medical problem; in patients admitted in coma (>6 hours) to a general accident and emergency department, approximately 40% of the comas are due to drug ingestion with or without alcohol, 25% to hypoxic-ischemic insult secondary to cardiac arrest, 20% to stroke, and the remainder to general medical disorders. Primary neurologic events that cause coma include intracerebral hemorrhage, subarachnoid hemorrhage, pontine or cerebellar hemorrhage, and basilar artery thrombosis. Infarction in the territory of the middle cerebral artery rarely leads to sudden onset of coma.

Table 5.1   Causes of coma

Coma with intact brain stem function, no meningism, and no lateralizing motor signs	
Toxins	Conversion reaction
Carbon monoxide	Infections (e.g., transmissible spongiform encephalopathy)
Methanol	Anoxic-ischemic encephalopathy
Lead	Respiratory causes
Cyanide	Hypoxia
Thallium	Hypercapnia
Alcohol	Electrolytes
Drug toxicity	Hyponatremia, hypernatremia
Sedatives	Hypercalcemia, hypocalcemia
Barbiturates	Hypermagnesemia
Tranquilizers	Diabetic causes
Opioids	Hypoglycemia
Psychotropics	Ketoacidosis
Amphetamines	Lactic acidosis
Others	Hyperosmolar nonketotic diabetic coma
Extrapyramidal causes	Renal causes (e.g., uremia)
Status dystonicus	Hepatic causes (e.g., hepatic encephalopathy)
Neuroleptic malignant syndrome	Endocrine causes
Seizures	Hypopituitarism
Status epilepticus	Hypothyroidism, hyperthyroidism
Postictal	Addison's disease
Postictal drug induced	Hashimoto's encephalopathy
Functional	Temperature
Psychiatric causes	Hypothermia
Catatonia	Hyperpyrexia

Table 5.1   Continued

Nutritional causes (e.g., Wernicke's
  encephalopathy)
Inborn errors of metabolism
  Hyperammonemia
  Aminoaciduria
  Organic aciduria
Others
  Porphyria
  Reye's syndrome
  Idiopathic recurrent stupor
**Coma with meningism (± intact brain
      stem function and lateralizing
      signs)**
Infection
  Meningitis
  Encephalitis
Vascular (e.g., subarachnoid hemorrhage)
**Coma with intact brain stem function
      and lateralizing signs**
Asymmetric lateralizing signs
  Vascular
  Infarction
    Ischemia
    Embolic: cardiac, large vessel, fat
    Hypoperfusion/hypotension
  Hemorrhage
    Extradural
    Subdural
    Subarachnoid
    Intracerebral (primary or secondary)
    Congophilic amyloid angiopathy
    Angioimmunoblastic lymphoma
  Vasculitis
  Venous thrombosis
  Mitochondrial disease
  Hypertensive encephalopathy
  Eclamptic toxemia

Endocarditis
  Bacterial
  Liebman-Sachs
  Marantic
Infection
  Abscess
  Subdural empyema
  Creutzfeldt-Jakob disease
Tumor
White matter
  Multifocal leukoencephalopathy
  Adrenoleukodystrophy
  Multiple sclerosis
  Leukoencephalopathy associated
      with chemotherapy/radiotherapy
  Acute disseminated
      encephalomyelitis
  Acute hemorrhagic leukoencephalitis
Symmetric lateralizing signs
  Diffuse axonal brain injury
  Bilateral subdural hematoma/empyema
  Vascular: multiple infarcts due to
    Fat emboli
    Cholesterol emboli
    Disseminated intravascular coagulation
    Thrombotic thrombocytopenic purpura
    Vasculitis
**Coma with signs of focal brain stem
      dysfunction**
Herniation syndrome
Intrinsic brain stem disease
Advanced metabolic/toxic encephalopathy
Others (e.g., central pontine myelinolysis)
Vascular
  Vertebrobasilar occlusion, dissection
  Posterior fossa hemorrhage/hematoma
Tumor (e.g., posterior fossa)

ASSESSMENT OF COMA

For information about the assessment of coma see Table 5.2.

Resuscitation and Emergency Treatment

Cardiopulmonary Resuscitation

Although the underlying cause of coma must be treated as soon as possible, rapid and effective cardiopulmonary resuscitation is the most pressing aspect of emergency treatment of the comatose patient if secondary cerebral damage is to be

Table 5.2   Assessment of coma

Resuscitation and emergency treatment	Oculovestibular
Medical assessment	Corneal reflex and facial movements
Establish level of consciousness	Bulbar
Eye opening	Cough
Motor response	Gag
Verbal output	Respiratory pattern
Identify brain stem activity	Motor function
Brain stem reflexes	Involuntary movements
Pupils	Seizures
Eye movements	Muscle tone
Spontaneous	Motor responses
Oculocephalic	Tendon reflexes

avoided. A patent airway must be established by placing the patient in the left lateral position, introducing an oral airway, or performing endotracheal intubation. Coma owing to a variety of causes results in disordered respiration and often leads to hypoxemia and hypercarbia that requires assisted ventilation. Similarly, hypotension causes cerebral hypoperfusion and further cerebral ischemia. Appropriate resuscitation with intravenous fluids or inotropic drugs, or both, must be effected as rapidly as possible [5].

Blood Tests

During resuscitation, blood should be taken for estimation of electrolytes (especially sodium, glucose, and urea) and full blood count. Other tests, such as toxicology screen, anticonvulsant drug levels, and ammonia, should be performed as appropriate.

Drug Treatment

After baseline blood samples are taken, 50% glucose, 25 ml, should be given intravenously. If possible, glucose level should be tested, providing there is no delay. The potential harmful results of giving glucose to a patient with cerebral ischemia are far outweighed by the benefits of rapid treatment of hypoglycemia. Administration of glucose should be preceded by the intravenous injection of 50–100 mg thiamine to prevent the precipitation of Wernicke's encephalopathy in alcoholic patients. If narcotic or benzodiazepine overdose is suspected, naloxone or flumazenil, respectively, should be given [6–8].

Further Acute Management

Further management of the unconscious patient includes adequate treatment of seizures [9]; correction of electrolyte and acid-base disturbances; and supportive therapy, including adequate nutrition and physiotherapy [10,11].

Medical Assessment

History

Obtaining as detailed and accurate a history as possible is essential. This must include any information about the previous history and circumstances of the acute event. In particular, information must be sought from family members, witnesses, and the paramedical staff who were called to the scene. The patient's personal belongings must be examined for any clue about pre-existing treatment (e.g., steroids) or disease (e.g., diabetes), and a search should be made for any evidence of alcohol or drug ingestion. It may be necessary to telephone family members or the primary care physician. A history of pre-existing neurologic disease should be sought. There may be known epilepsy, structural central nervous system disease, or neuromuscular disorders. The patient may have a history of a pre-existing general medical disorder in which a secondary neurologic event occurred; for example, psychiatric, cardiac, endocrine, or metabolic disease. It is important to establish any history of a predisposing event; for example, previous trauma, pyrexia, prodromal symptoms such as headache, neck stiffness, ataxia, epilepsy, or previous episodes of coma [12–14]. Coma may present as failure to awake after general anesthesia. This may be associated with pre-existing neurologic disease (e.g., previous poliomyelitis, muscular dystrophy, or motor neuron disease), a neurologic complication of general medical disorders (e.g., cardiogenic emboli or metabolic encephalopathy), or a primary neurologic event (e.g., subarachnoid hemorrhage or meningitis).

Examination

It is necessary to undertake an urgent and detailed general medical examination of the patient in coma [4,15]. The general appearance of the patient, when discovered and on admission, may give important clues to the etiology of the coma. His or her breath may smell of alcohol, ketones, or hepatic or renal fetor. Examination of the mucous membranes may show evidence of cyanosis, anemia, jaundice, or carbon monoxide intoxication. Bruising in the mastoid and orbital regions may suggest temporal, orbital, or basal skull fractures, as may blood in the external auditory meatus. Opiate intoxication is suggested by needle track marks in the antecubital fossa. Relevant skin lesions include a purpuric-petechial rash of meningococcal septicemia or other causes of sepsis, including *Pseudomonas*, *Staphylococcus*, or endocarditis. Maculopapular lesions suggest viral meningoencephalitis, endocarditis, or fungal infection, and a vesicular rash may suggest herpes simplex or varicella; barbiturate intoxication is associated with bullous lesions. Petechiae and ecchymosis suggest abnormal coagulation from a variety of causes, including trauma, corticosteroid use, abnormal coagulation from liver disease or anticoagulants, disseminated intravascular coagulation, or thrombotic thrombocytopenic purpura. Hyperpigmentation may suggest Addison's disease, porphyria, disseminated malignant melanoma, and chemotherapy. Human immunodeficiency virus is suggested by Kaposi's sarcoma, anogenital herpetic lesions, oral candidiasis, or lymphadenopathy.

Disorders of temperature should be sought. Hyperpyrexia is usually caused by systemic sepsis, but the absence of sepsis does not exclude the possibility, particularly in the elderly or in the immunosuppressed. Other causes include thyrotoxic crises, heat stroke, drug toxicity, and malignant hyperpyrexia. Primary neurogenic hyperpyrexia is unusual and associated with subarachnoid or hypothalamic lesions. Hypothermia may cause coma directly but is usually associated with environmental (accidental hypothermia) or metabolic causes, endocrine disorders (hypopituitarism, hypothyroidism), drugs (alcohol, barbiturate), and Wernicke's encephalopathy; it is rarely associated with central disorders in the region of the diencephalon.

Hypertension is a feature of subarachnoid hemorrhage and raised intracranial pressure. Hypertensive crisis can lead to disturbed consciousness. Hypotension can lead to reduced cerebral perfusion, coma, and irreversible cerebral injury; it is associated with hypovolemia owing to hemorrhage, myocardial infarction, cardiac tamponade, septicemia, intoxication, diabetes mellitus, and Addison's disease. Tachycardia results from a tachyarrhythmia, hypovolemia, pyrexia, toxins, and drug intoxication. Bradycardia can result from bradyarrhythmias, raised intracranial pressure, and drugs. Irregularity of the pulse may be caused by atrial fibrillation.

Meningism suggests infective or carcinomatous meningitis, central or tonsillar herniation, or subarachnoid hemorrhage. It has been suggested that meningism is unusual in deep coma whatever its cause and that its presence suggests a less severe disturbance of consciousness [16]; it is certainly true that the assessment of meningism is difficult in patients who have been intubated. Characteristic patterns of respiration are associated with coma, particularly that caused by cerebral herniation or metabolic and toxic conditions, including drug overdose, acidosis, and diabetic and hepatic disease.

Fundal examination may show evidence of retinopathy owing to diabetes or hypertension. Papilledema may suggest raised intracranial pressure, hypertensive retinopathy, or carbon dioxide retention. Subhyaloid hemorrhage may suggest subarachnoid hemorrhage. Otoscopic examination may show evidence of otorrhea or hemotympanum from a basal skull fracture. Rhinorrhea is suggested by the presence of glucose in the watery nasal discharge.

Cardiac examination can show the presence of an arrhythmia and cardiac or valvular disease, suggesting endocarditis or a possible embolic source. Examination of the abdomen may show evidence of an ileus or increased bowel motility. Hepatomegaly caused by cardiac failure, portal hypertension, or secondary carcinomatous deposits may be present. Lymphadenopathy may indicate infection, neoplasia, collagen vascular disorders, or sarcoidosis.

Level of Consciousness: Coma Score

In the assessment of the depth of coma, the patient should be tested using visual, auditory, and painful stimuli of increasing intensity. Noxious stimuli should be presented bilaterally in cranial nerve and limb territories. The patient's eyelids should be held open and the patient asked to move his or her eyes in a horizontal and vertical plane to exclude preservation of volitional control of these movements as occurs in the locked-in syndrome.

The Glasgow Coma Scale (GCS) is the most widely used scale to assess the level of consciousness. It was introduced to assess the severity and progression of traumatic brain injury but has been increasingly applied to determining the level of coma regardless of etiology. It has proved an extremely valuable and reproducible scale that can be easily applied by medical and nursing staff. The GCS has many limitations, however; in particular, it excludes assessment of many important neurologic functions, requires regular and consecutive observations to be effective, is limited to the best response in a single limb and therefore cannot reflect asymmetry, and has poor reliability in nonexperienced observers, particularly as the level of maximal auditory, visual, and noxious stimuli can vary between observers. Finally, in intubated patients or those with swollen eyes, full assessment cannot be undertaken. Furthermore, the scale represents the addition of ordinal values that are not equal and are not independent of each other. For these reasons, a total GCS score makes little sense and is not a reliable predictor of outcome. Nonetheless, the GCS has provided an extremely valuable focus that has emphasized the importance of intensive observation of the comatose patient, allowing rapid intervention with deterioration in conscious level [17–22].

Other scales have been introduced to improve the sensitivity and prognostic reliability of bedside assessment of coma. The Innsbruck Coma Scale is similar to the GCS in that it is composed of ordinal measures aggregated together [23]. The criticisms of its validity are therefore similar, but the scale does extend the range of observations and can be used in intubated patients. As with other scales, it is reliable in predicting poor outcome after trauma. More recently, the Reaction Level Scale has been advocated; it has the advantage of being ordinal without having the need to aggregate the scores, but it does depend entirely on limb motor responses [24].

Assessment of Neurologic Function

Pupillary Responses

When light is shone on one eye, it causes constriction of the pupil of that eye (*direct response*) as well as in the other eye (*consensual response*). Pupillary light reflexes are mediated by the retinal ganglion cells, which respond to overall changes and project to the pretectal area of the tegmentum ventral to the superior colliculus. An infraneural connection exists between the pretectal nuclear complex and the Edinger-Westphal nucleus (parasympathetic) of the oculomotor nerves. From the Edinger-Westphal nucleus, pupilloconstrictor fibers travel in the oculomotor nerve and synapse in the ciliary ganglion. Preganglionic fibers run in the short ciliary nerves to innervate the smooth muscles of the pupillary sphincter. The consensual response occurs because a proportion of retinal ganglion cell input to the brain stem is crossed. The ciliospinal reflex consists of bilateral pupillodilation in response to painful cutaneous stimulation. This reflex tests the integrity of the sympathetic pathways in lightly comatose patients. The synapse between afferent pain pathways and efferent pupillodilatory pathways lies in the cervical spinal cord, however, and if the reflex is absent it is of limited value in assessing brain stem function. If bilaterally present, however, it suggests a metabolic cause of coma. A unilaterally present ciliospinal reflex suggests a possible third nerve lesion or pre-existing Horner's syndrome [16].

Normal pupillary size in the comatose patient depends on the level of illumination and the state of autonomic innervation. It is important to ensure adequate illumination and, if necessary, to examine the pupils with a magnifying glass. Pre-existing ocular or neurologic injury can fix the pupils or result in pupillary asymmetry. Local and systemic medication can affect pupillary function (e.g., topical ophthalmologic preparations that contain acetylcholinesterase inhibitor, used in the treatment of glaucoma, result in miosis). When topical mydriatics are used, the pupil is often of larger diameter (8 mm) than would be owing to third nerve compression (5–6 mm). The effects of mydriatic agents placed by the patient or a prior observer may wear off unevenly, resulting in pupillary asymmetry.

The pupillary response indicates the functional state of the afferent and efferent pathways. The presence of equal, light reactive pupils indicates that the afferent (II) and efferent (III) pathways and the midbrain tegmentum are all intact. Normal pupillary reaction to light in a comatose patient with other signs of midbrain dysfunction is strongly suggestive of a metabolic rather than structural cause of the coma. Lesions above the midbrain (i.e., involving the diencephalon) may involve the descending sympathetic pathways, causing a unilateral or bilateral Horner's syndrome with small, reactive pupils, anhidrosis, and enophthalmos. Similar pupillary changes may be noted in toxic or metabolic coma. The effects of midbrain lesions depend on their site. Dorsal tectal or pretectal lesions interrupt the pupillary light responses but spare the response to accommodation. This leads to slightly dilated pupils that do not respond to light but spontaneously and rhythmically fluctuate in size (hippus) and dilate to ciliospinal reflex. Tegmental lesions involve the third nerve nucleus and interrupt both sympathetic and parasympathetic pathways to the eye. The pupils are midposition, irregular, possibly asymmetric, and fixed to light but respond to accommodation. Fascicular lesions of the third nerve are usually bilateral and produce external oculomotor paresis accompanied by fixed pupillary dilatation. Peripheral third nerve lesions usually result from uncal herniation, causing the nerve to be compressed against the posterior cerebral artery at the tentorial notch. A sluggishly reactive pupil may be an early sign of uncal herniation, followed by fixed pupillary dilatation (due to sparing of the sympathetic pathways) associated with extraocular motor abnormalities. Unilateral third nerve lesions can also cause an efferent pupillary defect in which a light stimulus elicits a consensual but not a direct response. Thus, the afferent limb of the reflex (optic nerve) is intact but the ipsilateral efferent limb (third nerve) is damaged. Pontine lesions in the tegmentum interrupt the descending sympathetic pathways and produce bilaterally pinpoint pupils; the response to direct light is preserved, but the small extent of constriction may make this difficult to observe and magnification may be required. Lesions of the medulla and ventrolateral cervical spine may involve the descending sympathetic tracts, leading to an ipsilateral Horner's syndrome with ptosis and constricted pupils that react to light [25].

Pupillary Asymmetry

Asymmetry in pupillary size or reactivity may be due to dilatation (mydriasis) of one pupil, such as with a third nerve palsy, or constriction of the other (miosis), as occurs in Horner's syndrome. A sluggishly reactive pupil may be one of the first signs of uncal herniation, soon to be followed by dilation of that pupil and, later, complete third nerve palsy.

Pupillary Effects of Drugs

Anticholinergic agents, applied either locally or given systemically during anesthesia or cardiopulmonary resuscitation, cause fixed, dilatated pupils, as does glutethimide toxicity. Other agents that can cause poorly reactive pupils include barbiturates (the pupillary light reflex is usually retained), succinylcholine, and aminoglycoside antibiotics. Narcotics cause miosis with a sluggish and small constriction to light [26].

Oculomotor Disorders

The position of the eyes at rest, the pattern of spontaneous eye movements, and the presence of oculocephalic and oculovestibular reflexes indicate oculomotor function and the pattern of brain stem or higher cortical involvement. Normal ocular motility depends on the integrity of a large portion of the cerebellum, cerebrum, and brain stem. The preservation of normal ocular motility indicates that normal functioning pathways in a large proportion of brain stem from the vestibular nuclei at the pontomedullary junction to the oculomotor nucleus in the midbrain are intact [27,28].

The primary ocular position may be either dysconjugate, conjugate in the midline, or deviated in a conjugate manner. Dysconjugate deviation of the eyes is common and, in the absence of pre-existing strabismus, generally indicates loss of voluntary control of eye movements, implying that a reduced level of consciousness causes a lack of fusional control. It may represent a horizontal phoria that is normally compensated by fusion/vergence stimuli, which are lost in stupor and coma. However, oculomotor cranial nerve palsies occur frequently in comas of varying etiologies [29]. Third nerve palsies are the most common and are a consequence of primary midbrain lesions or a manifestation of transtentorial herniation. Complete third nerve palsy causes pupillary dilatation, ptosis, and deviation of the eye downward and laterally. Lesions of the medial longitudinal fasciculus are common in comatose patients and lead to an internuclear ophthalmoplegia with isolated failure of ocular adduction (ipsilateral to the medial longitudinal fasciculus lesion) in the absence of pupillary changes and with normal vertical eye movements. Trochlear nerve palsy is usually the result of trauma and gives rise to a vertical tropia. Bilateral abducent palsy may be induced by raised intracranial pressure and nerve damage at the petroclinoid ligament and produces inward deviation and failure of abduction [30].

Skew deviation is a condition of unilateral hypertropia and may be encountered in stupor and coma. It is associated with otolithic, cerebellar, or brain stem lesions. Tonic horizontal conjugate deviation of patients' eyes is common and the direction of deviation depends on the level of the lesion. In lesions between the frontal eye fields and the oculomotor decussation in the midbrain, patients' eyes deviate to the side of the lesion and thus away from the side of the hemiparesis. Below the decussation, for example, at the level of the pons, patients' eyes deviate away from the lesion side, and thus look toward the hemiparesis. Peripheral vestibular lesions in coma lead to conjugate tonic deviation of patients' eyes to the ipsilateral side. Conjugate horizontal deviation can be overcome by vestibular stimuli, however, which can drive patients' eyes across the midline. Intermittent horizontal deviation is usually due to seizure activity that is aversive to the cortical focus, although postictal gaze palsy can deviate patients' eyes to the side of the focus. Tonic downward deviation of patients' eyes is associated with thalamic hemorrhage and dorsal midbrain lesions, causing tectal compression, although a similar deviation can be seen in metabolic or in psychogenic coma. Tonic upward deviation may occur transiently in seizures or oculogyric crises in encephalitis lethargica. Prolonged tonic upward deviation usually occurs as a consequence of extensive hypoxic-ischemic damage and carries a poor prognosis. Conjugate lateral eye deviation is usually the result of an ipsilateral lesion in the frontal eye fields but may be caused by a lesion anywhere in the pathway from the ipsilateral eye fields to the contralateral parapontine reticular formation (lateral gaze center).

Spontaneous Eye Movements

Roving eye movements consist of slow, random, lateral to-and-fro movements and can be conjugate or dysconjugate. Their presence implies that oculomotor nuclei and their connections are relatively intact; coma is caused by a metabolic or toxic cause or bilateral lesions above the brain stem. Slow, spontaneous, alternating, roving horizontal deviation of the eyes (3–5 Hz; ping-pong gaze) is usually associated with diffuse bilateral hemispheric or peduncular vascular disease.

Conjugate Vertical Eye Movements

Conjugate vertical eye movements are separated into different types according to the relative velocities of the downward and upward phases [31–36] (Table 5.3).

Vertical nystagmus is caused by an abnormal pursuit or vestibular system and describes vertical deviation of the eyes from the primary position, with a rapid immediate return to the primary position. It differs from ocular bobbing in that there is no latency between the corrective saccade and the next slow deviation. Ocular myoclonus/downward nystagmus occurs after damage to the lower brain stem in the region of the inferior olive. The ocular movements, which can be rotatory or circular, move with the same beat as the palatal myoclonus.

Horizontal nystagmus occurring in comatose patients suggests an irritative or epileptogenic supratentorial focus. Nystagmus owing to an irritative focus rarely occurs alone without other motor manifestations of seizures. In addition, there may be movements of the patient's eye, eyelid, face, jaw, or tongue and electroencephalographic evidence of status. Unilateral nystagmoid jerks in a horizontal or rotatory fashion are associated with mid or lower pontine damage. Optokinetic nystagmus is only present when afferent visual pathways to the visual cortex and the connections to the brain stem oculomotor systems are intact. It is absent in stupor and coma, and its presence suggests either a slight disturbance of consciousness or functional coma.

Repetitive divergence is characterized by eyes initially in midposition or slightly divergent at rest. They then slowly deviate out and become fully divergent for a brief period before returning to the primary position and repeating the cycle. This occurs in metabolic encephalopathy (e.g., hepatic encephalopathy).

Table 5.3   Rhythmic involuntary vertical eye movements in coma

Syndrome	Causes	Findings
Ocular bobbing	Acute pontine lesion Metabolic and toxic Extra-axial posterior fossa masses	Rapid downward jerks of both eyes followed by a slow return to the mid- position Paralysis of both reflex and spontaneous horizontal eye movements
Monocular/paretic bobbing	—	Coexisting oculomotor palsy alters the appearance of typical bobbing.
Atypical bobbing	Anoxia	Ocular bobbing when lateral eye move- ments are preserved
Ocular dipping (inverse ocular bobbing)	Diffuse cerebral anoxia After status epi- lepticus	Spontaneous eye movements in which an initial slow downward phase is followed by a relatively rapid return Reflex horizontal eye movements are preserved
Reverse ocular bobbing	Nonlocalizing Metabolic Viral encephalitis Pontine hemorrhage	Slow initial downward phase, followed by a rapid return that carries the eyes past the midposition into full upward gaze; then eyes slowly return to mid- position

Vertical movements associated with convergence and divergence usually suggest dorsal midbrain lesions.

Vestibulo-Ocular Reflexes

Oculocephalic Component

The horizontal and vertical vestibulo-ocular reflexes (VORs) are based in a three-neuron pathway linked to structures in or adjacent to the pons (horizontal VOR) and rostral to the region of the oculomotor nucleus in the midbrain (vertical VOR). The function of the VOR is to provide compensatory eye movements to stabilize the eye in space. The physiologic basis is the neuronal activity, which arises predominantly in the semicircular canal, and, to a lesser extent, the otoliths. The VOR is therefore what determines ocular movements after stimulation of the vestibular apparatus. This includes mechanical rotation of the patient's head and caloric irrigation. After rotation of the patient's head, irrespective of the axis of rotation, his or her eyes will normally remain fixed with respect to space. The presence of quick phases indicates an intact brain stem oculomotor system and excludes a significant depression of the level of consciousness. Asymmetries of the VOR point to localized lesions within the brain stem, such as with medial longitudinal fasciculus, abducens, or oculomotor lesions [37,38].

The oculocephalic response is tested by sudden passive rotation of the patient's head in both directions laterally and flexion and extension of his or her neck while the motion of his or her eyes is observed (Table 5.4). This maneuver should not be

Table 5.4   Oculocephalic responses

Rotation	Responses	Causes
Horizontal	Eyes remain conjugate	Normal with reduced level of consciousness
	No movement in either eye	Low-brain stem lesion
		Peripheral vestibular lesion
		Drugs
		Anesthesia
	Eyes move appropriately in one direction but do not cross the midline in the other	Gaze palsy (unilateral lesion in pontine gaze center)
		Pontine lesion
	One eye abducts but the other fails to adduct	Third nerve palsy
		Internuclear ophthalmoplegia (lesion of the median longitudinal fasciculus)
	One eye adducts but the other fails to abduct	Sixth nerve palsy
Vertical	Eyes remain conjugate and maintain fixation (move in direction opposite head movement)	Normal with reduced level of consciousness
	No movement in either eye	Low brain stem lesion
		Peripheral vestibular lesion
		Drugs
		Anesthesia
	Only one eye moves	Third nerve palsy
	Loss of upward gaze	Pretectal or midbrain tegmental compression

Source: Adapted from JO Harris, JR Berger. Clinical Approach to Stupor and Coma. In WG Bradley, RB Daroff, GM Fenichel, CM Marsden (eds), Neurology in Clinical Practice. London: Butterworth, 1991.

performed on any patient until the stability of his or her neck has been adequately assessed. When supranuclear influences on the oculomotor nerves are removed, the patient's eyes maintain their fixation on a point in the distance when his or her head is turned. In the normal oculocephalic response, the patient's eyes move conjugately in a direction opposite to the direction of movement of his or her head. Cranial nerve palsies predictably alter the response of this maneuver.

Oculovestibular Component

The oculovestibular response is usually tested by applying cold water to the tympanic membrane (Table 5.5). This is best done with the patient's head tilted 60 degrees backward from the horizontal to allow maximum stimulation of the lateral semicircular canal, which is most responsive for reflex lateral eye movements. After a careful check to make sure the ear canal is patent and the tympanic membrane is free of defect, 60 ml ice-cold water is slowly injected into one canal. Iced water caloric stimulation may sometimes be a more effective vestibular stimulus than the oculocephalic response, producing tonic deviation of the patient's eyes toward the irrigated ear.

Table 5.5   Oculovestibular responses

Test	Response	Cause
Cold water instilled into the right ear	Nystagmus with slow phase to right and fast phase to left	Normal
	No response	Obstructed ear canal
		Dead labyrinth
		Low brain stem lesion
	Tonic deviation toward stimulated side (slow phase to right, no fast phase)	Supratentorial lesion with intact pons
		Toxic/metabolic
		Drugs
		Structural lesion above brain stem
	Dysconjugate response	Brain stem lesion (usually in region of medial longitudinal fasciculus)
	Downbeat nystagmus	Horizontal gaze palsy
	Vertical eye deviation	Drug overdose
Warm water instilled into left ear after no response to cold	Slow phase to right, fast phase to left	Peripheral eighth nerve lesion
		Labyrinthine disorder on right

Source: Adapted from JO Harris, JR Berger. Clinical Approach to Stupor and Coma. In WG Bradley, RB Daroff, GM Fenichel, CM Marsden (eds), Neurology in Clinical Practice. London: Butterworth, 1991.

Cold water results in a change in the baseline firing of the vestibular nerves and slow (tonic) conjugate deviation of the comatose patient's eyes toward the stimulated ear. In an awake person, the eye deviation is corrected, with a resultant nystagmoid jerking of his or her eye toward the midline (fast phase). Warm-water irrigation produces reversal of flow of the endolymph, which causes conjugate eye deviation with a slow phase away from the stimulated ear and a normal corrective phase back toward the ear. Simultaneous cold-water application (to both ears) results in slow downward deviation, whereas simultaneous warm-water application causes upward deviation. False-negative or misleading responses on caloric testing occur with pre-existing inner ear disease, vestibulopathy (e.g., ototoxic drugs), vestibular paresis, and drug effects. Oculovestibular stimulus provides additional information concerning neural pathways and is more effective in distinguishing functional coma from that caused by structural lesions than the oculocephalic maneuver.

Effects of Drugs on Eye Movements

Unlike the response to pupillary light, eye movements are particularly sensitive to the effects of metabolic disturbances or drugs that can alter or abolish reflex responses. All kinds of eye movements may be affected by drugs, although smooth pursuit, accommodation, vergence, and eccentric gaze-holding are particularly susceptible to drug effects. As coma deepens, roving eye movements disappear first, followed by VORs, initially to head movements and then to caloric stimulation.

Fifth Cranial Nerve

In the examination of a comatose patient, the response in the ophthalmic division of the trigeminal nerve (V1 corneal response) is most helpful. The patient's eyes are usually closed, but if both the afferent and the efferent limbs of the reflex are intact, the patient blinks either spontaneously or in response to stimuli (blinking occurs bilaterally because of the crossover of afferent fibers centrally). Spontaneous blinking implies intact pontine reticular formation, and reflex blinking (in response to bright light and sound) implies intact visual and auditory pathways. Blinking induced by a bright light is probably mediated by the superior colliculus and remains even in the presence of occipital damage. Absence of blinking on one side only is indicative of unilateral nuclear, fascicular, or peripheral facial dysfunction. In a comatose patient with a lesion at the level of the pons, afferent impulses along the fifth cranial nerve are interrupted and no blink reflex is observed (absent corneal reflex). However, in some cases there is no blink on the stimulated side but a blink is observed on the contralateral side (consensual response). In such cases, absence of the blink response reflects ipsilateral efferent motor damage. The corneal reflex has a higher threshold in comatose patients and may be totally lost with deep sedation. There may be decreased corneal sensitivity (e.g., V nerve lesion, ipsilateral lateral pontomedullary lesions, or contralateral parietal lesions), or impaired eye closure (e.g., seventh nerve or low pontine lesions). In the latter case, the stimulus can induce deviation of the patient's jaw to the opposite side (corneopterygoid reflex) and, given an intact upper pons and midbrain, his or her eyes may roll upward (Bell's phenomenon). The eyelids may remain tonically retracted due to failure of levator inhibition in some cases of pontine infarction. The patient's jaw jerk may be brisk, and the presence of jaw clonus suggests metabolic encephalopathy

Seventh Cranial Nerve

The seventh cranial nerve supplies the muscles of facial expression. It can be assessed by observing the patient's grimace. A grossly asymmetric grimace suggests impairment of either the seventh cranial nerve nucleus or its axons or a lesion somewhere along the descending corticobulbar fibers, which are destined to supply the seventh cranial nerve nuclei. Lesions at a pontine level can damage facial nerve nuclei and produce ipsilateral complete facial weakness. Upper motor neuron lesions produce contralateral facial weakness and tend to spare the forehead and orbicularis oculi muscles because of the bilateral cortical representation. A deeply comatose patient may not grimace in response to a noxious stimulus, which does not necessarily imply weakness but may imply depressed sensory function [39].

Bulbar Function

The clinical assessment of bulbar function in patients with an altered level of consciousness is unreliable. Airway protection may be impaired despite the presence of palatal movement and a pharyngeal reflex. Symptoms and signs of glossopharyngeal and vagus nerve dysfunction must be sought. These include loss of pharyngeal sensation and of sensation over the posterior third of the tongue (ninth cranial nerve), impaired speech and swallowing, palatal weakness (manifest as reduced palatal and uvular excursion in the pharyngeal reflex), tracheal sensory loss as evidenced by absence of distress, lack of lacrimation, and poor cough response to tracheal stimulation or tracheal intubation [18].

Respiration

Abnormal patterns of rate and rhythm in coma reflect impaired automatic ventilatory control [40]. Many of these patterns were first described by Plum and Posner [1] as manifestations of progressive central brain stem herniation and were considered to have fairly precise localizing values patterns. However, these phenomena are now seen less commonly because controlled ventilation is instituted earlier in patients with neurogenic respiratory insufficiency. Primary central neurogenic hyperventilation is considered to be present if rapid, regular hyperventilation persists in the face of alkalosis, elevated Po_2, and low Pco_2 and in the absence of any pulmonary or airway disorder. It is extremely rare, and the few cases in the literature have been associated with either lymphoma or infiltrating glioma. However, hyperventilation in the seriously ill patient is common and is usually caused by intrinsic pulmonary involvement leading to ventilation-perfusion ratio mismatch, pulmonary shunting, and increased vagally mediated reflexes. In apneustic breathing, sustained inspiratory cramps with a prolonged pause at full inspiration or alternating brief end-inspiratory and expiratory pauses occur. The pattern has been associated with bilateral tegmental infarcts or demyelinating lesions in the pons. In cluster breathing, respiration occurs in irregular bursts separated by variable periods of apnea; the regularity and decrescendo-crescendo pattern of Cheyne-Stokes respiration are absent, and the cycle time is much shorter. Cluster breathing reflects a high medullary or low pontine lesion.

Ataxic respiration is characterized by a completely irregular respiratory cycle of variable frequency and tidal volume alternating with periods of apnea; it is particularly associated with medullary compression owing to rapidly expanding lesions and may be an important sign of impending respiratory arrest. Intractable hiccups may be the result of structural or functional disturbances of the medulla or afferent or efferent connections with the respiratory muscles. They may be associated with structural lesions of the medulla, including infarction in the territory of the posteroinferior cerebellar artery, tumor, tuberculoma, abscess, syrinx, hematoma, and demyelination. The development of hiccups in this context may anticipate the development of irregularities of the respiratory rhythm culminating in respiratory arrest. Cheyne-Stokes respiration is a pattern of periodic breathing in which phases of hyperpnea regularly alternate with apnea. The breathing waxes from breath to breath in a smooth crescendo and then, once a peak is reached, wanes in an equally smooth decrescendo. It is nonspecific and may be a sign of bilateral subcortical dysfunction or may be seen in coma caused by metabolic disturbance or as an early sign of increased intracranial pressure. It is also seen in patients with cardiac disease.

Motor Responses

Examining the motor responses involves assessment of (1) resting posture of the patient's limbs and head, (2) involuntary movements, and (3) spontaneous movements (purposeful or nonpurposeful) and response to external stimuli.

Decorticate posture refers to flexion at the elbows and wrists with shoulder adduction and internal rotation and extension of the lower extremities. When unilateral, it is contralateral to the hemispheric lesion. It is a poor localizing feature, as it can result from lesions in many locations, although usually above the brain stem. It generally indicates that the structures below the diencephalon are intact but that dysfunction of the thalamus or cerebral hemispheres is occurring. *Decerebrate response* refers to bilateral extensor posture with extension of the lower extremities and adduction and internal rotation of the patient's shoulders and extension at his or her elbows and wrists. It is usually caused by lesions of the bilateral midbrain or pons. Less commonly, severe metabolic encephalopathy (e.g., owing to hypoglycemia or liver failure) or bilateral supratentorial lesions involving the motor pathways may produce a similar pattern. Severe metabolic (e.g., anoxic) disorders give rise to decerebrate rigidity, which is characterized by extension and pronation of the upper extremities and forcible plantar flexion of the patient's foot. Brought about by painful stimuli, opisthotonus develops intermittently with hyperextension of the patient's trunk and hyperpronation of his or her arms. Spontaneous extension and internal rotation of the patient's arms and legs may signify a disturbance at a higher pontine or midbrain level. Abnormal extension of the patient's arms with weak flexion of his or her legs usually indicates damage to the pontine tegmentum. With even lower lesions involving the medulla, total flaccidity ensues. Posturing may occur spontaneously or in response to external stimuli, such as pain, or even be set off by such minimal events as the patient's own breathing. These postures, although common, may be variable in their expression because of other associated or more rostral brain stem damage [41].

Tone

The symmetry of tone is more important than the absolute level. A flaccid arm and leg on one side and normal tone on the other strongly suggest a hemiparesis on the flaccid side. Muscle tone and asymmetry in muscle tone are helpful in localizing a focal structural lesion and can help in differentiating metabolic from structural coma. Acute structural damage above the brain stem usually results in decrease in flaccid tone. In older lesions, tone is generally increased. Metabolic insults usually cause a symmetric decrease in tone. A grasp reflex may be found on one side, signifying a degree of lateralization, which indicates frontal lobe disturbance. Plucking or clutching movements of the coma patient's limbs indicate intactness of the corticospinal pathways and imply that the coma cannot be deep.

Involuntary Movements

Tonic-clonic or other stereotyped movements signal generalized seizures or epilepsia partialis continua. *Myoclonic jerking*, which refers to nonrhythmic jerking movements in single or multiple muscle groups, is seen with anoxic encephalopathy or other metabolic comas; for example, hepatic encephalopathy. Generalized myoclonic status is seen in approximately 40% of survivors from postanoxic coma and is highly predictive of permanent vegetative state or death [42,43]. Myoclonic seizures typically lack a tonic component and typically involve facial muscles and other axial structures. Touch, tracheal suction, or loud hand-clapping can precipitate the jerks. Myoclonic status should be distinguished from a single myoclonic jerk or other types of generalized seizures. Some patients may recover from postanoxic coma associated with myoclonic status and be left with multifocal action myoclonus and stimulus-sensitive myoclonus (Lance Adams syndrome), however, which may continue to improve with time and is only rarely associated with persistent or severe additional neurologic deficit [44]. Rhythmic myoclonus must be distinguished from epileptic movements and is usually a sign of brain stem injury. Cerebellar fits result from intermittent tonsillar herniation. Cerebellar fits are characterized by a deterioration in the level of arousal, opisthotonus, respiratory rate slowing and irregularity, and pupillary dilatation.

Painful Stimuli

Motor responses to painful stimuli should be tested, although the pattern of response may vary depending on the site and nature of stimulation [45]. Reflex flexor response to pain in the upper extremity consists of adduction of the patient's shoulder, flexion of his or her elbow, and pronation of his or her arm. *Triple flexion response in the lower extremities* refers to reflex withdrawal with flexion of the hip and knee and dorsiflexion at the ankle in response to painful stimuli on the patient's foot or lower extremity. It is not helpful in localization. Spinal reflexes are reflexes that are mediated at the level of the spinal cord and are not dependent on the functional integrity of the brain or brain stem. The plantar reflex may be extensor in coma from any cause, including drug overdose and postictal states.

MECHANISMS OF COMA

Cerebral Herniation

To cause coma directly, supratentorial lesions must affect both cerebral hemispheres. Supratentorial lesions with mass effect (e.g., hemispheric tumors, subdural or intracerebral hemorrhage, and massive infarcts) cause a secondary impairment of consciousness by compressing the diencephalon and upper brain stem structures [1,15].

When the intracranial pressure of the supratentorial compartment reaches a certain level, the brain substance is squeezed downward through the tentorial opening. Depending on the supratentorial location of the mass and the size of the tentorial opening, either one of two different syndromes can result.

Uncal Herniation

Classically, early signs of third nerve and midbrain compression are present. The pupil initially dilates as a result of third nerve compression but later returns to midposition with midbrain compression that involves the sympathetic and parasympathetic tracts. Lateral extracerebral or temporal lobe masses push the mesial temporal lobe (uncus or parahippocampal gyrus) between the ipsilateral aspect of the midbrain and the free edge of the tentorium. As the tongue of herniated tissue compresses the third cranial nerve and posterior cerebral artery downward, the ipsilateral pupil becomes progressively dilatated and responds sluggishly to light. The posterior cerebral artery, pinched against the tentorial edge by the herniated hippocampal gyrus, becomes occluded, giving rise to a hemorrhagic mesial occipital infarction. The herniated hippocampus also pushes the midbrain against the rigid edge of the dura on the opposite side of the tentorial opening. This rigid structure carves out a notch (Kernohan's notch) in the lateral aspect of the midbrain, interrupting the cerebral peduncles (particularly those fibers that project to the patient's leg) on the side opposite the original temporal lobe lesion. This results in a hemiparesis ipsilateral to the original lesion and the third nerve lesion (Kernohan's notch phenomenon). The hemiparesis is thus a false localizing sign. At this point, anteroposterior elongation and downward displacement of the midbrain cause tearing of the paramedian perforating vessels that feed the midbrain tegmentum. The consequent infarction and hemorrhage (Duret hemorrhages) that involve this structure make recovery virtually impossible. The pupil that was larger may become a little smaller as the sympathetic pathway is damaged in the midbrain, whereas the other pupil becomes midsized and unresponsive. Oculomotor paresis appears, first in the patient's eye that was originally involved and shortly afterward in his or her other eye.

Survivors of tentorial herniation may be left in a locked-in or vegetative state and may demonstrate oculomotor nerve dysfunction, internuclear ophthalmoplegia, vertical gaze paresis, pretectal signs, homonymous hemianopia or blindness, parkinsonism and other extrapyramidal syndromes, or spastic leg weakness.

Central Herniation

Unlike uncal herniation, impairment of consciousness occurs early in central herniation. The earliest signs are mild impairment of consciousness with poor concentration, drowsiness, unexpected agitation, small but reactive pupils, loss of the fast phase on caloric testing, poor or absent reflex vertical gaze, and unilateral corticospinal tract signs. Unlike temporal masses, frontal, parietal, and occipital masses first compress the diencephalon, which, as the supratentorial pressure increases, shifts downward and buckles over the midbrain. Subsequent flattening of the midbrain and pons in the rostrocaudal direction causes elongation and rupture of the paramedian perforating arteries that feed these structures, resulting in infarction and hemorrhage in the tegmentum of the midbrain and pons. The classic clinical picture reflects an orderly progression of brain stem damage reflecting rostrocaudal deterioration. The early diencephalic state is characterized by impairment of attention, somnolence, sighing, and yawning. Roving eye movements occur, and VOR elicits rapid eye movements and nystagmus. Paratonia may be present. During the late diencephalic stage, the patient is not rousable with Cheyne-Stokes respiration. The pupils are small and reactive and roving eye movements are lost, but VOR elicits full and conjugate deviation, although there may be mild limitation of upgaze with tectal involvement. Painful stimuli provoke decorticate posturing. In the pontine stage, there is progressive tachypnea and temperature oscillations. The pupils are midsized, unequal, and irregular. VOR elicits restricted vertical eye movements. Bilateral dysfunction of third nerve nuclei can lead to impairment of adduction. Progressively, eye movements are lost completely. Painful stimuli evoke decerebrate posturing with the subsequent development of decerebrate rigidity. The medullary state is agonal with apnea, hypotension, and irregularity of the pulse [46].

Early depression of the level of alertness in a patient with an acute hemispheric mass lesion may be more related to distortion of the brain by horizontal displacement than to transtentorial herniation with brain stem compression. Ropper [47,48] showed that horizontal displacement of the pineal body of 0–3 mm from the midline was associated with alertness, 3–4 mm with drowsiness, 6.0–8.5 mm with stupor, and 8–13 mm with coma.

With extratemporal masses, the perimesencephalic cistern was often widened, suggesting that the space was not filled by herniated temporal lobe. Ropper further determined horizontal and vertical components of brain displacement on coronal magnetic resonance imaging in patients with acute supratentorial masses. Brain displacement near the incisura increased from 3 mm in awake patients to 6–13 mm in stuporous and comatose patients and remained predominantly horizontal. Uncal herniation did not appear to be the immediate cause of brain stem compression but is accompanied by prominent lateral distortion above the tentorium. Thus, it is possible that most patients with acute unilateral masses have upper brain stem distortion owing predominantly to horizontal shift and rotational torsion at or above the tentorium rather than vertical descent.

Other Forms of Herniation

Subfalcine herniation occurs when an expanding hemisphere (usually the cingulate gyrus) is displaced across the intracranial cavity and under the falx. This can lead to compression of the anterior cerebral artery and secondary infarction and edema.

In upward herniation, lesions that compress the upper brain stem can cause upward transtentorial herniation of the tectum of the midbrain and of the anterior cerebellar lobules, giving rise to signs of midbrain dysfunction with small, asymmetric, and fixed pupils; vertical ophthalmoplegia; abnormal VORs; a brain stem respiratory pattern; decerebrate posturing; and coma. Upward herniation can lead to compression of the vein of Galen, raising supratentorial venous pressure, or cause compression of the superior cerebellar arteries, resulting in infarction of the superior cerebellum. Causes include tumor or hemorrhage in the pons, cerebellum, or the region of the fourth ventricle.

Tonsillar herniation occurs when the inferior medial part of the cerebellar tonsils is downwardly displaced into the foramen magnum. This can occur as a consequence of a posterior fossa mass lesion leading to progressive medullary compression characterized by stiff neck, vomiting, skew deviation of the eyes, respiratory irregularities, coma, and death. The condition may present with a subacute or relapsing foramen magnum syndrome caused by a lesion, including tumors (meningioma, neurofibroma, glioma, or metastases) or Arnold-Chiari malformation.

Distinction of Toxic and Metabolic Coma from Structural Coma

It is generally possible to distinguish metabolic encephalopathy from structural causes on the basis of clinical examination. The medical history may indicate the presence of a metabolic abnormality, and onset is more likely to be acute in the presence of a structural lesion. Metabolic or toxic disorders usually cause coma without lateralizing or brain stem signs, whereas structural lesions may be indicated by asymmetric motor signs. Metabolic encephalopathy is also favored by the presence of involuntary limb movements (tremor, myoclonus, and asterixis), abnormalities of the respiratory pattern (hypo- or hyperventilation), and the presence of acid-base disturbances. The level of consciousness tends to fluctuate and be lighter in patients with metabolic disorders. However, these clinical features are merely indicators; structural lesions, such as subarachnoid hemorrhage, cortical venous thrombosis, bilateral subdural hematoma, or multifocal central nervous system disease (vasculitis, lymphoma, meningitis, or hematoma), may present with bilateral, symmetric signs, and metabolic disorders (e.g., hypoglycemia) may present with focal signs [49].

Psychogenic Unresponsiveness

Patients with psychogenic unresponsiveness can be distinguished by history, examination, and, if necessary, investigations. Often, atypical factors occur in the history and, occasionally, obvious psychiatric precipitating factors. Examination reveals inconsistent volitional responses, particularly on eyelid opening, when spontaneous roving eye movements are present and pupillary constriction occurs. Oculovestibular stimulation with cold stimulus shows preservation of the fast phase away from the stimulated side. Finally, electroencephalography shows responsive alpha rhythms.

OUTCOME FROM COMA

It is not possible to assess the prognosis of a patient in coma with complete accuracy, but a number of clinical factors help to guide the observer in predicting the likely outcome. Coma associated with drug and alcohol ingestion generally carries a good prognosis for recovery, providing the patient has no severe underlying disorder, has received adequate systemic support while in coma, and has had no secondary insult from hypoxia or hypoperfusion as a consequence of cardiac or respiratory arrest or aspiration pneumonia.

The prognosis for a patient in traumatic coma is more favorable than that for a patient at a similar level of coma from nontraumatic causes. Trauma patients are usually younger, and continued improvement may occur despite prolonged periods of coma and severe disability. The most important predictive features for survival in patients with coma caused by severe head injury of more than 6 hours' duration are depth of coma (as defined by the GCS, pupillary responses, eye movements, and motor responses) and patient age [50–56]. The extent of injury, presence of skull fracture, hemispheric damage, or extracranial injury do not seem to be important. However, these factors are less effective in predicting disability in survivors. It has been suggested that secondary insults, such as intracranial hypertension and low cerebral perfusion pressure, may be associated with a higher mortality and increase in severe disability [49,57].

The prognosis for patients in nontraumatic coma is poor and depends on several important factors [58–60]:

1. *Etiology*: Patients in coma owing to structural cerebral disease (e.g., cerebrovascular disease or subarachnoid hemorrhage) carry the poorest prognosis, with only 7% achieving moderate or good recovery. The outlook for hypoxic ischemic insults is a little better in published studies, but it is increasingly apparent that patients who are resuscitated out-of-hospital after cardiac arrests but remain in coma from hypoxic insults carry a very poor prognosis. The best outlook is in patients with coma caused by metabolic or toxic insults, in whom 35% achieve a moderate or good recovery [61].

2. *Depth of coma*: When determined by GCS augmented by vestibulo-ocular and corneal reflexes, this is a sensitive guide to outcome. At 24 hours, if there is no eye opening, vocal response, or motor function, the patient has a 6% chance of making a moderate or good recovery. In the presence of eye opening, grunting, and limb flexion to noxious stimuli, chances of moderate or good recovery are 20%.

3. *Duration of coma*: Nontraumatic coma that lasts for more than 1 week is said to carry only a 3% prospect of good recovery whereas a shorter duration (<6 hours) is associated with a 15% prospect of good recovery.

It must be emphasized that many of these findings relate to studies from the 1980s or earlier. It seems possible that with better techniques of intensive care, physiologic measurement, and cerebral protection these data are no longer accurate and should be used as a general guide only [62,63].

VEGETATIVE STATE

Diagnosis, prognosis, and management of the vegetative state have received considerable attention in Europe and the United States since the early 1990s [64]. This has been partly because of legal rulings on individual, highly publicized cases [65,66] but also because a series of professional bodies have attempted to establish guidelines on clinical and ethical aspects of management [67–72]. In a comprehensive and valuable review, the American Multi-Society Task Force on Persistent Vegetative State [71,72] sought to clarify the situation by summarizing information on the available literature concerning prognosis to facilitate consensus management recommendations [73].

Patients in a vegetative state appear to be awake with their eyes open but show no evidence of awareness of self or environment; are unable to interact with others; and have no evidence of sustained, reproducible, purposeful, or voluntary behavioral responses to visual, auditory, tactile, or noxious stimuli [74]. Patients exhibit no evidence of language comprehension and expression. Patients are able to breathe spontaneously, and gag, cough, sucking, and swallowing reflexes are usually present. Sleep-wake cycles are preserved as are the hypothalamic and brain stem autonomic responses. Bladder and bowel incontinence occurs, but cranial nerve (pupillary, vestibulo-ocular, corneal, and gag), spinal, and primitive reflexes are variably preserved. Inconsistent nonpurposive movements, facial grimacing, smiling and frowning, chewing, swallowing, bruxism, vocalization, grasping, and inconsistent auditory and oculomotor orientating reflexes to peripheral sounds or movement can occur. The diagnosis of the vegetative state is not tenable if any degree of voluntary movement, sustained visual pursuit, consistent and reproducible visual fixation, or response to threatening gestures is present [71,72,75].

The vegetative state usually develops after a variable period of coma; it may be partially or totally reversible or may progress to a persistent or permanent vegetative state or death. Persistent vegetative state (PVS) is defined as a vegetative state that has continued for at least 1 month. This definition does not imply permanency or irreversibility. Vegetative states are caused by acute cerebral injuries, degenerative and metabolic disorders, or developmental malformations. The first is by far the largest and most important group and can be subdivided into traumatic (e.g., traffic accidents or direct cerebral injury) and nontraumatic (e.g., hypoxic-ischemic encephalopathy, stroke, central nervous system infection, tumor, or toxic insult).

Pathology

No single pathologic pattern of brain damage that produces the vegetative state exists. After hypoxic brain damage, generalized or predominantly parieto-occipital loss of the cortical ribbon (caused by neuronal loss in layers 3 and 5) can occur, as well as severe necrosis of the thalamus, caudate nucleus, hippocampus, and Purkinje cells of the cerebellum. After trauma, the lesions are more complex, with diffuse axonal injury disconnecting the largely intact cerebral cortex and thalamus from other parts of the brain. In other cases, similar patterns to those of hypoxic brain damage are shown.

Andrews [76,77] has emphasized the difficulties in diagnosing the vegetative state. In the presence of profound disability (paralysis, spasticity, or dysphasia, or all), the patient may only be able to demonstrate awareness through specific motor acts (e.g., nonverbal gesture or specific movement). Diagnosis of vegetative state requires multiple observations, repeated for short periods over a considerable amount of time using standardized assessments and clear criteria for recording responses. It is important to ensure that the assessments are undertaken with the subjects in good general health and with any sedating drugs withdrawn. The patients should also be in a good nutritional state, in an optimal seating position, and well rested.

Two dimensions of recovery from vegetative states exist: recovery of awareness and recovery of voluntary motor function. Recovery of awareness can occur without functional recovery, but functional recovery cannot take place without recovery of awareness. The Multi-Society Task Force emphasized that the most important factors in determining the outcome of PVS include the patient's age and the etiology and duration of PVS. Overall, the available data indicate that the mortality for adults in PVS after an acute brain injury is 70% at 3 years and 84% at 5 years. Death is associated with pulmonary or urinary tract infections, respiratory failure, and sudden death of unknown causes.

The Multi-Society Task Force estimated the outcome probability at 12 months for patients who remained in PVS 3 and 6 months after the initial insult. In adults with PVS 3 months after traumatic injury, approximately one-third recover by 12 months and more than half are severely disabled. After 6 months in PVS, approximately 12% of patients recover to severe disability and 4% to moderate disability or good recovery. The outcome is worse after nontraumatic insults: After 3 months in PVS, approximately 7% of patients recover, generally with severe disability, and no patients recovered after 6 months in PVS. In children, the data are limited: Although the outcome for traumatic PVS at 12 months seems to be better than that for adults, there is little difference between children and adults for nontraumatic insults. On the basis of these data, it was concluded that a PVS can be judged to be permanent 12 months after a traumatic injury and 3 months after a nontraumatic insult in adults and children. Although occasionally a verified recovery has been reported, after these times such recovery is virtually always associated with severe disability [76,77].

What are the implications of these findings for the management of patients in coma or a vegetative state after acute brain injury? At the onset, it is appropriate to provide aggressive medical treatment when the prognosis remains uncertain. This includes the provision of adequate hydration and nutrition (via nasogastric tube or gastrostomy), airway protection, and appropriate attention to posture, contractures, and skin, bowel, and bladder care. It is important to ensure that stimulation and rehabilitation are available as soon as the patient's condition is stabilized [77], but the role of coma arousal programs remains unproved.

Once the diagnosis of PVS is established, continuing treatment is justified if, as the British Medical Association Ethics Committee states, "it makes possible a decent life in which a patient can reasonably be thought to have a continued interest" [78]. The level of treatment depends on clinical assessment by the physician and discussion with the patient's family or surrogate decision-makers. The role of high-technology treatments (e.g., mechanical ventilation, dialysis, cardiopulmonary resuscitation) and routine medications (e.g., antibiotics) or other commonly ordered treatments (e.g., supplementary oxygen) can only be determined in the context of the individual case.

A Royal College of Physicians Working Party has recommended that the term *continuing vegetative state* be used when the vegetative state continues for more than 4 weeks and it becomes unlikely that the condition is part of the recovery phase from coma. A patient in a continuing vegetative state enters a permanent vegetative state when the diagnosis of irreversibility can be established with a high degree of clinical certainty. The Working Party has recommended that the diagnosis be made when the patient has been in a continuing vegetative state after head injury for more than 12 months or after other causes of brain damage for more than 6 months. The diagnosis at birth can be made only in infants with anencephaly and hydranencephaly. For children with other severe malformations or acquired brain damage, observation for more than 6 months is recommended until lack of awareness can be established.

Diagnosis requires an established cause for the condition; the exclusion of persisting effects of sedative, anesthetic and neuromuscular blocking agents; and the exclusion of reversible metabolic factors. The diagnosis can only be made after the patient has been examined separately by two medical practitioners experienced in assessing disturbances of consciousness. The most important role of the medical practitioner in making the diagnosis is to ensure that the patient is not sentient and, in this respect, the views of nursing staff, relatives, and caregivers are of considerable importance and help.

Both medical and legal authorities have advised that, in some circumstances, it may be legitimate and ethically acceptable to withdraw life-sustaining treatment, including tube feeding, when the patient's condition is irreversible. When the diagnosis of permanent vegetative state has been established and it is accepted that further therapy will merely prolong an insentient life for the patient, the situation should be communicated sensitively to the relatives, who must then be given time to consider the possibility of withdrawing artificial means of administering food and fluid. In the United Kingdom at present, the courts require that the decision to withdraw nutrition and hydration, resulting in the inevitable death of the patient, should be referred to the court before any action is taken. The decision to withdraw other life-sustaining medication, such as insulin for diabetes, may also need to be referred to the courts, because the legal situation is uncertain. However, the decision not to intervene with cardiopulmonary resuscitation or not to prescribe antibiotics, dialysis, or insulin is a clinical decision.

Minimally Responsive State

Minimally responsive patients are no longer in a coma or vegetative state but demonstrate low-level behavioral responses that are consistent with severe neurologic impairment and disability. Patients who are minimally responsive are able to demonstrate some level of awareness of environmental stimuli or some behavioral response to command consistent with the presence of cognitive function. This response may be intermittent or incomplete, and the examining clinician must take into account the frequency and context of the behavioral response to interpret its meaning or significance.

LOCKED-IN SYNDROME

Locked-in syndrome can be described as a supranuclear tetraplegia associated with horizontal conjugate gaze palsy and the preservation of vertical eye movements with synergistic elevation of the upper eyelids when looking upward. Vertical eye movements may be slow and incomplete. Consciousness and awareness of the environment are preserved, but the patient is anarthric and, in the complete form of the syndrome, is only able to communicate by eye movements. The condition is associated with interruption of the pyramidal tract fibers in the ventral pons, leading to a loss of voluntary control below the level of the lesion. Interruption of corticobulbar fibers that innervate (crossed or uncrossed) the motor nuclei of the cranial nerves causes a supranuclear paralysis of the lower cranial nerves. The condition is often incomplete, with preservation of some degree of horizontal gaze and facial, tongue, and limb movements. Involuntary phenomena include ocular bobbing, crying, laughing, trismus, oral automatisms, pain reaction, facial grimacing, yawning, palatal myoclonus, and sighing [79].

Munschauer and associates [80] described a patient with locked-in syndrome owing to infarction of the basal pons. This condition led to loss of voluntary control, with normal carbon dioxide responses but preservation of respiratory modulation to emotional stimuli, including laughing, coughing, and anxiety. These findings imply that descending limbic influences on automatic respiration are anatomically and functionally independent of the voluntary respiratory system. It was suggested that such a descending pathway, mediating limbic control of respiration, lay either in the pontine tegmentum or lateral basis pontis. A similar dissociation between volitional and emotional control of facial movements has also been noted.

The most frequent cause of locked-in syndrome is occlusion of the vertebrobasilar artery, usually predominantly in the rostral or middle segments. Pontine hemorrhage or embolic disease can also cause the condition. Other causes have been described in which the lesion was situated in the pontine tegmentum, basis pontis, or mesencephalic region at the level of the cerebral peduncles. Cases of locked-in syndrome owing to bilateral internal carotid artery lesions have also been described. The etiologies of nonvascular cases have included central pontine myelinolysis, trauma, encephalitis, tumor, pontine abscess, multiple sclerosis, and heroin abuse. "Peripheral" lesions (i.e., severe neuropathy such as Guillain-Barré syndrome) can cause an apparent locked-in syndrome with severe limb, facial, and bulbar paresis, although respiration is frequently affected because of respiratory muscle weakness.

By definition, all of these patients, although severely restricted in motor function, are conscious and aware of the environment around them. This is reinforced by their ability to communicate using residual motor function. Because they are alert, it is important to establish a consistent form of communication to be used with them. Furthermore, functional recovery is possible in both vascular and nonvascular groups, and it is therefore necessary to introduce an aggressive rehabilitation program as early as possible to allow the patient to achieve the highest possible level of recovery as soon as possible. The prognosis for most patients in locked-in syndromes is poor, however, with severe residual disability being the usual outcome. The mortality is high, with most deaths occurring in the first 4 months, either from extension of the lesion or from respiratory complications (pneumonia, respiratory arrest, or pulmonary embolus).

BRAIN STEM DEATH

Death has been defined as "the irreversible loss of the capacity for consciousness with irreversible loss of the capacity to breathe" [81–85]. The irreversible cessation of brain stem function (brain stem death) produces this clinical state and is therefore equivalent to the death of the individual. The clinical diagnosis of brain stem death can only be considered if the following conditions pertain:

1. There should be no doubt that the patient's condition is caused by a known etiology that has caused irremediable brain damage.
2. Complicating metabolic, acid-base, electrolyte, and endocrine disorders must be excluded.
3. The patient has no history of drug intoxication with depressant drugs (e.g., hypnotics, tranquilizers, alcohol).
4. The patient has had no recent exposure to neuromuscular blocking agents.
5. Primary hypothermia has been excluded as a cause of the coma (temperature >35°C).

The diagnosis can only be considered if the patient is being maintained on a ventilator because spontaneous respiration has ceased. To establish the diagnosis, the patient must be in a coma with no response to stimulation. The diagnosis depends on the absence of all brain stem reflex activity as established by the following conditions:

1. Pupils are fixed in diameter and do not react to sharp changes in light intensity. The pupils may be between midposition (4 mm) and dilatated (9 mm), but if they are dilatated, it is important to ensure that there has been no drug intoxication or exposure to mydriatics.
2. No VORs. A caloric test should be undertaken as described earlier with several minutes of observation. It is necessary to exclude labyrinthine disease, sedatives, and anticonvulsants. The oculocephalic reflexes should also be absent but should only be tested if there is no instability of the cervical spine.
3. Facial motor responses should be absent. There should be no corneal reflex to touch, no jaw reflex, and no motor response within a cranial nerve distribution to deep pressure in the cranial nerve territory. There must be no decerebrate or decorticate posturing but spinal movements may be seen [86].
4. Absence of pharyngeal and tracheal reflex response to bronchial stimulation. The patient does not respond after stimulation of the posterior pharyngeal wall and does not cough after bronchial suction using a catheter passed down the trachea.
5. No respiratory movements occur despite a Pco_2 above 50 mm Hg (6.7 kPa). (This test must be undertaken with the patient adequately oxygenated by delivering oxygen through a catheter into the tracheal tube [87].)

The United Kingdom Code of Practice recommends that the tests be carried out by two medical practitioners who have expertise in this area. One should be a consultant and one a consultant or senior registrar. The duration between the two sets of tests has not been specified but is usually less than 24 hours.

The patient may continue to show vegetative responses, including spontaneous movements of the limbs and trunk (occasionally respiratory-like), sweating, tachycardia, labile blood pressure, and the presence of deep tendon reflexes and a positive Babinski sign. In the United Kingdom, confirmatory tests, including electroencephalography, angiography, and transcranial Doppler, are not part of the standard diagnostic criteria.

118   *Critical Care Neurology*

REFERENCES

 1. Plum F, Posner JR. Diagnosis of Stupor and Coma. Philadelphia: Davis, 1983.
 2. Zeman AZJ, Grayling AC, Cowey A. Contemporary theories of consciousness. J Neurol Neurosurg Psychiatry 1997;62:549.
 3. Niedermeyer E. Consciousness: function and definition. Clin Electroencephalogr 1994;25:86.
 4. Bates D. Medical Coma. In RAC Hughes (ed), Neurological Emergencies (1st ed). London: British Medical Journal, 1994;1–27.
 5. Hughes RAC, Bihari D. Acute neuromuscular respiratory paralysis. J Neurol Neurosurg Psychiatry 1993;56:334.
 6. Gueye PN, Hoffman JR, Taboulet P, et al. Empiric use of flumazenil in comatose patients: limited applicability of criteria to define low risk. Ann Emerg Med 1996;27:730.
 7. Weinbroum A, Rudick V, Sorkine P, et al. Use of flumazenil in the treatment of drug overdose: a double-blind and open clinical study in 110 patients. Crit Care Med 1996;24:199.
 8. Doyon S, Roberts JR. Reappraisal of the "coma cocktail." Dextrose, flumazenil, naloxone, and thiamine. Emerg Med Clin North Am 1994;12:301.
 9. Shorvon SJ. Tonic clonic status epilepticus. J Neurol Neurosurg Psychiatry 1993;56:125.
10. Berek K, Schinnerl A, Berek A, et al. Does the cause of coma influence treatment? Lancet 1994;344:195.
11. Ropper AH, Kennedy SK. Neurological and Neurosurgical Intensive Care (3rd ed). Rockville, MD: Aspen, 1988.
12. Tinuper P, Montagna P, Plazzi G, et al. Idiopathic recurring stupor. Neurology 1994;44:621.
13. Rothstein JD, Guidotti A, Tinuper P, et al. Endogenous benzodiazepine receptor ligands in idiopathic recurring stupor. Lancet 1992;340:1002.
14. Tinuper P, Montagna P, Cortelli P, et al. Idiopathic recurring stupor: a case with possible involvement of the gamma-aminobutyric acid (GABA)ergic system. Ann Neurol 1992;31:503.
15. Harris JO, Berger JR. Clinical Approach to Stupor and Coma. In WG Bradley, RB Daroff, GM Fenichel, CM Marsden (eds), Neurology in Clinical Practice. London: Butterworth, 1991;43–64.
16. Fisher CM. The neurological examination of the comatose patient. Acta Neurol Scand 1969;45 (suppl 4):1.
17. Teasdale G, Jennett B. Assessment of coma and impaired consciousness. A practical scale. Lancet 1974;2:81.
18. Moulton C, Pennycook AG. Relation between Glasgow coma score and cough reflex. Lancet 1994;343:1261.
19. Bhatty GB, Kapoor N. The Glasgow Coma Scale: a mathematical critique. Acta Neurochir 1993; 120:132.
20. Adnet F, Baud F. Relation between Glasgow Coma Scale and aspiration pneumonia. Lancet 1996; 348:123.
21. Rowley G, Fielding K. Reliability and accuracy of the Glasgow Coma Scale with experienced and inexperienced users. Lancet 1991;337:535.
22. Starmark J-E, Stålhammer D, Holmgren E, Rosander B. A comparison of the Glasgow Coma Scale and the Reaction Level Scale (RLS85). J Neurosurg 1988;69:699.
23. Benzer A, Mitterschiffthaler G, Marosi M, et al. Prediction of non-survival after trauma: Innsbruck Coma Scale. Lancet 1991;338:977.
24. Johnstone AJ, Lohlun JC, Miller JD, et al. A comparison of the Glasgow Coma Scale and the Swedish reaction level scale. Brain Injury 1993;7:501–506.
25. Larson MD, Muhiudeen I. Pupillometric analysis of the "absent light reflex." Arch Neurol 1995;52:369.
26. Gray AT, Krejci ST, Larson MD. Neuromuscular blocking drugs do not alter the pupillary light reflex of anesthetized humans. Arch Neurol 1997;54:579.
27. Buettner UW. Ocular Motor Dysfunction in Stupor and Coma. In U Buettner, TH Brandt (eds), Ocular Motor Disorders of the Brain Stem. Ballière's Clinical Neurology (1st ed, Vol 2). London: Ballière Tindall, 1992;289–300.
28. Leigh RJ, Zee DS. The Neurology of Eye Movement (2nd ed). Philadelphia: Davis, 1991.
29. Daroff RB, Troost BT. Supranuclear Disorders of Eye Movements In JS Glaser (ed), Neuro-Ophthalmology. Hagerstown, MD: Harper & Row, 1978;201–218.
30. Keane JR. Bilateral ocular motor signs after tentorial herniation in 25 patients. Arch Neurol 1986;43:806.
31. Keane JR. Pretectal pseudobobbing. Five patients with "V"-pattern convergence nystagmus. Arch Neurol 1985;42:592.
32. Drake ME, Erwin CW, Massey EW. Ocular bobbing in metabolic encephalopathy: clinical, pathologic and electrophysiological study. Neurology 1982;32:1029.

33. Keane JR. Acute vertical ocular myoclonus. Neurology 1986;36:86.
34. Ropper AH. Ocular dipping in anoxic coma. Arch Neurol 1981;38:297.
35. Rosenberg ML. Spontaneous vertical eye movements in coma. Ann Neurol 1986;20:635.
36. Brusa A, Firpo MP, Massa S, et al. Typical and reverse bobbing: a case with localising value. Eur Neurol 1984;23:151.
37. Buettner VW, Zee DS. Vestibular testing in comatose patients. Arch Neurol 1989;46:561.
38. Leigh RJ, Hanley DF, Munschauer FE, Lasker AG. Eye movements induced by head rotation in unresponsive patients. Ann Neurol 1984;15:465.
39. Keane JR, Baloh RW. Posttraumatic cranial neuropathies. Neurol Clin 1992;10:849.
40. Howard RS, Newsom Davis J. The Neural Control of Respiratory Function. In A Crockard, R Hayward, JT Hoff (eds), Neurosurgery—the Scientific Basis of Clinical Practice (2nd ed). Oxford, UK: Blackwell Scientific, 1992;318–336.
41. Greenberg DA, Simon RP. Flexor and extensor postures in sedative drug-induced coma. Neurology 1982;32:448.
42. Wijdicks EFM, Parisi JE, Sharbrough FW. Prognostic value of myoclonus status in comatose survivors of cardiac arrest. Ann Neurol 1994;35:239.
43. Wijdicks EFM, Young GB. Myoclonus status in comatose patients after cardiac arrest. Lancet 1994;343:1642.
44. Morris HR, Howard R, Brown P. Early myoclonic status and outcome following cardio-respiratory arrest. J Neurol Neurosurg Psychiatry 1998;64:267.
45. Wijdicks EFM. Temporomandibular joint compression in coma. Neurology 1996;46:1774.
46. Ropper AH. The opposite pupil in herniation. Neurology 1990;40:1707.
47. Ropper AH. Lateral displacement of the brain and level of consciousness in patients with acute hemispheral mass. N Engl J Med 1986;314:953.
48. Ropper AH. A preliminary MRI study of the geometry of brain displacement and level of consciousness with acute intracranial masses. Neurology 1989;39:622.
49. Chen R, Bolton CF, Young B. Prediction of outcome in patients with anoxic coma: a clinical and electrophysiologic study. Crit Care Med 1996;24:672.
50. Kane NM, Rowlands K, Nelson RJ, Moss T. Oculographic findings in traumatic unconsciousness: prognostic implications. J Neurol Neurosurg Psychiatry 1995;59:450.
51. Van de Kelft E, Segnarbieux F, Candon E, et al. Clinical recovery of consciousness after traumatic coma. Crit Care Med 1994;22:1108.
52. Combes P, Fauveage B, Colonna M, et al. Severe head injuries: an outcome prediction and survival analysis. Intensive Care Med 1996;22:1391.
53. Jennett B, Bond M. Assessment of outcome after severe brain injury. Lancet 1975;1:480.
54. Levy DE, Caronna JJ, Singer BH, et al. Predicting the outcome from hypoxic-ischemic coma. JAMA 1985;253:1420.
55. Mueller-Jensen A, Neuwzig H-P, Emskoetter T. Outcome prediction in comatose patients: significance of reflex eye movement analysis. J Neurol Neurosurg Psychiatry 1987;50:389.
56. Jennett B, Teasdale G. Aspects of coma after severe head injury. Lancet 1977;2:878.
57. Hamel MB, Goldman L, Teno J, et al. Identification of comatose patients at high risk for death or severe disability. SUPPORT investigators. Understand prognoses and preferences for outcomes and risks of treatments. JAMA 1995;273:1842.
58. Bates D, Caronna JJ, Cartilidge NEF, et al. A prospective study of nontraumatic coma: methods and results in 310 patients. Ann Neurol 1977;2:211.
59. Levy DE, Bates D, Caronna JJ, et al. Prognosis in non-traumatic coma. Ann Intern Med 1981;94:293.
60. Bates D. Defining prognosis in medical coma. J Neurol Neurosurg Psychiatry 1991;54:569.
61. Costa B, Candido J, Girbal A, et al. Coma of vascular etiology: evaluation and prognosis. Neurol Res 1992;14(suppl 2):100.
62. Krieger D, Adams HP, Schwarz S, et al. Prognostic and clinical relevance of pupillary responses, intracranial pressure monitoring, and brainstem auditory evoked potentials in comatose patients with acute supratentorial mass lesions. Crit Care Med 1993;21:1944.
63. Garcia-Larrea L, Artru F, Bertrand O, et al. The combined monitoring of brain stem auditory evoked potentials and intracranial pressure in coma. A study of 57 patients. J Neurol Neurosurg Psychiatry 1992;55:792.
64. American Neurological Association Committee on Ethical Affairs. Persistent vegetative state: report of the American Neurological Association Committee on Ethical Affairs. Ann Neurol 1993;33:386.
65. Dyer C. High court rules doctors can stop feeding Tony Bland. BMJ 1992;305:1312.
66. Angell M. After Quinlan: the dilemma of the persistent vegetative state. N Engl J Med 1994;330:1524.

67. Andrews K. Patients in the persistent vegetative state: problems in their long term management. BMJ 1993;306:1600.
68. BMA Medical Ethics Committee. Discussion paper on treatment of patients in persistent vegetative state. London: British Medical Association, 1992.
69. Institute of Medical Ethics working party on the ethics of prolonging life and assisting death. Withdrawal of life-support from patients in a persistent vegetative state. Lancet 1993;337:96.
70. BMA Medical Ethics Committee. BMA guidelines on treatment decisions for patients in a persistent vegetative state. London: BMA, 1994.
71. The Multi-Society Task Force on PVS. Medical aspects of the persistent vegetative state (1st part). N Engl J Med 1994;330:1499.
72. The Multi-Society Task Force on PVS. Medical aspects of the persistent vegetative state (2nd part). N Engl J Med 1994;330:1572.
73. Quality Standards Subcommittee of the American Academy of Neurology. Practice parameters: assessment and management of patients in the persistent vegetative state. Neurology 1995;45:1015.
74. Howard RS, Miller DH. The persistent vegetative state. BMJ 1995;310:341.
75. Jennett B, Plum F. Persistent vegetative state after brain damage: a syndrome in search of a name. Lancet 1972;1:734.
76. Andrews K. Recovery of patients after four months or more in the persistent vegetative state. BMJ 1993;306:1597.
77. Andrews K. Managing the persistent vegetative state. BMJ 1992;305:486.
78. Jennett B. Letting vegetative patients die. BMJ 1992;305:1305.
79. Patterson JR, Grabois M. Locked in syndrome: a review of 139 cases. Stroke 1986;17:758.
80. Munschauer FE, Mador MJ, Ahuja A, Jacobs L. Selective paralysis of voluntary but not limbically influenced automatic respiration. Arch Neurol 1991;48:1190.
81. Quality Standards Subcommittee of the American Academy of Neurology. Practice parameters for determining brain death in adults. Neurology 1995;45:1012.
82. Wijdicks EFM. Determining brain death in adults. Neurology 1995;45:1003.
83. Working Group of The Royal College of Physicians. Criteria for the diagnosis of brain stem death. J R Coll Physicians Lond 1995;29:381.
84. Marks SJ, Zisfein J. Apneic oxygenation to apnea tests for brain death. Arch Neurol 1990;47:1066.
85. Pallis C, Harley DH. ABCs of Brainstem Death (2nd ed). London: British Medical Journal, 1996.
86. Ropper AH. Unusual spontaneous movements in brain-dead patients. Neurology 1984;34:1089.
87. Lang CJG. Apnea testing by artificial CO_2 augmentation. Neurology 1995;45:966.

6

Convulsive and Nonconvulsive Status Epilepticus in the Intensive Care Unit and Emergency Department*

Kenneth G. Jordan

Despite the availability of potent medications and the popularization of strict treatment protocols [1,2], status epilepticus (SE) remains a life-threatening condition. Mortality and neurologic sequelae approach 30% in adults within 6 months of the first episode. These poor outcomes are the result of SE itself, side effects of treatment, and the progression of underlying neurologic disease [3]. At least 13 forms of SE have been described. Proper therapy for one may be inappropriate for another, and clinical differentiation may be difficult [4] (Table 6.1).

This review focuses on generalized convulsive status epilepticus (GCSE) and nonconvulsive status epilepticus (NCSE) in the neuroscience intensive care unit (NICU) and in the emergency department (ED). Studies in the early and mid-1990s, have suggested that the incidence, clinical features, and prognosis of SE in these venues differ in important ways from those of earlier community-based studies [5–8]. This chapter begins with a presentation of two cases, one from the NICU and the other from the ED. These provide clinical contexts for subsequent discussions of the definition, diagnosis, pathophysiology, and prognosis of SE. These discussions are followed by recommendations for management strategies, including pharmacologic agents.

CASE PRESENTATIONS

Status Epilepticus in the Neuroscience Intensive Care Unit

A 57-year-old woman underwent successful clipping of a right posterior communicating artery aneurysm within 24 hours of a subarachnoid hemorrhage. Postoperatively, it was difficult to rouse her and she had a mild left hemiparesis. A

---

*Parts of this chapter are based on a review by the author. Status epilepticus. A perspective from the neuroscience intensive care unit. Neurosurg Clin N Am 1994;5:671–686.

Table 6.1   Classification of status epilepticus

Primarily generalized convulsive status
   Tonic-clonic status
   Myoclonic status
   Clonic-tonic-clonic status
Secondarily generalized convulsive status
   Tonic-clonic status with partial onset
   Tonic status
Simple partial status
   Partial motor status, including epilepsy partialis continuans
   Partial sensory status
   Partial status with vegetative or autonomic symptoms
   Partial status with cognitive symptoms
   Partial status with affective symptoms
Complex partial status
Absence status or petit mal status
Pseudo–status epilepticus

Source: Modified from GO Walsh, AV Delgado-Escueta. Status epilepticus. Neurol Clin 1993;11:835.

computed tomographic (CT) scan of the brain revealed a small subacute infarction in the right temporal lobe. A transcranial Doppler study showed normal middle cerebral artery velocities. Blood determinations for routine studies were normal.

On the second postoperative day, the patient remained unresponsive. Rhythmic jerking of her left arm developed followed by a generalized convulsive seizure. Prophylactic phenytoin had been given preoperatively, and levels were measured at 6.5 mg/ml. The patient was treated with 4 mg intravenous lorazepam and 750 mg phenytoin. She sustained no further convulsions but remained unresponsive. On the third postoperative day, a repeat CT scan showed no new cerebral lesions. Lumbar puncture revealed no recurrent hemorrhage and no meningitis. On the morning of the fourth postoperative day, electroencephalography was performed and showed NCSE arising from the right temporal region with secondary generalization (Figure 6.1). Close neurologic examination revealed nystagmoid ocular jerks to the left and small-amplitude rhythmic movements of her left thumb. Additional intravenous diazepam, phenytoin, and high doses of phenobarbital failed to suppress the electroencephalographic seizure activity. Treatment for refractory SE was initiated.

Status Epilepticus in the Emergency Department

At 11:30 PM, a 76-year-old woman on theophylline for chronic obstructive pulmonary disease became bewildered, had incoherent speech, and experienced a generalized convulsive seizure. The patient had three more generalized convulsive seizures during paramedic transport and arrived comatose at the ED at 12:05 AM. The ED physician administered 4 mg lorazepam intravenously concurrent with intravenous fosphenytoin, 20 mg/kg at 150 mg/min. Upper airway obstruction developed, and the patient was intubated. Still comatose, she had a CT brain scan at 1:30 AM that was normal. By 3:00 AM, the patient was still unresponsive.

Figure 6.1 Continuous electro-encephalogram (EEG) of stupor-ous patient treated "successfully" for generalized convulsive seizures. The tracing demon-strates a nonconvulsive enceph-alographic seizure arising from the right temporal region and spreading to become generalized. In the intensive care unit, contin-uous EEG showed these seizures to be recurring, indicating non-convulsive status epilepticus. (Reprinted with permission from KG Jordan. Status epilepticus. A perspective from the neuroscience intensive care unit. Neurosurg Clin N Am 1994;5:671–686.)

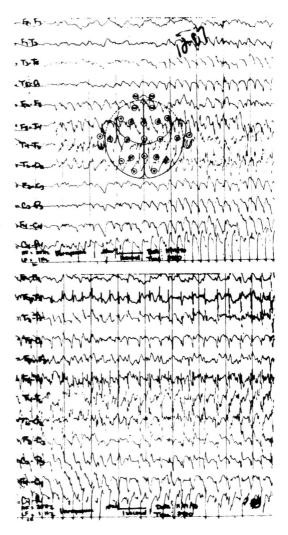

An electroencephalogram (EEG) was obtained at 3:45 AM and showed general-ized NCSE (Figure 6.2A). Intravenous midazolam, 8 mg, temporarily stopped the seizure activity, but active epileptiform discharges continued (Figure 6.2B). The patient was placed on a midazolam drip and admitted to the NICU.

DEFINITION AND DIAGNOSIS OF STATUS EPILEPTICUS AND NONCONVULSIVE STATUS EPILEPTICUS

The classic definition of *SE* is "a condition characterized by an epileptic seizure that is sufficiently prolonged or repeated so as to produce a fixed and lasting

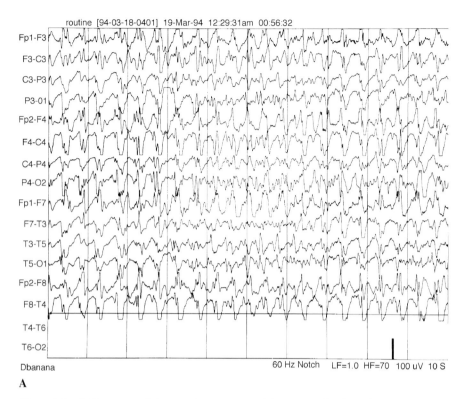

routine [94-03-18-0401] 19-Mar-94 12:29:31am 00:56:32

Dbanana   60 Hz Notch   LF=1.0 HF=70 100 uV 10 S

A

Figure 6.2   **A.** Electroencephalogram shows nonconvulsive status epilepticus after "therapeutic" doses of intravenous lorazepam and fosphenytoin. The record shows highly rhythmic, 2.5-Hz sharp and polysharp–slow wave discharges in a generalized distribution (channels 15 and 16 were nonfunctional). **B.** As the ictal discharges decrement, they assume a polyspike wave morphology. Intravenous midazolam was administered at the beginning of this record, with rapid cessation of seizure activity. Sharp wave and triphasic sharp wave activity persisted (channels 11, 12, 15, and 16 were nonfunctional).

epileptic condition" [9]. Previously, the duration of such a condition was considered to be 60 minutes, but more recent data have shortened the definition time to 30 minutes [10]. In convulsive seizures, visual observation usually suffices to establish the diagnosis (this is not always the case; see Differential Diagnosis of Status Epilepticus). In contrast, nonconvulsive seizures (NCS) produce altered mentation or behavior with only subtle or absent motor components. For this reason, NCS must be defined by EEG rather than clinical criteria. A 1996 study proposed diagnostic criteria based on continuous EEG (CEEG) monitoring of ICU patients with NCS [6]. These criteria combine previously published morphologic and frequency EEG characteristics, called *primary criteria*, with selective but widely accepted clinical observations, called *secondary criteria* [6,11,12] (Table 6.2). To qualify as NCSE, the ictal EEG episodes must be continuous or recurrent for longer than 30 minutes without improvement in the patient's clinical state and with no return to a pre-

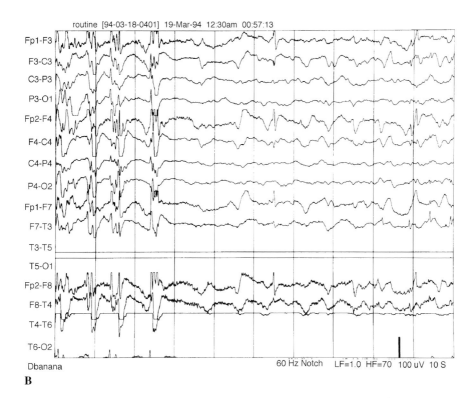

routine [94-03-18-0401] 19-Mar-94 12:30am 00:57:13

Dbanana   60 Hz Notch   LF=1.0 HF=70   100 uV   10 S

B

ictal EEG pattern between seizures. Although no universally accepted definition for NCSE exists, this description is compatible with SE criteria applied to
convulsive seizures [2,13] and is in agreement with published criteria for complex partial SE [14,15].

NCSE can develop as the result of incomplete treatment of GCSE, as the natural consequence of prolonged GCSE, or from neuromuscular blocking agents
that eliminate convulsions but not cerebral seizures. It can also be the de novo
presentation of SE.

PATHOPHYSIOLOGY OF GENERALIZED
CONVULSIVE STATUS EPILEPTICUS AND
NONCONVULSIVE STATUS EPILEPTICUS

Some studies have shown that experimental GCSE follows a predictable
sequence of five stages that are definable by distinct EEG patterns [16,17]. A
similar evolution of EEG stages has been described in humans [18]. The initial pattern is that of isolated seizures followed by merging seizures, leading to
continuous ictal activity. A flattening of interictal background is then seen, culminating in generalized periodic epileptiform discharges (Figure 6.3, Table 6.3).

Table 6.2   Electroencephalographic criteria for epileptic seizures

Guideline: To qualify, at least one of primary criteria 1–3 and one or more of secondary criteria 1–4, with discharges >10 secs
Primary criteria
1. Repetitive generalized or focal spikes, sharp waves, spike-and-wave, or sharp-and-slow wave complexes at more than three per second
2. Repetitive generalized or focal spikes, sharp waves, spike-and-wave, or sharp-and-slow wave complexes at less than three per second and secondary criterion 4
3. Sequential rhythmic waves and secondary criteria 1, 2, and 3 with or without 4
Secondary criteria
1. Incrementing onset: increase in voltage and/or increase or slowing of frequency
2. Decrementing offset: decrease in voltage or frequency
3. Postdischarge slowing or voltage attenuation
4. Significant improvement in clinical state and baseline electroencephalogram, or both, after antiepileptic drug

Source: Reprinted with permission from GB Young, KG Jordan, GS Doig. An assessment of nonconvulsive seizures in the intensive care unit using continuous EEG monitoring: an investigation of variables associated with mortality. Neurology 1996;47:84.

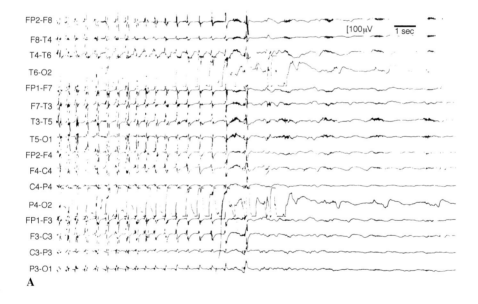

A

Figure 6.3   Sequential electroencephalographic pattern in generalized convulsive status epilepticus: (**A**) discrete seizures, (**B**) continuous ictal activity, and (**C**) periodic epileptiform discharges on a flat background. (Reprinted with permission from DM Treiman, NY Walton, B Kendrick. A progressive sequence of electroencephalographic changes during generalized convulsive status epilepticus. Epilepsy Res 1990;5:51–57.)

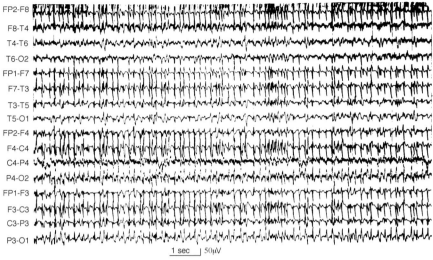

B

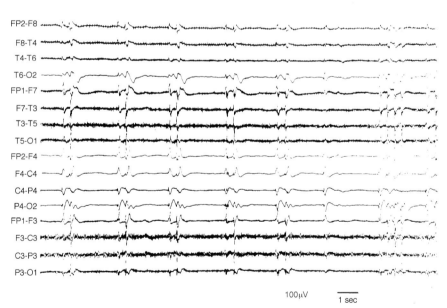

C

Table 6.3   Electroencephalographic and clinical correlation in generalized convulsive status epilepticus

Stage	Electroencephalographic features	Typical clinical manifestations*
1	Discrete seizures with interictal slowing	Tonic-clonic convulsions; hypertension and hyperglycemia common
2	Waxing and waning of ictal discharges	Low- or medium-amplitude clonic activity with rare convulsions
3	Continuous ictal discharges	Slight, but frequent, clonic activity; can be confined to the eyes, face, or hands
4	Continuous ictal discharges punctuated by flat periods	Rare episodes of slight clonic activity; hypotension and hypoglycemia can occur
5	Periodic epileptiform discharges on a flat background	Coma without other manifestations of seizure activity (electromechanical dissociation)

*The clinical manifestations can vary depending on the underlying anatomic abnormality and the patient's medications and underlying systemic disease.

Source: Reprinted with permission from CWJ Chang, TP Bleck. Status Epilepticus. In KG Jordan (ed), Neurological Critical Care. Neurologic Clinics. Philadelphia: Saunders, 1995;535.

Lothman [19] has distilled much of the seminal work by major researchers and summarized the systemic and cerebral pathophysiology that correspond to these stages of SE (Figure 6.4). Within the first 30 minutes, the duration of discrete EEG seizures lengthens with recurring generalized clonic convulsions. Associated hypertension, hyperglycemia, and hyperlactatemia producing a severe metabolic acidosis exists. Cerebral metabolic oxygen requirements and glucose utilization increase dramatically. The delivery of these substrates is provided by mobilized glycogen stores and a marked increase in cerebral blood flow. Brain lactate concentration also rises, as a result of a combination of elevated systemic lactate and cerebral anaerobic metabolism.

After 30 minutes of GCSE, the EEG discharges merge, leading to continuous ictal activity. Motor convulsions become less prominent and are replaced by subtle, low-amplitude rapid movements such as face and eyelid twitches or rhythmic ocular movements. Depending on the degree of "subtlety" of these movements, this clinical stage has been considered "subtle" GCSE [18], or part of the spectrum of NCSE [7,20].

Motor manifestations may subsequently become absent. The patient appears obtunded with no clinical signs to suggest seizure activity, even though ictal activity persists on the EEG (NCSE). Systemically, normotension and normoglycemia are usual although hypotension and hypoglycemia can occur. Blood lactate and pH normalize. At this stage, there is a tendency toward hyperthermia and hypoxemia. Cerebral blood flow drops below metabolic demand, brain glucose concentrations fall, and the production of high-energy phosphates declines [21].

Studies of experimental SE by Kreisman and associates [22] support a 30- to 60-minute transition period during which metabolic demand outstrips the supply of substrate. Microelectrodes monitored local cerebral Po_2 and measured the reduction-oxidation ratio of targeted cytochrome oxidases. In early seizures, increases in cortical Po_2 and oxidation of cytochrome A and A_3 were found. After 30–40 minutes of SE in several different animal species, transition from sufficient

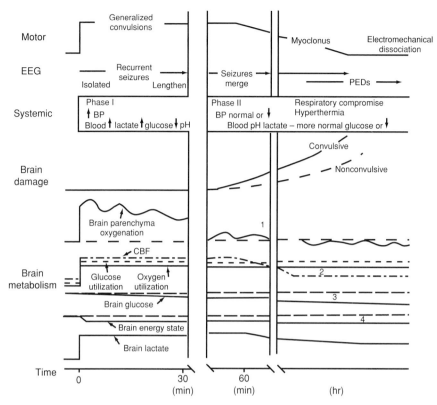

Figure 6.4 Summary of physiologic and electroencephalographic changes in status epilepticus (SE). Events are plotted against time. The critical transition period occurs at approximately 30 minutes after the onset of SE. Note that nonconvulsive SE does cause brain damage albeit at a slower rate than convulsive SE. Specific injurious effects on brain metabolism include (1) drop in brain parenchyma oxygenation at 30 minutes, (2) reduction of cerebral blood flow (CBF) below glucose and oxygen utilization, (3) depletion of brain glucose, and (4) decline in the energy state of the brain. (EEG = electroencephalogram; BP = blood pressure; PEDs = periodic epileptiform discharges.) (Reproduced with permission from EW Lothman. The biochemical basis and pathophysiology of status epilepticus. Neurology 1990;40[suppl 2]:13–23. Copyright © by Advanstar Communications, Inc., which retains all rights to this figure.)

to insufficient cerebral oxygenation was found, as determined by low Po_2 and reductive shift of cytochrome A and A_3. These findings held true under various anesthetic and anticonvulsant regimens [23]. The end point of these cellular changes was neuronal necrosis.

Although some controversy exists [24], many reports now support the view that in SE epileptic brain damage can occur without motor convulsions [24–26]. The purported mechanisms of neuronal death include excitotoxin-induced calcium-mediated cellular necrosis, cytotoxic free-radical production by uninhibited metabolic activity, osmotic lysis of neurons from uncontrolled depolarization, and gene induction leading to apoptotic cell death [19,27]. Emphasizing the danger

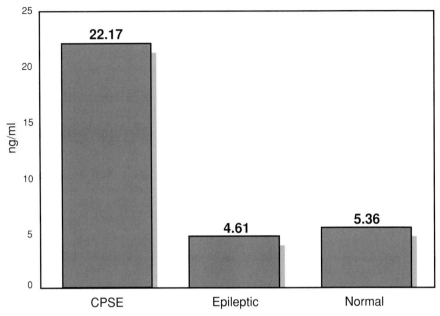

Figure 6.5 Comparison of serum neuron-specific enolase (s-NSE) in patients with the complex partial status epilepticus (CPSE) form of nonconvulsive status epilepticus compared to those of normal and nonconvulsing epileptic control subjects. s-NSE is a marker of neuronal damage. The significantly elevated s-NSE levels in the CPSE patients suggest brain damage from unremitting epileptic brain activity. (Data from CM DeGiorgio, PS Gott, AL Rabinowicz, et al. Neuron-specific enolase, a marker of acute neuronal damage, is elevated in complex partial status epilepticus. Epilepsia 1996;37:606–609.)

of unremitting NCSE, some biochemical evidence has demonstrated that it increases serum neuron-specific enolase (s-NSE), a marker of neuronal damage. NSE is an intracellular glycolytic enzyme with specific intraneural and intraglial isoenzymes [28]. In patients with NCSE, s-NSE levels were four times higher than those of normal and epileptic control subjects (Figure 6.5). Levels greater than 22 ng/ml were significantly associated with poor outcomes [29,30]. Histopathologic studies show that the areas of the brain most vulnerable to epileptic damage are the middle layers of the cortex, the hippocampus, the thalamus, and the cerebellum.

STATUS EPILEPTICUS IN ACUTE BRAIN INSULTS

In the NICU, patients may experience metabolic, structural, or both kinds of acute brain insults (ABIs). These can occur as the cause of patients' admission, complication of their illness, or an iatrogenic problem. Hyponatremia is common as a cause of seizures in the NICU. Usually, for seizures to occur, the serum sodium

Table 6.4 Etiology of nonconvulsive status epilepticus in 49 neuroscience
intensive care unit patients

Remote symptomatic	Number of patients (n = 25)	Acute symptomatic	Number of patients (n = 24)
Previous cerebral infarction	7	Multiorgan failure	5
Previous idiopathic seizure disorder	6	Anoxic-ischemic encepha-lopathy	5
Previous meningioma	4	Subarachnoid hemorrhage from berry aneurysm	5
Unruptured arteriovenous malformation	3	Intracerebral hemorrhage	3
Remote trauma	3	Encephalitis	2
Uncertain	2	Theophylline toxicity	1
Uncertain	2	Cerebral metastases	1
		Cerebrospinal fluid leak	1
		Meningitis	1

Source: Reprinted with permission from GB Young, KG Jordan, GS Doig. An assessment of nonconvulsive seizures in the intensive care unit using continuous EEG monitoring: an investigation of variables associated with mortality. Neurology 1996;47:86

level must drop relatively acutely below 120–125 mEq/liter. The seizures are usually caused by cerebral intracellular fluid shifts from extracellular hypo-osmolality. Hypocalcemia, hypomagnesemia, hyperglycemia, and hypoglycemia can also cause seizures in the ICU. Although these imbalances are potentially correctable if treated promptly, they have the potential of causing irreversible cerebral injury.

Some of the medications commonly prescribed in the ICU can decrease seizure threshold, particularly in patients with renal insufficiency. Potentially epileptogenic agents include lidocaine, imipenem, ciprofloxacin, penicillin derivatives, amitriptyline, phenothiazines, theophylline, and cyclosporine. Seizures can also occur as a result of withdrawal from prescribed medications, including morphine, propoxyphene, midazolam, and meperidine. Risks of seizures caused by alcohol and barbiturate withdrawal and cocaine and amphetamine use are well recognized [31].

Although withdrawal of antiepileptic medication is widely believed to be the most common precipitating factor for SE, more than half of the reported cases result from cerebral infarction, head trauma (HT), meningitis, intracranial hemorrhage, acute cerebral hypoxia, hypoglycemia, drug toxicity, and alcohol or illicit substance withdrawal [2,32,33]. Even in patients with epilepsy of "idiopathic" type or caused by remote brain injury, a new ABI is the precipitating event in approximately 25% of those who present with SE [34,35]. Among patients with no history of epilepsy, 59% with SE had ABIs, with a mortality of 54% [35].

Early convulsive seizures occur in 10–27% of patients with various forms of ABI [36]. In NICU patients diagnosed with NCSE by ICU-CEEG monitoring, half had an underlying ABI [8] (Table 6.4). In a separate ICU-CEEG study [5], among 124 monitored patients, seizures occurred in 35%. The large majority of the seizures were NCS. Of 43 patients, 75% sustained NCSE. NCS occurred in all diagnostic categories of ABI, including in 22% of patients with spontaneous intracranial hemorrhage (7 of 32 patients), 54% with postcraniotomy brain tumor (6 of 11 patients), 28% with HT (two of seven patients), 26% with cerebral infarction (11 of 43 patients), and 56% with GCSE who were admitted to the NICU after their convulsions were "controlled" (9 of 16 patients) [5].

The phenomenon of persisting NCSE in GCSE patients has been reported by Fagen and Lee [37]. Some studies support the view that this is not uncommon. DeLorenzo and associates [38] used CEEG prospectively to monitor GCSE patients. They found that 12% of 170 patients developed NCSE after their convulsions stopped. The NCSE patients were comatose and showed no clinical signs of convulsive activity. Clinical detection of NCSE could only be determined by CEEG monitoring. In a Veterans Administration cooperative study [39], 20% of patients who presented with overt GCSE continued to have ictal discharges on their EEGs after their convulsions had ceased. In most instances, treatment had converted GCSE into focal ictal discharges without clinical signs. No further treatment would have been given had the EEG not revealed this treatment failure. As full loading doses of anticonvulsants were routinely administered in this study, this percentage probably underestimates the true incidence of GCSE patients persisting in NCSE after receiving treatment or in whom treatment was assumed to be "successful."

Other investigators have pointed out the frequent occurrence of NCS and NCSE in patients with cerebral injuries. Grand'Maison and associates [40] found a 55% incidence in patients with ABIs or subacute lesions and a 67% incidence in patients with chronic lesions. Young and colleagues [6] found that nearly half of their cases of NCS occurred in the context of an ABI. Using ICU-CEEG, Vespa and coworkers [41] prospectively studied 20 patients with moderate to severe HT and identified seizures in five patients (25%), four of whom had NCS. In a follow-up report [42], these authors identified seizures in 9 of 56 HT patients (16%), in seven of whom (78%) NCS developed. These data indicate that among patients with ABI, seizures occur more commonly than was previously reported and may go unrecognized because they commonly take the form of NCS and NCSE.

DURATION, DELAY IN DIAGNOSIS, AND MORTALITY OF STATUS EPILEPTICUS

The longer SE continues, the more resistant it becomes to treatment and the more neuronal damage it causes [43]. In animal models, the risk of permanent brain damage is directly related to the duration of SE [44]. Towne and associates [45] found that patients with SE lasting more than 1 hour had a higher mortality than those with SE of shorter duration. Without CEEG, however, these authors could not determine the actual duration of the seizures or the incidence of NCSE. Lowenstein and Alldredge [33] reviewed a decade of clinical experience with GCSE and found a time-dependent response to intervention. Among 154 patients, treatment begun within 30 minutes of onset was associated with an 80% response to first-line anticonvulsants. Of patients in SE for 2 or more hours before treatment, only 40% responded to first-line medications. DeGiorgio and colleagues [28] found that s-NSE levels increased with the duration of SE, suggesting that the degree of neuronal injury was time dependent (Figure 6.6).

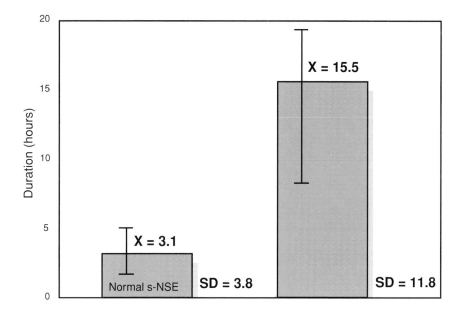

Figure 6.6 As the duration of status epilepticus (SE) increases, serum neuron-specific enolase (s-NSE) levels increase. After 15 hours of SE, mean s-NSE levels were fivefold higher than normal values seen in patients with SE of 3 hours' or less duration. (SD = standard deviation.) (Reprinted with permission from CM DeGiorgio, JD Correale, PS Gott, et al. Serum neuron-specific enolase in human status epilepticus. Neurology 1995;45:1136.)

Studies have demonstrated that the diagnosis of NCSE tends to be delayed or even protracted. In the Veterans Administration cooperative study cited earlier [39], patients in NCSE were in status longer than were patients in overt GCSE. One month after presentation, the NCSE patients had a mortality that was twice as high as the GCSE group (60% vs. 30%). In addition, approximately two-thirds of GCSE patients were controlled with first-line treatment, whereas this treatment was successful in only one-third of NCSE patients. Young and associates [6] found that in NCSE, mortality is more strongly linked to duration and delay in diagnosis than to etiology (Table 6.5). Some of the patients in their series were obtunded for hours before an EEG was performed, leading to the diagnosis of NCSE.

Prolonged delays to diagnosis of NCSE have been found in the ED. One study indicated that only 25% of patients with NCSE were controlled within 3 hours of initiation of treatment and only 50% were controlled by 5 hours. In four patients, it took more than 2 days to halt NCSE [8]. Kaplan [7] also noted significant delays in the ED diagnosis and treatment of NCSE. Both these studies found that family members often misinterpreted the signs and symptoms of NCSE and delayed calling for medical assistance. The major delaying factor, however, was misdiagnosis of NCSE by ED medical personnel. Among 30 cases, Jordan and associates [8] found that 60% were misdiagnosed as postictal, 13.5%

Table 6.5   Statistical significance of variables associated with mortality in nonconvulsive status epilepticus (NCSE)*

Analysis	Significance
Univariate	
Etiology	
Remote symptomatic: 4 of 25 patients (16%) vs. acute symptomatic: 11 of 24 patients (46%)	$p = .009$, OR = 6.0
Nonconvulsive seizures only vs. NCSE	$p = .002$, OR = 10.0
Seizure duration	
<10 hrs: 3 of 30 patients (10%) died vs. 10–20 hrs: two of six patients (33%) died vs. >20 hrs: 11 of 13 patients (85%) died	$p = .0006$, OR = 1.093/hr
Delay to diagnosis	
<0.5 hr: 5 of 14 patients (36%) died vs. >1 hr but <24 hrs: 7 of 18 patients (39%) died vs. ≥24 hrs: six of eight patients (75%) died	$p = .00001$
Multivariate logistic regression	
Only:	
Seizure duration	$p = .0057$, OR = 1.131
Delay to diagnosis	$p = .0351$, OR = 1.039/hr

OR = odds ratio.

*With univariate analysis, etiology, nonconvulsant seizures only versus NCSE, seizure duration, and delay to diagnosis each showed statistically significant impact on mortality. With multivariate logistic regression analysis, however, only seizure duration and delay to diagnosis were associated with increased mortality.

Source: Based on data from GB Young, KG Jordan, GS Doig. An assessment of nonconvulsive seizures in the intensive care unit using continuous EEG monitoring: an investigation of variables associated with mortality. Neurology 1996;47:83–89.

as transient ischemic attacks or stroke, and 13.5% as metabolic encephalopathy. Kaplan [7] found a similar spectrum of misdiagnosis, but in addition, 39% of his patients were believed to have psychiatric disorders that caused their altered behaviors.

POSSIBLE SYNERGISTIC BRAIN DAMAGE FROM COMBINED STATUS EPILEPTICUS AND ACUTE BRAIN INSULTS

Accumulating evidence exists that patients with combined SE and ABIs are at risk for compounded brain damage. Arboix and associates [46] found that seizures during a first-ever stroke were an independent prognostic factor for in-hospital mortality. Waterhouse [47] found that the mortality of acute stroke plus SE was three times higher than in stroke alone. In DeGiorgio's report [28] the highest s-NSE levels were found in patients with combined SE and ABIs. In their study of acute HT, Vespa and colleagues [42] found good outcomes in only one of nine (11%) head trauma patients who had concurrent seizures versus 21 of the 45 (47%) who did not have seizures. Jordan and coworkers [8] found that the combination of prolonged NCSE and ABIs exponentially raised the mortality, with an odds ratio of 23 to 8 of acute over remote brain injury. Young and asso-

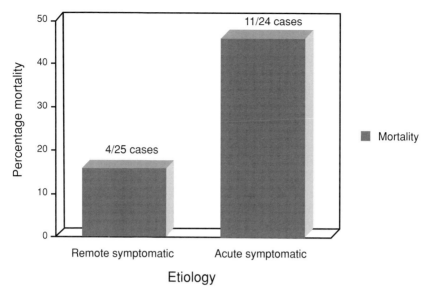

Figure 6.7 The compounded effect on mortality of nonconvulsive status epilepticus and acute brain injury (ABI). Compared to patients with remote symptomatic etiologies, those with acute symptomatic etiologies (ABI) showed a threefold increase in mortality. As described in the text and shown in Table 6.5, the magnitude of this difference was not owing to etiology alone. ($p = .009$, odds ratio = 6.0.) (Based on data from GB Young, KG Jordan, GS Doig. An assessment of nonconvulsive seizures in the intensive care unit using continuous EEG monitoring: an investigation of variables associated with mortality. Neurology 1996;47:83.)

ciates [6] found that the difference in death rates between NCSE patients with remote (16%) versus acute (45%) brain injuries was significant ($p = .0089$), with an odds ratio of 6.0 of acute over remote (Figure 6.7). In Jordan and colleagues' ED study [8], severe disability or death was seen in 75% of NCSE patients with, versus 28% without, coexisting ABI (Table 6.6).

These findings are consistent with the accepted concept of secondary neurologic insult described by Miller and Becker [48]. Acutely injured neurons are more likely than intact neurons to suffer irreversible injury or cell death when exposed to comparable ischemic, metabolic, or hypoxic insults [49]. This is relevant to defining the width of the therapeutic "time window" within which SE patients should be treated to prevent permanent neuronal injury. Patients with combined SE and ABIs may have a significantly narrower time window than SE patients without ABIs. Accelerated intervention may be necessary to preserve function and improve outcome in these patients.

DIFFERENTIAL DIAGNOSIS OF STATUS EPILEPTICUS

Not every instance of motor convulsive activity is caused by GCSE. Patients in the ICU exhibit a wide variety of nonepileptic involuntary and semipurposeful

Table 6.6   Outcome of nonconvulsive status epilepticus based on etiology and delay to diagnosis

Etiology (no.)	Percent outcome and mean delay (D)			
	% Good	D (min)	% Poor	D (min)
Acute symptomatic* (12)	25	73	75	140
Remote symptomatic (18)	72	160	28	222

*Acute symptomatic (AS) is equivalent to the term *acute brain insult* used in the text. Note that, among these patients, poor outcomes (death and invalidism) were three times more common than among the remote symptomatic (RS) patients, even though delay to diagnosis of AS patients was 37% shorter than that of RS patients. This supports a synergistic increase in mortality when AS is combined with nonconvulsive status epilepticus.
Source: Data based on KG Jordan, GB Young, GS Doig. Delays in emergency department (ED) diagnosis and treatment of nonconvulsive status epilepticus (NCSE). Neurology 1998;50(suppl 1):A243.

movements that can be difficult to distinguish from epileptic motor activity. These movements include tremor or tremulousness, periodic struggling movements, tetanic spasms, rigors owing to sepsis, rigidity owing to neuroleptic malignant syndrome, myoclonic jerks, ischemic tremors, medication-induced involuntary movements, hemiballism, tonic head or eye deviations, and decerebrate or decorticate posturing. Occasionally, these nonictal movements are assumed to be SE, leading to mistaken initiation of therapy. Clinical observation may not resolve the issue of whether these movements are ictal, and an EEG can be essential for accurate diagnosis and management.

Psychogenic SE is another relatively common cause of misdiagnosis. In one epilepsy center, 20% of patients who presented to the ED with intractable generalized convulsive seizures proved to have psychogenic seizures and several had psychogenic GCSE. Many of these patients were inappropriately treated with intravenous anticonvulsant drugs and maintained on unnecessary polypharmacy regimens. Some were even intubated and placed in pentobarbital coma [50,51]. Clues to psychogenic GCSE include out-of-phase limb movements, verbal or motor responsiveness during bilateral jerking, absence of autonomic signs, and prompt alertness on cessation of shaking. Pelvic thrusting may be seen with some psychogenic seizures. Studies have shown, however, that clinical features are not reliable in distinguishing GCSE from psychogenic GCSE [50]. For example, out-of-phase limb movements and pelvic thrusting can be features of frontal lobe seizures. Psychogenic GCSE can simulate GCSE closely enough that only concurrent EEG can distinguish between them.

NCSE poses the converse dilemma: Not all patients with SE convulse. In most series, the clinical features are subtle, ambiguous, and nonspecific [2,7,20,52]. Common findings include coma or obtundation, psychomotor retardation, drowsiness, inattentiveness, aphasia, limb posturing, abnormal eye movements, cortical blindness, automatisms, delusions, paranoia, and agitation. In the unresponsive patient, suspicion of NCSE should be raised if one or more of the following is observed: ocular deviation or nystagmoid eye movements, periodic facial or eyelid twitching, or unexplained fluctuations in responsiveness.

Attempts to classify NCSE have included absence SE, complex partial SE, partial somatosensory SE, prolonged ictal aphasia, elementary visual SE, and autonomic SE. As yet, however, there is no generally accepted classification of NCSE subtypes [6,7,52].

SEQUENCE OF DIAGNOSTIC TESTS FOR STATUS EPILEPTICUS AND NONCONVULSIVE STATUS EPILEPTICUS

Most published SE treatment protocols are algorithms based on a 30- to 60-minute time window from seizure onset. As has been shown, most patients come to medical attention beyond this time window. Those with concurrent ABI may be at particular risk for experiencing early and irreversible brain damage. In addition, SE presenting as NCSE is not uncommon and frequently leads to delays in diagnosis that adversely affect outcome. Recurring or persisting automatisms that would be identified in a clinic or office are often overlooked or misinterpreted in the ICU or ED context. Many ED physicians, intensivists, and nursing personnel do not fully appreciate the extent to which concurrent neurologic deficits can mask or distort typical epileptic movements and make them subtle and ambiguous. In the ICU, most patients receive sedation, neuroleptic medication, neuromuscular blocking agents, or prophylactic anticonvulsants, one or more of which can modify the expected clinical signs of SE.

For these reasons, the sequence of the diagnostic studies that are usually ordered in patients with suspected SE should be reassessed. The case presentations illustrate that individuals with unexplained mental status changes are usually sent initially for a CT scan of the brain, subsequently have various blood studies done, and, thereafter, may have a lumbar puncture performed to exclude meningitis or hemorrhage. Time elapses as results are obtained. In the case studies, these delays took more than 3 days in the ICU and more than 3½ hours in the ED. During this time, ongoing NCSE exacted a potentially irreversible toll on the patients' cerebral function. An emergency EEG, on the other hand, can quickly identify patients with de novo NCSE, those in NCSE after treatment for GCSE, those who are postictal, those in metabolic-based coma, and even those who have focal brain injury. For this level of care to be achieved, 24-hour EEG availability and its timely use are necessary, as are rapid and accurate interpretation. In the past, the cost and logistics of this level of service were limiting factors. Modern technology allows digital EEG printouts to be faxed to the neurologist for interpretation, however, and even allows real-time or near real-time EEGs to be sent via modem to the neurologist. An emergency EEG need not be a full 30-minute study, because the specific clinical question can usually be answered with only 10–15 minutes of recording. This is less time than it usually takes the CT technician or CT transport team to ready the patient for a CT scan. If a structural lesion is suspected or revealed by the EEG, a CT scan can be obtained quickly. Interposing an emergency EEG should have no adverse impact on the patient's care. The additional information can be crucial at times, such as in the diagnosis of NCSE. In addition, long before cerebral infarction appears on the CT scan, the EEG can show slowing or amplitude attenuation within minutes of the onset of the infarction. Epileptogenic activity in an area of cerebral hemorrhage can lead to the early and appropriate use of anticonvulsant medication preventing secondary neuronal damage. Relevant blood studies can easily be obtained before or concurrently with the EEG. It is my impression that, in NICU and ED patients, greater availability and more diligent use of emergency EEG can eliminate ambiguity, accurately target therapy, and prevent potentially harmful delays in patients with SE and NCSE [53].

CLINICAL MANAGEMENT OF STATUS EPILEPTICUS

In 1993, the Epilepsy Foundation of America's Working Group on Status Epilepticus (EFAWG) published a consensus statement on the treatment of GCSE [2]. More than 90 expert reviewers, including myself, contributed to this statement. The following guidelines are based on this document, with some referenced additions and modifications.

Immediate Systemic Requirements

Respiratory System

Maintaining ventilation and oxygenation is a fundamental necessity, but its adequacy may be overlooked or erroneously assumed in the emergent treatment of GCSE. Sustained hypoxemia can potentiate neuronal damage from SE and must be avoided. Airway management is best accomplished by rapid control of seizures. The patient's head and mandible should be placed in the cardiopulmonary resuscitation (sniff) position. The airway should be suctioned to prevent obstruction by secretions or vomitus. Oxygen, 100%, should be administered by nasal cannula or bag–valve mask ventilation. If ventilation is ineffective, prompt endotracheal intubation should be considered. Occasionally, laryngeal spasm as a concomitant of GCSE can produce sufficiently severe upper airway obstruction as to be life-threatening. Additionally, intubating a patient with convulsive motor activity or tonic masseter contraction may be impossible. In this situation, convulsions can be stopped temporarily with a high dose of short-acting barbiturates, and prompt muscle relaxation can be achieved with short-acting neuromuscular blocking agents such as succinylcholine. After intubation, a nasogastric tube should be placed to relieve gastric distention. This improves diaphragmatic excursion and reduces the risk of aspiration.

Terminating convulsive movements with neuromuscular blocking agents does nothing to control cerebral seizure activity. Administering an effective and rapidly acting antiepileptic drug remains a top priority.

Cardiovascular System

During SE, cerebral autoregulation is severely impaired, making cerebral perfusion directly dependent on systemic mean arterial pressure. Although hypertension is commonly seen during the early stages of GCSE, hypotension is frequently late in its course. Additionally, some patients may have hypotension early as a result of profuse vagotonic discharges or as a side effect of intravenous antiepileptic medications. Hypotension should be scrupulously avoided because it endangers the balance of cerebral oxygen delivery and oxygen consumption. Adequate and reliable venous access must be achieved early. Administration of crystalloid or colloid solutions for volume expansion may be sufficient to maintain mean arterial pressure, but vasopressors should be administered without delay, if necessary.

SE can cause bradyarrhythmias or tachyarrhythmias, which may be life-threatening [54]. During SE, myocardial oxygen requirements may increase, running the risk of coronary ischemia. Therefore, electrocardiographic monitoring is a mandatory part of emergency SE management.

Thermoregulation

Increased body temperature, sometimes to a striking degree, can occur in patients with SE as a result of increased motor activity, autonomic dysfunction, or both. Sustained hyperpyrexia increases the risk of excitotoxic neuronal necrosis [19]. Therefore, core temperature must be closely monitored and appropriate cooling measures applied to keep it at normal or slightly hypothermic levels.

Metabolic Balance and Screening for Drug Toxicity

When SE is caused by hyponatremia, hypocalcemia, or other dysmetabolic states, it may be refractory to anticonvulsant treatment but usually responds to correction of the metabolic abnormality. Therefore, electrolyte levels must be tested and reported as soon as possible. In their study of 217 patients with SE, Barry and Hauser [34] found metabolic derangements to be the most common acute causes. These included uremia, hyperglycemia, and hyponatremia as the leading abnormalities. In a series of NCSE in the NICU [5], hyponatremia and theophylline toxicity were common causes. In patients in whom theophylline is used, an emergency level should be obtained because, even at therapeutic levels, it can trigger SE. This is particularly true in patients with chronic cerebral lesions [55]. Theophylline toxicity may require hemofiltration for control of seizures and cardiac arrhythmias. Cocaine- and alcohol-related SE are cited as common causes, particularly in series from public hospitals [33]. Cocaine toxic SE can be associated with dangerous levels of hypertension and hyperpyrexia.

Specific Antiepileptic Therapy

The longer SE continues, the more difficult it is to control. A large amount of experimental data indicate that the risk of permanent brain damage is directly related to the duration of SE [19]. Clinical corroboration of this evidence is now available [6,33]. Therefore, the agents selected to stop SE must act promptly, safely, and predictably.

No ideal drug for treating GCSE exists, and numerous treatment algorithms have been published [56,57]. Several studies have compared various first-line agents in the treatment of GCSE [1,58,59]. The available data support the use of lorazepam, a diazepam-phenytoin combination, or phenobarbital as the preferred medication in GCSE. Lorazepam has a long duration of therapeutic action, ranging from 12 to 24 hours. It is administered in a 0.1-mg/kg dosage range up to a maximum of 8–10 mg. In 88% of patients with GCSE, lorazepam stops convulsions within 3–10 minutes [57]. Phenytoin does not necessarily have to be infused shortly thereafter; however, this is frequently done because phenytoin is commonly selected for long-term therapy. Lorazepam has been found to be as effective as a diazepam-phenytoin combination. Diazepam has an effective duration of only 25–50 minutes. Because of its high lipid solubility, diazepam quickly redistributes to other fatty tissues, causing a fall in brain and serum concentrations. As a result, SE frequently recurs if diazepam is relied on as monotherapy. For this reason, intravenous phenytoin is administered concurrently through a separate intravenous route to prevent recurrent seizures. Diazepam is given in a 0.15- to 0.25-mg/kg dosage range, usually to a maximum of 20 mg. The EFAWG protocol suggests a rate of administration of 5 mg per minute, but I and others [57] suggest a slower rate of infusion, no faster than 2 mg per minute. Relying on phenytoin as the sole first-line agent is unwise because, when administered at the recommended maximum rate of 50 mg per minute to decrease the risk of hypotension and arrhythmias, a loading dose takes at least 20 minutes to infuse. It may take another 30 minutes for sufficient brain levels to be obtained to stop convulsions.

A controlled study comparing phenobarbital with diazepam-phenytoin concluded that phenobarbital is rapid, effective, and safe and has some practical advantages over the combination approach [58]. Intravenous phenobarbital is given at a rate of 100 mg per minute for a total dose of 20 mg/kg. Using aliquots of 5–10 mg/kg at 10- to 15-minute intervals may avoid the need to administer the entire 1–2 g phenobarbital. After infusing 750 mg phenobarbital, we usually intubate the patient because of the high likelihood of ventilatory suppression.

A suggested treatment timetable for GCSE published by the EFAWG is presented in Table 6.7. The availability of fosphenytoin provides an attractive alternative for intravenous phenytoin. I recommend its use, particularly in patients who have difficult venous access or unstable cardiac arrhythmias, or when rapid administration is required. Unlike phenytoin, fosphenytoin can be given intramuscularly and can be rapidly infused intravenously. It also has less cardiotoxicity because, unlike phenytoin, it is water soluble and does not contain propylene glycol in solution. Patients who continue to seize after recommended doses of lorazepam or diazepam, phenytoin, and phenobarbital have refractory SE and require rapid intervention with anesthetic doses of medication and intensive monitoring.

Treatment of Refractory Status Epilepticus

In approximately 9–12% of patients with GCSE, treatment with sequentially administered first-line medications fails and they enter refractory SE [10,60]. NCSE proves refractory to initial treatment in approximately 30% of patients [20].

Table 6.7 A suggested timetable for the treatment of status epilepticus

Time* (min)	Action
0–5	Diagnose status epilepticus by observing continued seizure activity or one additional seizure.
	Give oxygen by nasal cannula or mask; position patient's head for optimal airway patency; consider intubation if respiratory assistance is needed.
	Obtain and record vital signs at onset and periodically thereafter; control any abnormalities as necessary; initiate ECG monitoring.
	Establish an IV line: Draw venous blood samples for glucose levels, serum chemistries, hematology studies, toxicology screens, and determinations of antiepileptic drug levels.
	Assess oxygenation with oximetry or periodic arterial blood gas determinations.
6–9	If hypoglycemia is established or a blood glucose determination is unavailable, administer glucose; in adults, give 100 mg thiamine first, followed by 50 ml 50% glucose by direct push into the IV line; in children, the dose of glucose is 2 ml/kg 25% glucose.
10–20	Administer either 0.1 mg/kg lorazepam at 2 mg/min or 0.2 mg/kg diazepam at 5 mg/min by IV line; if diazepam is given, it can be repeated if seizures do not stop after 5 mins; if diazepam is used to stop the status, phenytoin should be administered next to prevent recurrent status.
21–60	If status persists, administer 15–20 mg/kg phenytoin at no faster than 50 mg/min in adults and 1 mg/kg/min in children by IV line; monitor electrocardiogram and blood pressure during the infusion; phenytoin is incompatible with glucose-containing solutions—the IV line should be purged with normal saline before the phenytoin infusion.
>60	If status does not stop after 20 mg/kg phenytoin, give additional doses of 5 mg/kg to a maximal dose of 30 mg/kg.
	If status persists, give 20 mg/kg phenobarbital by IV line at 100 mg/min; when phenobarbital is given after a benzodiazepine, the risk of apnea or hypopnea is great and assisted ventilation is usually required.
	If status persists, give anesthetic doses of drugs such as phenobarbital or pentobarbital; ventilatory assistance and vasopressors are virtually always necessary.

*Time starts at seizure onset. Note that a neurologic consultation is indicated if the patient does not wake up, convulsions continue after the administration of a benzodiazepine and phenytoin, or confusion exists at any time during evaluation and treatment. I suggest infusing diazepam at no faster than 2 mg per minute.

Source: Reprinted with permission from Epilepsy Foundation of America. Treatment of convulsive status epilepticus: recommendations of the Epilepsy Foundation of America's Working Group on Status Epilepticus. JAMA 1993;270:854.

As was documented under Status Epilepticus in Acute Brain Insults, GCSE not uncommonly evolves to NCSE after apparently "adequate treatment" stops the convulsions [5,37–39]. Therefore, in any patient who is not fully awake after treatment for GCSE, EEG testing is required to document cessation of cerebral seizure activity. This level of care requires 24-hour EEG availability and its timely use (see Sequence of Diagnostic Tests for Status Epilepticus and Nonconvulsive Status Epilepticus).

Several anticonvulsant medications have been recommended for refractory SE. The most frequently used and well-documented agent is pentobarbital, given as a high-dose intravenous infusion. Use of this intervention requires familiarity with its side effects and intensive hemodynamic monitoring. Different protocols have been recommended, and no single optimal regimen has emerged [61–63]. Suggestions have ranged from using the minimal dose needed to stop overt clinical seizures to inducing deep anesthesia with electrocerebral inactivity [64]. Continuous EEG is necessary to guide the degree of cerebral suppression. It is not yet established how much "suppression" is required for successful treatment or whether any particular protocol makes a difference. It is my practice to administer the lowest dose necessary to produce cessation of EEG epileptiform activity for 12–24 hours and then to gradually lighten the coma under EEG guidance.

Before initiation of pentobarbital coma, all patients must be intubated, because all become apneic at therapeutic levels. In addition, all patients become hypotensive and require increased volume infusion. For this reason, central venous access and monitoring with a central venous pressure or pulmonary artery catheter as well as intra-arterial blood pressure monitoring are strongly recommended. The use of dopamine, dobutamine, and other pressors is commonly required. Regular monitoring of temperature, oxygenation, and fluid balance is necessary. Maintenance of adequate nutrition is challenging because peristalsis is slowed.

Pentobarbital treatment exposes the patient to significant risks, some of which are life-threatening. Among the published reports of pentobarbital coma for refractory SE, the mortality is 39% [10]. Many of these deaths were directly related to the cause of SE but, in at least 3%, pentobarbital was implicated as a contributing factor.

Because of these problems, reports of using high-dose intravenous midazolam treatment have captured the attention of neurointensivists. Kumar and Bleck [65] have reported success using continuous intravenous midazolam in seven patients with SE. Other investigators reported similar benefits [66,67]. One protocol recommends a loading dose of 0.15 mg/kg followed by an infusion ranging between 0.05 and 0.5 mg/kg per hour or higher to achieve seizure control. In a report by Rivera and colleagues [67], treatment of 24 children in refractory SE produced prompt cessation of seizures in less than an hour. The lack of significant complications was exceptional. No child experienced cardiovascular or respiratory difficulties and none required intubation. Most clinicians, however, would not hazard such treatment without secure airway protection.

Chang and Bleck [10] have summarized the current view toward intravenous midazolam treatment for refractory SE: Intravenous infusion of midazolam should be instituted as soon as conventional agents have failed. Their group recommends it as a third-line agent after lorazepam and phenytoin, before high-dose intravenous pentobarbital is administered. Continuous EEG should be instituted as quickly as possible to detect NCSE. Because of tachyphylaxis to midazolam, frequent increases in its infusion rate may be needed to suppress seizure activity. The appropriate infusion rate is determined by CEEG monitoring to the desired end point. Hypotension and hypothermia, although less frequent with midazolam than with barbiturates, can still occur and require supportive treatment. Successful discontinuation of midazolam infusion is probably easier if the patient's circulating phenytoin and phenobarbital concentrations are maintained near maximal therapeutic levels. Gradual decreases in the infusion rate are preferable to the termination of midazolam therapy abruptly. Should high doses of intravenous midazolam fail to stop refractory SE within 1 hour, high-dose intravenous pentobarbital coma is initiated.

An interesting possible addition to the SE armamentarium is propofol. This is an intravenous lipid-based anesthetic agent with a shorter duration of action than midazolam. An initial bolus of 1–2 mg/kg is administered followed by a continuous infusion of 20–100 mg/kg per minute titrated to EEG seizure control. The major advantage of propofol is its rapid elimination time, usually permitting extubation within 1–2 hours after stopping the infusion. In one study, midazolam was four times more costly than propofol in controlling SE patients, mainly because patients receiving midazolam required prolonged ventilator support after the infusion was discontinued. It is too early to add propofol as a recommended agent in NCSE, but further studies are anticipated. Chang and Bleck [10] have provided a cogent discussion of various anticonvulsants that are available, their pharmacokinetics, and recommended order of administration. Table 6.8 summarizes their

Table 6.8 Suggested pharmacologic sequence for terminating status epilepticus

I. Terminate status epilepticus. Be aware that cessation of clinical seizures may not always mean that electrographic seizures are terminated. The patient may have progressed to nonconvulsive status epilepticus. Patients who do not respond to external stimuli within 15 mins after apparent cessation of seizures should undergo emergent electroencephalographic monitoring.
   A. Lorazepam, 0.05–0.20 mg/kg at 0.04 mg/kg/min. Onset should be within 5 mins; other medications should be used if no response is attained by that time. Typically, adult patients respond by a dose of 8 mg.
   If seizures persist:
   B. Fosphenytoin, 20 mg/kg at no more than 150 mg/min. Initial infusion should be slower at 75–100 mg/min and can be increased if hypotension or arrhythmias do not occur. An additional 5 mg/kg can be administered before advancing to another medication. If the patient is allergic to phenytoin, use phenobarbital, 10 mg/kg with a maximum infusion rate of 50 mg/min. Repeat with same dose if not controlled. (At this dose of phenobarbital, patient should be intubated.)
   If seizures persist: Transfer to critical care unit and intubate if not yet done.
   C. Midazolam bolus and drip, 0.2 mg/kg bolus with infusion of 0.1–2.0 mg/kg/hr to achieve seizure control by continuous electroencephalographic monitoring.
   If seizures still persist:
   D. Pentobarbital bolus and drip, 12 mg/kg at maximal rate of 0.2–0.4 mg/hr, followed by an infusion of 1.0–2.0 mg/kg/hr titrated to burst-suppression pattern on electroencephalogram. Patients may need intravascular invasive monitoring. If hypotension ensues, fluid and vasopressors should be used to maintain blood pressure.
II. Prevent recurrence of status epilepticus. Although seizures may stop after above therapy, patients should be placed on prophylactic anticonvulsants depending on seizure type (e.g., absence: valproic acid or ethosuximide; generalized tonic-clonic or partial: phenytoin, phenobarbital, carbamazepine, valproic acid, felbamate; generalized myoclonic: clonazepam). Often, patients with severe brain injury require more than one anticonvulsant at "toxic" levels.

Source: Modified from CWJ Chang, TP Bleck. Status Epilepticus. In KG Jordan (ed), Neurologic Critical Care. Neurologic Clinics. Philadelphia: Saunders, 1995;545.

recommendations, with which this author concurs and that can be compared with the EFAWG recommendations in Table 6.7. The availability of fosphenytoin establishes an attractive replacement for intravenous phenytoin and is used in this protocol, but phenytoin is less expensive and more widely available.

SUMMARY

Patients with GCSE and NCSE are commonly seen and may present to the ED or the NICU. NCSE is more common than GCSE in the NICU. In the ED, NCSE is more common than was previously recognized as a late sequela of prolonged GCSE, owing to partial treatment of GCSE or as a de novo presentation of SE. In the ED and NICU, SE combined with ABIs increases the risk for significant morbidity and mortality and may require more urgent intervention than standard published timelines.

Status epilepticus evolves sequentially through several stages, the end point of which is a condition of refractory SE, usually NCSE, leading to neuronal necrosis and permanent cerebral injury. The responsiveness of SE is time dependent. This makes early diagnosis and initiation of treatment essential. Published treatment algorithms stress a 30- to 60-minute time window from onset to complete cessation of seizures. In both the NICU and ED, however, significant delays in diagnosis and treatment occur, limiting the effectiveness of these algorithms. In both venues, data suggest the need for more timely and accurate diagnosis. A high clinical index of suspicion is necessary with recognition of the subtle and nonspecific clinical features of NCSE. In the ED, 24-hour EEG availability and its appropriate use are recommended. In the NICU, ICU-CEEG monitoring is necessary for the timely diagnosis of NCSE and management of refractory SE.

Clinical management of SE requires meticulous attention to ventilation and oxygenation, maintenance of adequate blood pressure, prevention of hyperthermia, and close monitoring for cardiac abnormalities. No single medication or combination of medications is ideal for controlling SE. Current knowledge and available data suggest that, excluding simple absence status, NCSE should be treated aggressively according to the same pharmacologic algorithm as GCSE. The knowledgeable and prompt use of intravenous lorazepam, a diazepam-phenytoin or diazepam-fosphenytoin combination, or phenobarbital is acceptable for first-line treatment as part of a systematic algorithm. Refractory SE has been treated conventionally with high-dose barbiturate coma. Some evidence suggests that high-dose intravenous midazolam, and perhaps propofol, may be useful alternatives.

REFERENCES

1. Leppik IE. Status epilepticus (SE): the role of benzodiazepines. Cleve Clin Q 1990;57(suppl):S39.
2. Epilepsy Foundation of America. Treatment of convulsive status epilepticus: recommendations of the Epilepsy Foundation of America's Working Group on Status Epilepticus. JAMA 1993;270:854.
3. Lederman RJ. Status epilepticus. Cleve Clin Q 1984;51:261.

4. Delgado-Escueta AV, Bajorek JG. Status epilepticus: mechanism of brain damage and rational management. Epilepsia 1982;23(suppl 1):S29.
5. Jordan KG. Nonconvulsive status epilepticus in the neuro ICU detected by continuous EEG monitoring. Neurology 1992;42(suppl 1):194.
6. Young GB, Jordan KG, Doig GS. An assessment of nonconvulsive seizures in the intensive care unit using continuous EEG monitoring: an investigation of variables associated with mortality. Neurology 1996;47:83.
7. Kaplan PW. Nonconvulsive status epilepticus in the emergency room. Epilepsia 1996;37:643.
8. Jordan KG, Young GB, Doig GS. Delays in emergency department (ED) diagnosis and treatment of nonconvulsive status epilepticus (NCSE). Neurology 1995;45(suppl 4):A346.
9. Gastau TH. Clinical and electroencephalographic classification of epileptic seizures. Epilepsia 1970;11:102.
10. Chang CWJ, Bleck TP. Status Epilepticus. In KG Jordan (ed), Neurologic Critical Care. Neurologic Clinics. Philadelphia: Saunders, 1995;529–548.
11. Gotman J. Automatic recognition of seizures in the EEG. Electroencephalograph Clin Neurophysiol 1982;54:530.
12. Gotman J. Computer Analysis during Intensive Monitoring of Epileptic Patients. In RJ Gumnit (ed), Intensive Neurodiagnostic Monitoring. Advances in Neurology (Vol 46). New York: Raven, 1987;249–269.
13. Rowan AJ, Scott DF. Major status epilepticus: a series of 42 patients. Acta Neurol Scand 1970;46:573.
14. Mayeux R, Luders H. Complex partial status epilepticus: case report and proposal for diagnostic criteria. Neurology 1978;28:957.
15. Treiman DM, Delgado-Escueta AV. Complex Partial Status Epilepticus. In AV Delgado-Escueta, CG Wasterlain, DM Treiman, RJ Porter RJ (eds), Status Epilepticus: Mechanisms of Brain Damage and Treatment. Advances in Neurology (Vol 34). New York: Raven, 1983;69–81.
16. Lothman EW, Bertram EH, Bekenstein JW, et al. Self-sustaining limbic status epilepticus induced by "continuous" hippocampal stimulation: electrographic and behavioral characteristics. Epilepsy Res 1989;3:107.
17. Treiman DM, Walton NY, Kendrick CKB. A progressive sequence of electroencephalographic changes during generalized convulsive status epilepticus. Epilepsy Res 1990;5:49.
18. Treiman DM, Walton NY, Wickboldt C, et al. Predictable sequence of EEG changes during generalized convulsive status epilepticus in man and three experimental models of status epilepticus in the rat. Neurology 1987;34:244.
19. Lothman EW. The biochemical basis and pathophysiology of status epilepticus. Neurology 1990;40(suppl 2):13.
20. Privitera M, Hoffman M, Layne Moore J, et al. EEG detection of nontonic–clonic status epilepticus patients with altered consciousness. Epilepsy Res 1994;18:155.
21. Holmes GL. Do seizures cause brain damage? Epilepsia 1991;32(suppl 5):S14.
22. Kreisman NR, LaManna JC, Rosenthal M, et al. Oxidative metabolic responses with recurrent seizures in rat cerebral cortex: role of systemic factors. Brain Res 1981;218:175.
23. Kreisman NR, Rosenthal M, Sik TJ, et al. Oxidative metabolic responses during recurrent seizures are independent of convulsant, anesthetic, or species. Neurology 1983;33:861.
24. Young GB, Jordan KG. Do nonconvulsive seizures cause brain damage? Yes. Arch Neurol 1998;55:117.
25. Meldrum BS, Brierley JB. Prolonged epileptic seizures in primates: ischemic cell change and its relation to ictal physiologic events. Arch Neurol 1973;28:10.
26. Meldrum BS, Vigouroux RA, Brierley JB. Systemic factors and epileptic brain damage: prolonged seizures in paralyzed, artificially ventilated baboons. Arch Neurol 1973;29:82.
27. Applegate CD, Pretel S, Piekut DT. Substantia nigra pars reticulata, seizures, and Fos expression. Epilepsy Res 1995;20:31.
28. DeGiorgio CM, Correale JD, Gott PS, et al. Serum neuron-specific enolase in human status epilepticus. Neurology 1995;45:1134.
29. Rabinowicz AL, Correale J, Bracht K, et al. Neuron-specific enolase is increased after nonconvulsive status epilepticus. Epilepsia 1995;36:475.
30. DeGiorgio CM, Gott PS, Rabinowicz AL, et al. Neuron-specific enolase, a marker for acute neuronal injury is increased in complex partial status epilepticus. Epilepsia 1996;37:606.
31. Wijdicks EFM. Neurology of Critical Illness. Contemporary Neurology Series No. 43. Philadelphia: Davis, 1995.

32. DeLorenzo RJ, Towne AR, Pellock JM, et al. Status epilepticus in children, adults, and the elderly. Epilepsia 1992;33(suppl 4):S15.
33. Lowenstein DH, Alldredge BK. Status epilepticus at an urban public hospital in the 1980s. Neurology 1993;43:483.
34. Barry E, Hauser WA. Status epilepticus: the interaction of epilepsy and acute brain disease. Neurology 1993;43:1473.
35. Barry E, Hauser WA. Status epilepticus and anti-epileptic medication levels. Neurology 1994;44:47.
36. Engle J. Seizures and Epilepsy. Philadelphia: Davis, 1989;112.
37. Fagen KJ, Lee SI. Prolonged confusion following convulsions due to generalized nonconvulsive status epilepticus. Neurology 1990;40:1689.
38. DeLorenzo RJ, Towne AR, Boggs JG, et al. Nonconvulsive status epilepticus following the clinical control of convulsive status epilepticus. Neurology 1997;48:A45.
39. Treiman DM, Meyers PD, Walton NY, et al. A comparison of four treatments for generalized convulsive status epilepticus. N Engl J Med 1998;339:792.
40. Grand'Maison F, Reiher J, Laduke CP. Retrospective inventory of EEG abnormalities in partial status epilepticus. Electroencephalogr Clin Neurophysiol 1991;79:264.
41. Vespa PM, Bergsneider M, Kelly DF, et al. Effect of early seizures on cerebral metabolism in severe brain trauma. J Clin Neurophysiol 1995;12:A104.
42. Vespa PM, Newar M, Hoyda DA, et al. Nonconvulsive and convulsive seizures in acute brain trauma: incidence and impact on outcome. Crit Care Med 1997;25(suppl):A22.
43. Walton NY, Treiman DM. Response of status epilepticus induced by lithium and pilocarpine to treatment with diazepam. Exp Neurol 1988;101:267.
44. Simon RP. Physiologic consequences of status epilepticus. Epilepsia 1985;26(suppl 1):S58.
45. Towne AR, Pellock JM, Ko D, et al. Determinants of mortality in status epilepticus. Epilepsia 1994;35:27.
46. Arboix A, Combs E, Massons J, et al. Relevance of early seizures for inhospital mortality in acute cerebral vascular disease. Neurology 1996;47:1429.
47. Waterhouse EJ. Mortality of status epilepticus in stroke. Epilepsia 1995;36(suppl 4):46.
48. Miller JD, Becker DB. Secondary insults to the injured brain. J R Coll Surg Edinb 1982;27:292.
49. Chesnut RM, Marshall LF. Analysis of the role of secondary brain injury in determining outcome from severe head injury. J Neurosurg 1990;72:360.
50. Gates JR, Ramani V, Whalen S, et al. Ictal characteristics of pseudoseizures. Arch Neurol 1985;42:1183.
51. Luther JS, McNamara JL, Carwile S, et al. Pseudo epileptic seizures: methods and video analysis to a diagnosis. Ann Neurol 1982;12:458.
52. Krumholz A, Sung GY, Fisher RS, et al. Complex partial status epilepticus accompanied by serious morbidity and mortality. Neurology 1995;45:1499.
53. Jordan KG. Continuous EEG and evoked potential monitoring in the neuroscience intensive care unit. J Clin Neurophysiol 1993;10:445.
54. Natelson BH, Chan Q. Sudden death: a neurocardiologic phenomenon. Neurol Clin 1993;11:301.
55. Bahls FH, Bird TD. Theophylline-associated seizures with "therapeutic" or low toxic serum concentrations: risk factors for serious outcomes in adults. Neurology 1991;41:1309.
56. Delgado-Escueta AV. The emergency treatment of status epilepticus. Merritt-Putnam Q 1983;1:3.
57. Walsh GO, Delgado-Escueta AV. Status epilepticus. Neurol Clin 1993;11:835.
58. Shaner DM, McCurdy SA, Herring MO, et al. Treatment of status epilepticus: a prospective comparison of diazepam and phenytoin versus phenobarbital and optional phenytoin. Neurology 1988;38:202.
59. Treiman DM, DeGiorgio CM, Ben-Menachen E, et al. Lorazepam versus phenytoin in treatment of generalized convulsive status: report of an ongoing study. Neurology 1985;35(suppl 1):284.
60. Jagoda A, Riggio S. Refractory status epilepticus in adults. Ann Emerg Med 1993;22:1337.
61. Lowenstein DH, Aminoff MJ, Simon RP. Barbiturate anesthesia in the treatment of status epilepticus: clinical experience in 14 patients. Neurology 1988;38:395.
62. Osorio I, Reed RC. Treatment of refractory generalized tonic clonic status epilepticus with pentobarbital anesthesia after high-dose phenytoin. Epilepsia 1989;30:44.
63. Van Ness PC. Pentobarbital and EEG burst suppression in treatment of status epilepticus refractory to benzodiazepines and phenytoin. Epilepsia 1990;31:61.
64. Tasker IC, Boyd SG, Harden A, et al. EEG monitoring of prolonged thiopentone administration for intractable seizures and status epilepticus in infants and young children. Neuropediatrics 1989;20:147.

65. Kumar A, Bleck TP. Intravenous midazolam for the treatment of refractory status epilepticus. Crit Care Med 1992;20:483.
66. Crisp CB, Gannon R, Knauft F. Continuous infusion of midazolam hydrochloride to control status epilepticus. Clin Pharm 1988;7:322.
67. Rivera R, Segnina M, Baltodano A, et al. Midazolam in the treatment of status epilepticus in children. Crit Care Med 1993;20:1994.

7
Current Management
of Acute Ischemic Stroke

Scott E. Kasner and Eric C. Raps

Therapy for acute ischemic stroke has four goals: restoration of cerebral blood flow (reperfusion), prevention of recurrent thrombosis (antithrombotic therapy), neuroprotection, and supportive care. All of these components have, to a greater or lesser extent, been the subject of rigorous clinical investigation, and research continues at a swift pace. The timing of these therapies is critical, and methods for improving the speed of initial evaluation are being studied. As nihilistic attitudes toward stroke therapy are replaced by proactive postures, a greater need for neurologists to act urgently and decisively has evolved. Specific expertise in acute diagnosis and therapy of ischemic stroke is essential for safe and effective management.

PATHOPHYSIOLOGY OF ACUTE ISCHEMIC STROKE

Experimental stroke models have demonstrated that an intricate series of events occurs after the onset of regional cerebral ischemia (Figure 7.1). Ischemia is a dynamic process that depends on severity and duration. The ischemic cascade begins within seconds to minutes after perfusion failure, rapidly creating a core zone of irreversible infarction and a surrounding area of potentially salvageable "ischemic penumbra" [1,2]. The ultimate target of acute stroke therapy is this territory at risk.

Within the ischemic neuron, protein synthesis halts as the cell attempts to conserve its declining energy stores. Membrane ion transport systems fail, and the neuron depolarizes. Membrane depolarization results in calcium influx, causing release of stored neurotransmitters. Glutamate, the major cerebral excitatory neurotransmitter, is released in large quantities and exacerbates the neuronal assault by further increasing intracellular calcium and by depolarizing other neurons in the penumbral zone. Other neurotransmitters, including glycine and dynorphin, can also amplify the injury. The massive calcium influx overstimu-

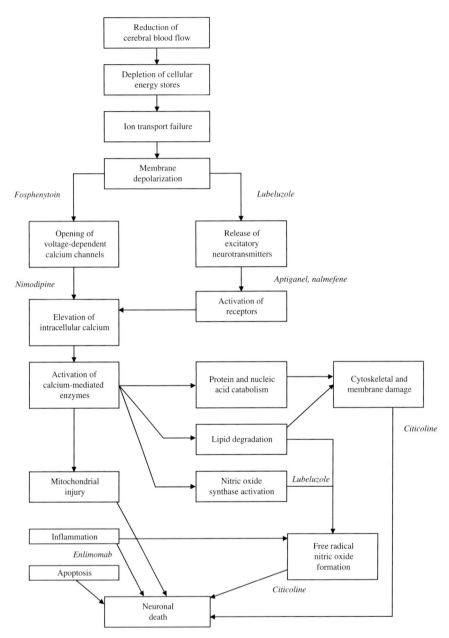

Figure 7.1   The "ischemic cascade." Multiple effects contribute to neuronal death after an ischemic injury. Several of these are the targets of putative neuroprotective agents (*italics*).

lates several enzymes, which become unregulated. This can lead to dysfunction of cellular homeostatic mechanisms, cytoskeletal components, mitochondria, and cell membranes. Consequently, free radicals and nitric oxide are liberated, contributing further to neuronal damage.

Over the next few hours to days, specific genes are activated within surviving ischemic neurons. Production of cytokines and cellular adhesion molecules is augmented, stimulating local inflammation and potentially impairing blood flow in the microcirculation. Finally, apoptotic genes are activated, resulting in further delayed cell death among the shrinking population of surviving neurons. Without effective intervention, the entire ischemic penumbra may eventually succumb and become part of the infarct core.

Based on current information regarding the mechanisms and course of ischemia, acute intervention must occur very early to preserve a substantial portion of brain tissue. Animal models of acute ischemic stroke suggest that reperfusion must occur within 3–6 hours and preliminary results from human imaging studies suggest a similar time frame [3]. Not surprisingly, the only proven effective therapy for acute stroke also mandates a 3-hour window for reperfusion. The time window for altering the course of the ischemic cascade is less well defined, but is also believed to be quite brief [4]. However, the cascade offers many targets for novel neuroprotective strategies.

INITIAL ASSESSMENT OF THE PATIENT WITH ACUTE ISCHEMIC STROKE

First contact with the acute stroke patient commonly occurs in the emergency department, where the initial focus is on the "ABCs" of oxygenation and hemodynamic stability. The history and physical examination are directed toward ascertaining specific stroke risk factors and etiologies, followed by localization of the ischemic territory. Alternative entities that mimic stroke must be considered and excluded to the extent allowed by the available information. Laboratory studies are ordered, including a complete blood cell count with platelets, electrolytes, glucose, and coagulation parameters if clinically indicated. Electrocardiography is performed to assess for evidence of arrhythmia or cardiac ischemia. Emergent computed tomography (CT) is performed to exclude intracerebral hemorrhage and early signs of cerebral ischemia. Based on these data, which can be obtained in less than 60 minutes [5–7], a treatment decision is reached.

Ideally, treatment of the patient with acute stroke would be directed toward the underlying pathophysiology. Five major etiologic categories of stroke exist: large artery atherothromboembolic disease, cardioembolism, small vessel thrombotic disease, other determined etiology (hypercoagulable state, dissection, vasculitis), and cryptogenic (unknown) [8]. Each of these stroke subtypes can hypothetically benefit from a distinct therapeutic maneuver. Early determination of stroke mechanism is difficult, however, and fewer than two-thirds of patients seen within the first 24 hours after symptom onset are correctly classified [9] (Table 7.1). Because both proven and potential therapies for acute stroke must commence during this window of uncertainty, the physician must select a treatment that has broad efficacy and safety.

Table 7.1   Accuracy of stroke subtype diagnosis in the first 24 hours after stroke onset

Initial stroke subtype	Large artery atherosclerosis	Cardio-embolism	Small vessel occlusion	Other etiology	Cryptogenic (undetermined)
Large artery atherosclerosis	**62**	14	7	2	15
Cardio-embolism	12	**69**	7	1	11
Small vessel occlusion	15	8	**66**	1	9
Other etiology	25	0	25	**50**	0
Cryptogenic (undetermined)	20	16	20	6	**39**

Final stroke subtype determined at 3 mos (%)*

*Appropriate correlations are indicated in boldface.

Source: Adapted from KP Madden, PN Karanjia, HP Adams, WR Clarke, and the TOAST Investigators. Accuracy of initial stroke subtype diagnosis in the TOAST study. Neurology 1995;45:1975.

Several imaging techniques can be used to characterize the acute vascular lesion. The gold standard is conventional catheter arteriography, which can demonstrate an acute occlusion of the intra- or extracranial circulation and often can detect an embolus lodged at a vascular bifurcation. After such a lesion is identified, therapeutic options, such as intra-arterial thrombolysis, angioplasty, or emergent surgery, may become relevant. Arteriography may require a relatively long period to obtain, however, potentially limiting its usefulness in a disease in which irreversible damage occurs quickly. The vasculature can also be evaluated noninvasively. Advances in CT technology have made CT-angiography available in many centers. CT-angiography uses a small amount of intravenous contrast to rapidly provide a three-dimensional view of the cervical and intracranial vessels. Alternatively, transcranial Doppler ultrasonography or magnetic resonance angiography can be used to detect occlusion or stenosis, but these techniques lack specificity. Moreover, these noninvasive methods can guide medical therapy but provide no acute therapeutic options by themselves.

The ability to identify at-risk cerebral tissue has considerable clinical relevance, because the presence of viable tissue may prove to be an appropriate indication for reperfusion or neuroprotective therapies. Positron emission tomography can be used to detect the presence of an ischemic but viable penumbra surrounding an infarcted core [10,11]. Infarcted tissue typically has low regional cerebral blood flow and low cerebral metabolic rates of oxygen consumption, whereas potentially viable tissue has a preserved oxygen extraction fraction despite poor perfusion. The mismatch between blood flow and aerobic metabolism ("misery perfusion") can ultimately result in necrosis. The time course of this process is poorly defined, although substantial volumes of brain tissue have been shown to remain potentially viable for as long as 17 hours after stroke [11].

If early reperfusion occurs, cerebral blood flow supply may exceed metabolic demand ("luxury perfusion"), and this may portend a better clinical outcome [10]. However, positron emission tomographic studies may be impractical in the hyper-acute setting because of the requirement for radioactive agents and the time needed for the imaging and data analysis. Single-photon emission CT may be more available, but this technique only demonstrates the perfusion defect associated with acute ischemia rather than the potentially viable penumbra [12].

Novel magnetic resonance techniques provide a rapid, high-resolution, and noninvasive means to evaluate the ischemic penumbra. The physics that forms the foundations for these modalities is beyond the scope of this discussion. Diffusion-weighted imaging reveals changes in infarcted tissue hours before any abnormality can be recognized on conventional CT or magnetic resonance imaging (Figure 7.2A). Qualitatively, hyperintensity on diffusion-weighted imaging is predictive of the extent of infarction [13], but some component of this may be reversible if early reperfusion occurs. Analysis of the quantitative data in the form of the apparent diffusion coefficient suggests that there may be a threshold that demarcates the permanently infarcted tissue, although this level is still unknown [1]. The maximal extent of the territory at risk may be better imaged with perfusion-weighted imaging (Figure 7.2B). This technique reveals the area of reduced cerebral blood flow and hence the region exposed to possible ischemic injury [14]. The difference between the perfusion defect and the diffusion defect then appears to represent penumbra. Because these techniques do not require a radioactive tracer, studies can be performed repeatedly to observe the fate of potentially viable tissue and its response to a specific therapy. This approach has been used in animal studies [3,15] and is being actively investigated in the clinical arena.

Current emergent stroke management uses crude tools to assess the patient; namely, the clinical examination, CT, and the clock. Consequently, acute therapy during the first few hours must largely be dictated by a "shoot first, ask questions later" paradigm. In the future, more refined techniques may allow for specific therapeutic approaches based on a rapid but thorough evaluation of the pathophysiology of the vascular lesion and the presence or absence of viable tissue. Rigid time windows for initiation of therapy may become less relevant [16], whereas neuroimaging may become of paramount importance.

REPERFUSION

Reperfusion after an acute vascular occlusion can be achieved by the administration of intravenous thrombolytic agents. Recombinant tissue plasminogen activator (t-PA) and streptokinase both have proven efficacy in acute myocardial infarction and are the most rigorously and extensively studied agents for thrombolysis in stroke. Based on the results of several major trials, however, only t-PA has a favorable risk-benefit profile in the treatment of stroke. Other agents, such as urokinase and prourokinase, remain the subject of clinical research. The newer derivative forms of t-PA are being studied in coronary disease, but no final data exist regarding their use in stroke.

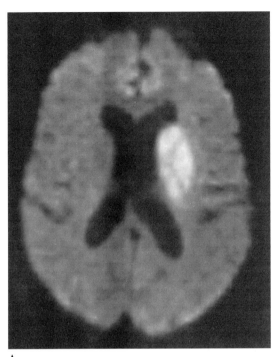

A

Figure 7.2   Novel magnetic resonance imaging techniques for acute ischemic stroke in the territory of the left middle cerebral artery. **A.** Diffusion-weighted imaging. **B.** Perfusion-weighted imaging. The ischemic penumbra may be represented by the territory that has impaired perfusion but retains normal diffusion characteristics.

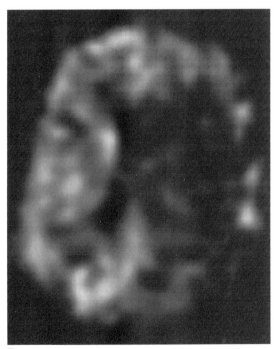

B

The specific choice of thrombolytic drug for acute stroke is dependent on a number of pharmacologic factors. Although both t-PA and streptokinase convert plasminogen into plasmin, which in turn causes cleavage of fibrin and ultimately results in lysis of a clot, they have distinct mechanisms of action. t-PA specifically activates plasminogen that is already bound to thrombus, while streptokinase activates unbound circulating plasminogen and results in systemic depletion of fibrinogen. The effects of streptokinase therefore last much longer and are less clot-specific than those of t-PA. t-PA was also shown to restore angiographic patency more rapidly than streptokinase in myocardial infarction studies [17]. In the treatment of acute myocardial infarction, streptokinase does not necessarily require the concurrent use of heparin because of its induction of a prolonged lytic state, but t-PA has a relatively brief effect and is typically administered with heparin [17]. Finally, streptokinase costs substantially less than t-PA. Many of these differences became particularly important when these agents were studied in acute ischemic stroke.

Timing of thrombolysis is critical. As was described in Pathophysiology of Acute Ischemic Stroke, ischemic brain tissue can be rescued only if it is reperfused before irreversible damage occurs. Furthermore, the risk of hemorrhage appears to increase as ischemic tissue becomes edematous [18,19]. In accord with experimental animal studies and preliminary human studies, the National Institute of Neurological Disorders and Stroke (NINDS) t-PA study limited the use of t-PA to within the first 3 hours after the onset of symptoms [20]. In the other trials of t-PA and streptokinase, patients were treated up to 6 hours after stroke onset.

Intravenous Thrombolytic Therapy

Tissue Plasminogen Activator

Two major trials investigated the effect of t-PA on acute ischemic stroke. The European Cooperative Acute Stroke Study (ECASS) was a randomized, prospective, multicenter, double-blind placebo-controlled study of 620 patients with acute ischemic hemispheric stroke [21]. Patients were randomly assigned to treatment with either intravenous recombinant t-PA, 1.1 mg/kg, or placebo within 6 hours of stroke onset. The primary end points were the Barthel index (a 100-point scale of independence with activities of daily living) and the modified Rankin scale (a 5-point scale of disability) at 90 days. t-PA had no significant benefit over placebo in the overall (intention-to-treat) analysis in the primary end points. However, 109 patients (17.4%) included in this analysis should not have been enrolled because of one or more exclusion criteria, and were therefore considered to have protocol violations. In the remaining patients, termed the *target population*, a significant improvement in outcome, as quantified by the Rankin scale, was demonstrated at 90 days. In addition, several secondary end points, including the combined Barthel and Rankin scores, speed of neurologic recovery, and length of hospital stay, were significantly improved by t-PA in both the intention-to-treat and target population analyses. Although t-PA–treated patients had a higher incidence of parenchymal intracerebral hemorrhage (19.8% vs. 6.5%; $p < .001$), no significant difference in mortality was seen at 30 days

Table 7.2   Criteria for acute ischemic stroke treatment with tissue plasminogen activator

Inclusion criteria
    Age >18 yrs
    Clinical diagnosis of ischemic stroke, with onset of symptoms within 3 hrs of initiation
        of treatment
    CT scan (noncontrast) without evidence of hemorrhage
Exclusion criteria
    Historical data
        Stroke or head trauma in previous 3 mos
        History of intracranial hemorrhage that can increase risk for recurrent hemorrhage
        Major surgery or other serious trauma in previous 14 days
        Gastrointestinal or genitourinary bleeding in previous 21 days
        Arterial puncture at a noncompressible site in previous 7 days
        Lumbar puncture in previous 7 days
        Pregnant or lactating woman
    Clinical presentation
        Rapidly improving symptoms
        Seizure at stroke onset
        Symptoms suggestive of subarachnoid hemorrhage, even if CT scan is normal
        Persistent systolic BP >185 mm Hg or diastolic BP >110 mm Hg, or aggressive
            therapy necessary to control BP
        Clinical presentation consistent with acute MI or post-MI pericarditis requires evalu-
            ation before treatment
    Computed tomography
        CT evidence of hemorrhage
        CT evidence of hypodensity and/or effacement of cerebral sulci in more than one-
            third of the middle cerebral artery territory
    Laboratory analysis
        Glucose <50 mg/dl or >400 mg/dl
        Platelets <100,000/μl
        On warfarin and prothrombin, time >15 secs
        On heparin within 48 hrs and partial thromboplastin, time is elevated

CT = computed tomographic; BP = blood pressure; MI = myocardial infarction.

between the t-PA and placebo groups (17.9% vs. 12.7%; not significant [NS]) in either analysis.

The majority of protocol violations were owing to CT exclusion criteria: major signs of early infarction, primary hemorrhage, or computed tomographic scan not readable or available. Patients in the protocol violation group who were treated with t-PA had a much higher incidence of hemorrhage and death than those given placebo. Based on differences between the intention-to-treat and target population groups, the ECASS investigators concluded that the use of t-PA within 6 hours cannot be recommended in an unselected population of stroke patients.

The NINDS t-PA Stroke Study was a randomized, prospective, multicenter, double-blinded, placebo-controlled study of 624 patients with acute ischemic stroke [20]. Individuals who met the inclusion and exclusion criteria (Table 7.2) were randomized to either intravenous t-PA, 0.9 mg/kg, or placebo within 3 hours of onset of symptoms. The study was partitioned in two, each part with a specific primary end point. Part 1 examined the effect of t-PA within 24 hours as

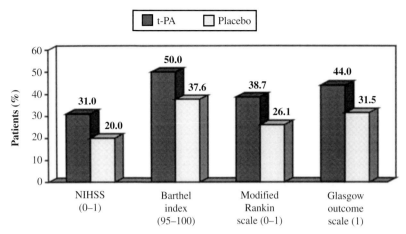

Figure 7.3 Three-month outcomes in the National Institute of Neurological Disorders and Stroke t-PA Stroke Trial. Intravenous tissue plasminogen activator (t-PA) resulted in a significant increase in the proportion of patients with minimal or no deficit at 3 months in terms of the National Institute of Health Stroke scale (NIHSS), Barthel index, modified Rankin scale, and Glasgow outcome scale.

measured by complete resolution of deficit or improvement of at least four points on the National Institute of Health Stroke scale (NIHSS, a 42-point scale of specific neurologic deficits), while outcome at 3 months was a secondary end point. Based on the analysis of part 1, part 2 was designed to assess the longer-term benefit of t-PA at 3 months as determined by a global statistic that reflected four outcome measures: the Barthel index, Rankin scale, Glasgow outcome scale, and NIHSS. Investigators remained blinded to the results of part 1 until both parts were completed. Part 1 did not demonstrate a significant effect of t-PA on the primary end point at 24 hours, although t-PA was associated with significant improvement in the median NIHSS at 24 hours in a secondary analysis, and outcome at 3 months was significantly improved. Part 2 demonstrated significant improvement in clinical outcome at 3 months in patients treated with t-PA. This benefit was observed in the global statistic and in each of its four individual measures (Figure 7.3). The odds ratio for a favorable outcome in the t-PA group was 1.7 (95% confidence interval, 1.2–2.8; $p = .008$). The absolute increase in the number of patients with minimal or no deficit in part 2 was 11% (relative benefit, 55%) by the NIHSS and 13% (relative benefit, 50%) by the Rankin scale. The benefit of t-PA was demonstrated regardless of whether the stroke etiology was large vessel occlusive disease, small vessel occlusive disease, or cardioembolism. Symptomatic intracerebral hemorrhage within the first 36 hours occurred significantly more often in the patients treated with t-PA than in those given placebo (6.4% vs. 0.6%; $p < .001$), but no significant difference in mortality was seen at 3 months (17% and 21%; NS), even when accounting for those patients with hemorrhagic complications.

The division of the NINDS t-PA trial into two parts has been a source of confusion. Each part was independent of the other and each had a unique hypothesis, but the methods were identical and the data were published together. It may have been expected that if thrombolysis was effective, it should have improved early outcome rather than only cause a late response at 3 months. The specific hypothesis of part 1, that t-PA would cause a four-point improvement on the NIHSS or complete resolution of symptoms within 24 hours, was not statistically significant. With the same data presented in an alternative format, however, a significant reduction in the median NIHSS was seen, from 12 to 8 (p <.02), a difference of four points. A similar benefit was observed in the 24-hour outcome of the patients in part 2 of the study. In addition, only 4% of the patients given placebo had complete resolution (NIHSS of 1 or less) at 24 hours, compared to 17% of t-PA–treated patients. The thrombolytic effects of t-PA are rapid, but the ultimate benefits of such therapy may not be immediately evident. Neurologic recovery is a slow process even after effective therapy.

The NINDS trial demonstrated that treatment with intravenous t-PA within 3 hours of stroke onset improved outcome at 3 months. However, the four outcome scales used in the study may not be familiar to many neurologists in practice. The definition of favorable outcome (minimal or no deficit) used in the study was quite stringent. On the NIHSS, a patient had to score 0 or 1, which would represent either an isolated mild facial droop, mild dysarthria, or slight arm drift, for example. On the Barthel index, a favorable score was considered to be 95 or 100, requiring the patient to be independent in all activities of daily living. To score 0 or 1 on the Rankin scale, the patient had to be able to return to all prestroke occupational, social, and personal functions. Finally, a score of 1 on the Glasgow outcome scale was scored only if the patient was able to return to a full and completely independent life.

Because of key differences between the NINDS and ECASS studies, direct comparisons are limited. The major difference was the time window. The use of t-PA is currently only recommended when therapy can be initiated within 3 hours. As suggested by the results in the target population of the ECASS study, however, careful selection of patients with appropriate computed tomographic criteria may eventually allow for treatment beyond 3 hours. Although the NINDS trial only excluded patients with hemorrhage, a retrospective analysis has suggested that major early infarct signs on CT scan (i.e., hypodensity in more than one-third of the middle cerebral artery territory) should be considered a contraindication to t-PA treatment, possibly in any time frame [18,19]. These early CT abnormalities may indicate that the time of onset is earlier than reported, or that the injured brain tissue is already beyond the point of potential recovery. The dangers related to more subtle CT changes are less clear, and these should not contraindicate t-PA therapy within the first 3 hours. Current trials of t-PA for acute stroke are evaluating a longer time window and exclude patients with major infarct signs to minimize the risk of hemorrhage (see Addendum). The ECASS trial also used a larger dose of t-PA than the NINDS study, which may also have contributed to the greater incidence of intracerebral hemorrhage. The ongoing ECASS-2 trial has shifted to the lower dosing regimen of the NINDS trial, 0.9 mg/kg, and continues to enroll patients within 6 hours after onset of stroke.

Streptokinase

Three major trials have demonstrated that streptokinase is neither beneficial nor safe for acute ischemic stroke treatment when given up to 6 hours after stroke onset. All three trials were randomized, prospective multicenter studies, and all three were terminated before completion because of unacceptably high mortality.

The Multicentre Acute Stroke Trial–Italy (MAST-I) enrolled 622 patients with acute ischemic stroke within 6 hours of onset [22]. Patients received either intravenous streptokinase (1.5 million units/day) or aspirin (300 mg/day) for 10 days, or both or neither. Neither streptokinase, aspirin, nor the combination significantly improved outcome. Streptokinase, either alone or with aspirin, caused a significant increase in the 10-day mortality compared with that of the control group (27% vs. 12%; p <.00001), although the incidence of hemorrhage with streptokinase alone (6%) was similar to that found with t-PA in the NINDS study.

The Multicentre Acute Stroke Trial–Europe (MAST-E) randomized 310 patients within 6 hours after onset of symptoms [23]. Patients received either intravenous streptokinase (1.5 million units) or placebo. The majority of patients also received concomitant treatment with heparin, many within the first 12 hours after administration of streptokinase or placebo. A nonsignificant trend toward less disability occurred, as measured by the Rankin scale, in patients who received streptokinase. Mortality was greater in those treated with streptokinase than in those given placebo, however, both at 10 days (34% vs. 18.2%; p = .002) and 6 months (46.8% vs. 38.3%; p = .13, NS).

The Australian Streptokinase Trial recruited 340 patients within 4 hours of onset of acute stroke [24]. Patients were randomized to either placebo or treatment with intravenous streptokinase (1.5 million units). Aspirin was also administered to all patients when possible. Of the three streptokinase trials, only the Australian Streptokinase included a hypothesis regarding the importance of the time frame: There may be a difference in efficacy between patients treated within 3 hours and those treated later. However, more than three-fourths of the patients were treated beyond 3 hours. Overall, streptokinase afforded no benefit with regard to outcome on the Barthel index at 3 months and was associated with a significantly increased risk of intracerebral hemorrhage (13.2% vs. 3% with placebo; p <.01). Mortality at 3 months was also significantly greater with streptokinase (36.2% vs. 20.5%; p <.05). However, these poor outcomes were predominantly attributable to treatment after 3 hours. Among the 70 patients treated within the 3-hour window, a notable trend was seen toward improved outcome without excess mortality.

Based on the results of these three trials, streptokinase should not be used in the treatment of acute stroke. The MAST-E study group suggested that this conclusion should also be extrapolated to the use of all thrombolytics for stroke, and the NINDS t-PA results might be a statistical aberration. However, direct comparisons between the streptokinase and t-PA studies are difficult because of several critical differences in study design. The prolonged and nonspecific systemic lytic effects of streptokinase probably contributed to the high risk of hemorrhage in the trials. Moreover, the dose of t-PA in the NINDS study was lower than the standard dose used for myocardial infarction, whereas the thrombolytic doses in all of the other four studies were likely too high. The 6-hour time window, without careful selection by computed tomographic criteria (as previously described with regard to the ECASS study), can also increase the risk of hemorrhagic transformation. Even the Australian Streptokinase Trial supported the importance of the first 3 hours. The concurrent use of heparin (either intravenously or subcutaneously) or aspirin in the MAST-E, MAST-I, and Australian Streptokinase trials probably contributed to hemorrhage in all of the streptokinase studies, whereas both t-PA trials prohibited the use of heparin and antiplatelet agents during the first 24 hours. The overall rate of intracranial hemorrhage (both symptomatic and asymptomatic) among patients treated with placebo in the MAST-E trial was dramatically higher than the rate of hemorrhage associated with placebo in the NINDS trial (43.5% vs. 3.5%) [23]. Much of this difference can be attributed to anticoagulation with heparin.

Conclusions: Intravenous Thrombolysis in Acute Ischemic Stroke

Intravenous thrombolysis is an effective therapy for acute stroke, but only one thrombolytic agent, t-PA, has proven efficacy and safety. Early and rapid assessment is essential, because treatment must be started within the first 3 hours after onset. Patient selection must rigidly adhere to the inclusion and exclusion criteria, and careful evaluation of the baseline computed tomographic scan is also important in minimizing the risk of intracranial hemorrhage. Finally, the use of anticoagulants and antiplatelet agents must be strictly avoided during the first 24 hours. Ongoing research seeks to improve safety and efficacy by identifying those patients who can benefit most while excluding those at greatest risk for hemorrhage.

Intra-Arterial Thrombolytic Therapy

Direct infusion of a thrombolytic agent into an occluded blood vessel is a potential alternative or adjunctive therapy to intravenous t-PA (Figure 7.4). When conventional cerebral angiography is performed within 6–12 hours after the onset of stroke, an acute arterial occlusion can be detected in more than 75% of patients [25,26]. Intra-arterial thrombolysis has proven efficacy in acute coronary, pulmonary, and peripheral vascular thromboembolic disease, but its role in acute ischemic stroke remains speculative. In principle, local intra-arterial therapy poses a smaller risk of systemic bleeding while delivering the medication directly to its target, theoretically making it safer and more effective than intravenous thrombolysis. However, the usefulness of intra-arterial therapy is limited by demands on personnel, technology, and the time window.

　The only prospective, controlled, randomized clinical trials to evaluate intra-arterial thrombolysis are still under way. The Prolyse in Acute Cerebral Thromboembolism Trial [27], initiated in 1996, is enrolling patients with ischemic stroke symptoms referable to the middle cerebral artery (MCA) who present within 6 hours of onset. After computed tomographic scan excludes hemorrhage, patients are evaluated by conventional angiography, and if a major occlusion of the MCA is confirmed, they are then randomized to intra-arterial infusion of recombinant prourokinase or placebo. All patients receive concomitant intravenous heparin. Prourokinase is the naturally occurring precursor to urokinase and is highly clot-specific, but is limited to investigational use at present.

　The Australian Urokinase Stroke Trial, also started in 1996, is enrolling patients with acute ischemic stroke in the posterior circulation within 24 hours of onset. If conventional angiography reveals an arterial thrombus in the vertebrobasilar system, patients are randomized to treatment with either intra-arterial urokinase plus intra-arterial heparin or to intra-arterial heparin alone.

Figure 7.4 Intra-arterial thrombolysis. **A.** An acute occlusion of
the left middle cerebral artery is
demonstrated by conventional
angiography (*arrow*). **B.** After local
intra-arterial infusion of urokinase,
the left middle cerebral artery is
recanalized (*arrow*).

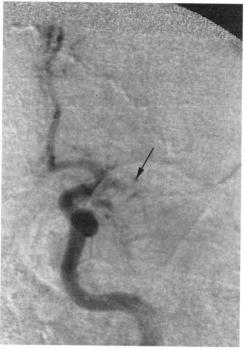

A

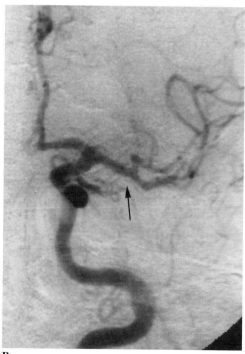

B

Both urokinase and t-PA are commercially available for intra-arterial use, although neither is currently indicated for selective use in the intracranial circulation. A number of small, uncontrolled series have been reported that describe the effect of intra-arterial urokinase or t-PA in acute ischemic stroke [28–32]. Because of the multiple differences in methods, however, no recommendations regarding the protocols can be made. The optimal patient population, time window, thrombolytic agent, and interventional approach are all unknown, as are the roles of concomitant anticoagulation and mechanical clot disruption [33,34]. In general, recanalization has been achieved in 50–70% of patients. The reported rate of intracerebral hemorrhage with intra-arterial therapy ranges from 2% to 11%, which is comparable to the 6% risk associated with intravenous t-PA, but the risk of systemic bleeding may be reduced.

If intra-arterial therapy is proved to be beneficial by prospective, controlled clinical trials, it will still need to overcome several obstacles before it becomes widely useful. A 1997 analysis determined the geographic availability of interventional neuroradiologists in the United States [35]. Based on the geographic data and the critical time windows required for acute stroke intervention, it appears that only 37% of the population would be eligible for intra-arterial therapy within 3 hours of stroke onset. If intra-arterial therapy has a longer time window, however, up to 96% of patients could be theoretically identified, transported, triaged, and treated in a 6-hour period. This model assumes that the interventional neuroradiology suite and personnel can be made ready in a relatively brief period, which may be quite difficult in busy centers and during off hours. Thus, the time thresholds for intra-arterial therapy should be better categorized to determine the therapy's applicability.

Because of the potential delays associated with intra-arterial thrombolysis, the Emergency Management of Stroke Investigators examined the effect of intravenous followed by intra-arterial t-PA [36]. This protocol could allow for early therapy while preparations are being made for intra-arterial thrombolysis. Thirty-five patients with acute ischemic stroke who presented within 3 hours of onset were randomized to receive either 0.6 mg/kg intravenous t-PA or placebo. Cerebral angiography was performed immediately after the intravenous dose, and if a clot was detected, patients from both groups were given intra-arterial t-PA. The intra-arterial dose was determined by the amount required to achieve angiographic patency, up to a maximum of 20 mg over 120 minutes. Comparable rates of patency were obtained in both groups: 67% for combined therapy and 60% for intra-arterial t-PA alone. Early clinical recovery was also similar in both groups, but severe hemorrhagic complications were more common in the group that received both intravenous and intra-arterial therapy. Combined therapy appears to be feasible, but whether it provides any added benefit remains to be demonstrated.

Revascularization Procedures

Restoration of cerebral blood flow is possible by emergent treatment of the underlying vascular abnormality. Carotid endarterectomy has proven efficacy in the treatment of severe symptomatic carotid stenosis, but it is usually performed at least several weeks after stroke. This procedure has been accomplished during the acute stages of stroke [37], but the risks and benefits of this aggressive approach are unknown. As with thrombolysis, it is likely that reperfusion after the first few hours of stroke is associated with an increased risk of hemorrhagic transformation. The requirements for angiography, preparation of the operating room, anesthesia, and the surgical approach to the internal carotid artery are formidable barriers to effective revascularization within the first 3–6 hours.

Angioplasty and stenting of the extracranial and intracranial cerebral vessels have become possible because of advances in microcatheter technology. This procedure is being compared to carotid endarterectomy as a secondary preventive therapy [38,39]. In the future, angioplasty may also be suitable for use in acute stroke. Several series have been reported describing both clinical and radiographic improvement in patients treated with emergent angioplasty [40]. Until the efficacy and safety of this technique can be demonstrated in nonacute situations, however, its role in urgent stroke therapy remains speculative.

ACUTE ANTITHROMBOTIC THERAPY

Prevention of progressive or recurrent thrombosis is believed to limit the potential cerebral injury caused by acute stroke. Anticoagulants and antiplatelet agents are commonly used during the acute period for this purpose. Despite their long-standing use in neurologic practice, their efficacy and safety are not well established, and few issues in clinical stroke management are more controversial. However, some studies have shed new light and new doubts on the roles of these traditional therapies.

Anticoagulation

Heparin

The majority of neurologists use heparin, but only a small fraction believe that it offers a proven benefit to patients with acute stroke [41]. Early administration of heparin has been advocated as a means to prevent propagation of an acute thrombus or recurrent embolism. Therefore, the usefulness of heparin has been postulated in a variety of clinical settings, including cardioembolism, stroke-in-evolution, acute partial stroke, and recurrent or crescendo transient ischemic attacks (TIAs).

The International Stroke Trial (IST) was the first major multicenter, randomized, controlled clinical trial to evaluate heparin in acute ischemic stroke [42]. This study enrolled 19,435 patients within 48 hours of stroke onset and made no specific requirements regarding stroke etiology, vascular distribution, or likelihood of progression at baseline. Patients received either 12,500 units of subcutaneous heparin twice a day, 5,000 units twice a day, or were assigned to "avoid heparin" for a course of 14 days or until hospital discharge, if sooner. Because this trial was performed simultaneously with an analysis of acute aspirin therapy (described in Antiplatelet Therapy: Aspirin), half of the patients also received aspirin. The rate of recurrent ischemic stroke, hemorrhagic stroke, or death at 14 days was 12.8% with heparin (either dose) and 13.3% without heparin, a nonsignificant difference. A relative reduction in the rate of ischemic stroke with heparin occurred that was completely counterbalanced by an increase in hemorrhagic stroke rate. These results of the IST contradict the routine use of heparin in the majority of patients with acute stroke.

The benefit of heparin in cardioembolism is more readily accepted. After a cardioembolic stroke, the risk of recurrent cerebral embolism is approximately 1% per day for the first 2 weeks after the event [43]. This risk appears to be similar for the major sources of cardioembolism, including atrial fibrillation, valvular disease, ventricular wall motion abnormalities, and dilated cardiomyopathy. The Cerebral Embolism Study Group showed that early anticoagulation with heparin can reduce this risk by approximately 60–70% [43]. Embolic infarcts are believed to have a relatively high rate of hemorrhagic conversion as a result of reperfusion injury, however, usually within the first 48 hours [44]. Consequently, if heparin is considered in a patient with acute cardioembolic stroke, a delay of at least 2 days and repeated neuroimaging may be advisable before initiation of this therapy. Acute anticoagulation with heparin is usually followed by warfarin therapy in patients with nondisabling, nonhemorrhagic cardioembolic stroke as secondary prevention.

The potential benefit of heparin in progressing stroke, or stroke-in-evolution, is unclear. No universal definition exists for stroke-in-evolution [45–47], and therefore interpretation of the conflicting literature is nearly impossible. Several different mechanisms can contribute to acute worsening of the neurologic deficit, including propagation of thrombus, recurrent embolism, cerebral edema, hemorrhagic transformation, toxic-metabolic factors, and delayed neuronal death or apoptosis. Heparin would only be expected to theoretically improve the first two of these mechanisms. The earliest trials of heparin for progressing stroke were performed during the pre-CT era and had numerous design flaws, but suggested that heparin was beneficial [48–51]. More recent but still uncontrolled studies have challenged the value of heparin in this setting [45,52]. Haley and associates [45] demonstrated that deterioration continued in up to half of the patients despite early heparin treatment. Some studies have suggested that progression is a more common complication of stroke in the vertebrobasilar system than in the carotid territory, although it remains uncertain whether heparin actually has a different effect in each vascular distribution [53,54].

In the extreme view, some neurologists note that it is impossible to determine which strokes will progress after initial diagnosis, and therefore recommend that nearly all patients with acute incomplete deficits be treated with heparin. In a double-blind, placebo-controlled trial, Duke and associates [55] randomized 225 patients with acute partial stable stroke to therapy with intravenous heparin or placebo for 7 days. The incidence and degree of progressive neurologic deficit were no different between the two groups, and no statistically significant difference in short- or long-term disability was found. Mortality was greater in the heparin-treated patients, but death predominantly occurred 3–12 months after stroke and appeared to be unrelated to acute treatment. These results suggest that heparin has no beneficial effect on acute partial stroke.

In patients with recent or multiple TIAs, the risk of cerebral infarction appears to be highest in the period immediately after the transient events, particularly during the first month. To minimize this risk, many neurologists consider the use of heparin appropriate while the underlying etiology is being investigated. However, no clinical data support the use of heparin as an effective therapy in patients with recent TIA. A population-based, retrospective study evaluated the effect of heparin in patients with recent (<30 days) TIA [56]. No significant differences were observed in the risk of death, stroke, or recurrent TIA between the 102 patients treated with heparin and the 187 patients who did not receive the drug. In a small randomized study, heparin was compared with aspirin (1,300 mg/day) in 55 patients with recent TIA [54]. Recurrent TIA occurred in equal proportions during an average treatment period of 5.5 days, but infarction was more common in the aspirin group. The study sample size was too small for meaningful statistical analysis. Crescendo TIA is a particularly ominous situation in which multiple TIAs occur during a brief period with increasing duration or severity of deficit. Again, conflicting data obscure the role of heparin [53,57], although it is frequently used in this potentially dire circumstance.

Beyond the question of the indication for heparin in the treatment of acute ischemic stroke lies the controversy regarding the optimal means of administration. Heparin can be administered by the intravenous or subcutaneous route, by infusion or by repeated doses, titrated to a therapeutic level by the partial thromboplastin time, or given as a fixed dose, each for a variable duration of therapy. Given the complete lack of data regarding these parameters, all decisions regarding the practical pharmacologic issues of acute heparinization are empiric. Many institutions use heparin dosing protocols to standardize such therapy [58], but none have been validated for use in ischemic stroke. Similarly, the risks of heparin in patients with acute stroke are poorly defined. Elevated blood pressure, elevated partial thromboplastin time, infarct size, patient age, and duration of therapy have all been implicated as risk factors for hemorrhage associated with heparin therapy, but only on the basis of anecdotal evidence.

Low-Molecular-Weight Heparin and Heparinoids

The fractionation of heparin produces low-molecular-weight heparins (LMWHs), which may be more effective in preventing thrombosis with an improved margin of safety [59,60]. Like standard heparin, LMWHs bind to antithrombin III to produce an anticoagulant effect. LMWHs cause less platelet inhibition, however, resulting in less bleeding. In addition, they have greater bioavailability and are easier to administer. Because the response to fixed-dose therapy is relatively consistent and predictable, LMWHs can be given as a single daily subcutaneous injection without laboratory monitoring in most cases.

A randomized, double-blind, placebo-controlled trial was performed in Hong Kong in 306 patients with acute ischemic stroke who presented within 48 hours of the onset of symptoms [61]. Patients were assigned to either high-dose LMWH (nadroparin), low-dose nadroparin, or placebo for a total of 10 days. Although outcome was no different at 3 months, the number of patients left dead or disabled at 6 months was significantly reduced among patients treated with the LMWH compared to placebo ($p = .005$). No significant difference was found among the groups with regard to hemorrhagic transformation of the infarction or acute bleeding complications. Ongoing studies have been unable to confirm these results.

Heparinoids are novel compounds that are believed to offer effective anticoagulation with minimal bleeding risk. The heparinoid ORG 10172 is a composite of heparin sulfate, dermatan sulfate, and chondroitin sulfate [62]. The Trial of ORG 10172 in Acute Stroke Treatment was a randomized, double-blind, placebo-controlled trial in which patients who presented within 24 hours of stroke onset were given a continuous intravenous infusion of the heparinoid or placebo for 7 days [62]. Preliminary analysis (presented at the European Stroke Conference in May 1997) failed to demonstrate a significant difference between patients treated with ORG 10172 and those given placebo in terms of recurrent stroke or clinical outcome at 3 months. However, there may have been a benefit among patients with stroke caused by large vessel atherosclerotic disease.

Ancrod

Ancrod, an enzyme extracted from the venom of the Malaysian pit viper, cleaves fibrinogen into components that neither aggregate nor clot. It has been used as an alternative to heparin in patients with heparin-induced thrombocytopenia. The Stroke Treatment with Ancrod Trial (STAT) is a placebo-controlled trial of 460 patients randomized within 3 hours of stroke onset to receive a continuous intravenous infusion of ancrod or placebo for 3 days. Preliminary studies and interim analyses have suggested that the risk of symptomatic intracerebral hemorrhage is less than 2.4%. Efficacy is not yet determined, but the study is nearing completion.

Antiplatelet Therapy: Aspirin

The value of early antiplatelet therapy in acute stroke had not been assessed until the 1990s. The largest trial to do so was the aspirin limb of the IST [42]. Performed in parallel with the heparin analysis described previously, 19,435 patients with acute ischemic stroke were randomly allocated to receive aspirin, 300 mg/day, or to avoid aspirin. Therapy was initiated within the first 48 hours of onset and continued for 14 days or until hospital discharge. Half of the patients in each group were also given subcutaneous heparin during this period. Aspirin reduced the risk of recurrent ischemic stroke from 3.9% to 2.8% ($p < .05$), a relative risk reduction of more than 20%, but had no effect on mortality. No significant increase was found in the rate of intracerebral hemorrhage in patients treated with aspirin (0.8% vs. 0.9%, NS). Overall, aspirin use offered a small but significant benefit when started within the first 48 hours after stroke onset.

In the Chinese Acute Stroke Trial [63], 21,106 patients with acute ischemic stroke were given either aspirin, 160 mg per day, or placebo within 48 hours after the onset of symptoms; this was continued for up to 4 weeks. Aspirin reduced the risk of recurrent ischemic stroke from 2.1% to 1.6% ($p = .01$) and mortality from 3.9% to 3.3% ($p = .04$). A nonsignificant trend toward a small increased risk of intracerebral bleeding in patients who received aspirin occurred. At the time of discharge from the hospital, approximately 11 fewer patients per 1,000 were dead or dependent among those treated with aspirin compared to placebo, comparable to the small but significant benefit found in the IST.

Conclusions: Antithrombotic Therapy in Acute Ischemic Stroke

Antithrombotic therapy is appropriate in many patients with acute stroke, but is absolutely contraindicated for at least 24 hours in all patients who are treated with intravenous t-PA. In patients without contraindications, the routine use of aspirin during the first 14 days after stroke will prevent approximately 11 recurrent strokes per 1,000 patients treated, and may improve mortality. The routine use of heparin in all patients may offer little or no benefit to most patients. Specific patient groups may benefit from acute heparin therapy, although the data to support this view remain limited. Newer antithrombotic therapies are on the horizon, but the results of several major trials are needed before these can be incorporated into clinical practice.

NEUROPROTECTION

The ischemic cascade can be interrupted at many junctures. The earliest events, including calcium influx, neurotransmitter release, and enzyme activation, are potential targets for hyperacute therapy. Later events, such as free-radical formation, gene expression, inflammation, and apoptosis, might be amenable to a longer time window of therapeutic intervention. In animal stroke models, several neuroprotective agents have shown efficacy when aimed at these targets. Preliminary studies in humans have been promising, and several agents are nearing U.S. Food and Drug Administration evaluation. None of these drugs has been proved to be safe and effective for acute stroke, however, and none are currently approved by the Food and Drug Administration for this purpose. Because of the vast number of potential neuroprotective agents, this review is limited to those that are nearly finished or have completed phase III trials (Table 7.3).

Calcium channel blockers were the first neuroprotective agents to be proposed. Nimodipine is a proven therapy for the ischemic complications associated with subarachnoid hemorrhage but provided no significant benefit for ischemic

Table 7.3   Neuroprotective agents in clinical trials

Drug	Time window (hrs)	Putative mechanism of action	Status
Aptiganel	6	Noncompetitive NMDA receptor antagonist	Completed, negative
Nalmefene	6	Kappa opiate antagonist, indirect glutamate antagonist	Completed, pending
Fosphenytoin	6	Ion channel blocker, indirect glutamate antagonist	In progress
Enlimomab	6	Inhibitor of intercellular adhesion molecule–1	Completed, negative
Lubeluzole	6–8	Inhibitor of glutamate release and nitric oxide toxicity	Completed, negative
Nimodipine	6	Calcium channel blocker	In progress
Citicoline	24	Membrane component analogue, free-radical scavenger	In progress

NMDA = *N*-methyl-D-aspartate.

stroke patients in a major study [64]. Nimodipine, 60, 120, or 240 mg per day or placebo for 21 days, was given orally to patients who presented within the first 48 hours after onset of symptoms. They had no difference in neurologic outcome or mortality compared with those given placebo, and high-dose nimodipine therapy was limited by significant hypotension. Post hoc analysis suggested benefit in those patients who were treated with 60 or 120 mg per day starting within the first 12 hours after onset, however, and further evaluation of nimodipine at lower doses and within a narrower time frame is under way. Because calcium entry is an early event in the ischemic cascade, it is likely that neuroprotection at this level will require very early intervention.

Glutamate is the major cause of excitatory neurotoxicity in stroke. Inhibition of glutamate release or binding at its receptors was shown to be neuroprotective in animals [65,66]. However, early human trials of glutamate receptor antagonists, such as MK-801, were limited by central side effects [67,68]. Newer, safer drugs have been developed more recently. Lubeluzole (Prosynap) inhibits glutamate release and the nitric oxide–mediated intracellular consequences of glutamate neurotoxicity and appeared to be safe and effective in small preliminary studies [69]. In a 1997 North American phase III trial, lubeluzole or placebo was given intravenously to 700 patients within 6 hours of stroke onset at a dose of 10 mg per day for 5 days [70]. Lubeluzole treatment caused significantly fewer patients to be dead or disabled at 3 months, and the side effect profile was minimal. However, a trial of lubeluzole conducted simultaneously in Europe and Australia did not find significant benefit [71]. Preliminary results from an additional phase III study again suggested no overall benefit of lubeluzole for acute stroke patients.

Aptiganel (Cerestat, CNS-1102) is a noncompetitive antagonist of the glutamate N-methyl-D-aspartate receptor. Although aptiganel was relatively well tolerated in early trials [72], a phase III trial for acute stroke within 6 hours of symptom onset was discontinued because of safety and efficacy concerns.

Other promising new agents for which phase III trials have been initiated include nalmefene (Cervene), a kappa opiate antagonist; and fosphenytoin (Cerebyx), an ion channel blocker, both of which also use a 6-hour time window, although their direct effects on the earliest stages of neuronal ischemia are unclear.

Enlimomab, an antibody directed against intercellular adhesion molecule–1, also offers a neuroprotective effect late in the course of ischemia in animal models [73]. Regional expression of intercellular adhesion molecule–1 promotes leukocyte adhesion and infiltration in the ischemic territory, resulting in enhanced tissue damage. A double-blind, randomized, placebo-controlled trial enrolled 625 patients within 6 hours of stroke onset and demonstrated worse outcome (higher mortality and morbidity) in enlimomab-treated patients. The poor outcome in the treatment group may in part be related to enlimomab-induced fever [74]. Similar anti-inflammatory compounds are the subjects of ongoing investigation.

The membrane component precursor, CDP-choline (citicoline), is believed to have a dual neuroprotective effect. Citicoline stabilizes neuronal membrane, promotes the synthesis of acetylcholine, and inhibits the formation of free radicals [75,76]. Preliminary studies demonstrated significant improvement in recovery at a dose of 500 mg orally per day for 6 weeks and no important side effects [77,78]. The phase III trial, completed in March 1997, showed no overall effect. However, patients with more severe strokes (NIHSS ≥8) may have benefited. A new citicoline trial includes patients who present within 24 hours of symptom onset with a minimum NIHSS score of 8.

At present, neuroprotective therapies remain a focus of clinical research. No specific medication can be recommended for limiting the damage caused by an acute stroke, although several potential neuroprotectants are available for other uses. Soon, clinical research studies will yield more compelling data in support of at least some of these agents, and it is likely that early intervention will be as important for neuroprotection as it is for reperfusion.

SUPPORTIVE CARE

Management of the patient with acute ischemic stroke depends in part on the clinical manifestations of the stroke, severity of the deficit, size and site of infarction, coexisting conditions, and patient and family issues. Nevertheless, several general factors are important for all patients, such as airway and oxygenation, blood pressure and hemodynamics, temperature, and blood glucose. In the most critically ill patients, specific therapies are indicated to control cerebral edema and elevated intracranial pressure (ICP).

Routine Care

Respiratory function must be evaluated immediately in all stroke patients. Although ventilatory drive is usually intact for the majority, notable exceptions are seen in stroke patients with medullary or massive hemispheric infarction. Similarly, the patient's ability to protect his or her airway from aspiration may be impaired, particularly in the acute setting. Endotracheal intubation and mechanical ventilation are necessary in these patients [79]. However, intubation and ventilation may be associated with alterations in hemodynamic parameters and ICP. Short-acting sedatives, such as thiopental and propofol, are preferable, as is rapid neuromuscular blockade with succinylcholine. Most stroke patients do not require such aggressive maneuvers, but supplemental oxygen should be provided to maintain the oxygen saturation above 95% [80].

Maintenance of adequate blood pressure is vital for all patients. Cerebral blood flow is dependent on cerebral perfusion pressure, which in turn is determined by the difference between mean arterial pressure and ICP. Hypertension is a common finding at the time of initial stroke presentation, even among patients without prior elevation in pressure. Rapid treatment of hypertension in this setting is believed to be detrimental and should generally be avoided, because the autoregulation of cerebral blood flow is impaired in the ischemic zone and a decline in mean arterial pressure can result in worsening ischemia [81]. Most patients will have spontaneous and gradual reductions of blood pressure during the first hours to days after stroke [81]. Anti-hypertensive therapy may be indicated in several instances: (1) before and during thrombolysis with t-PA, (2) after significant hemorrhagic conversion of the infarction, (3) in the presence of myocardial ischemia or aortic dissection, and (4) in association with hypertensive encephalopathy. Candidates for thrombolysis should only be treated with modest measures, such as topical nitropaste or one to two intravenous boluses of labetalol (10–20 mg), to maintain blood pressure below 185/110 mm Hg. If these attempts are not effective, t-PA should not be given. Definitive treatment is appropriate for the other indications and intravenous infusions of labetalol, nicardipine, or sodium nitroprusside may be necessary.

Careful volume replacement improves cardiac output and cerebral perfusion in many patients with acute stroke [82]. Additional fluid administration, or hypervolemic hemodilution, has been advocated as another method for increasing cerebral blood flow. Blood volume can be increased systemically, while reducing blood viscosity and increasing blood flow without a reduction in oxygen delivery. Animal models have suggested that reduction of the hematocrit to 30–33% is optimal [83]. This can be achieved with intravenous crystalloid or colloid plasma volume expanders. Hypervolemic hemodilution with saline is the least expensive of these therapies, but it does not remain in the intravascular bed for long, and large volumes can cause complications in patients with coexisting cardiac or renal disease. Randomized studies of dextran therapy have yielded mixed results [84–86], with the largest of these [86] showing no benefit. Additional investigation is required before hemodilution can be recommended for the majority of stroke patients. The advent of novel blood substitutes may dramatically enhance the possibilities for hemodilution therapy in the future. These agents are acellular fluids that can reduce serum viscosity and increase the oxygen-carrying capacity of blood. However, their role in clinical medicine is just beginning.

Hypothermia has been associated with improved outcomes from ischemic injury in animal models and during complex cardiac and neurosurgical procedures, but has not been adequately studied in acute stroke. Hypothermia can mitigate neurotransmitter toxicity, reduce neuronal metabolic demands (with relative sparing of cerebral blood flow), and improve cerebral edema [87]. On the other hand, fever or even mild hyperthermia is deleterious [88]. In a noninterventional study from 1996, a significant negative association was found with elevated body temperature on admission, such that the relative risk of severe disability or death increased by a factor of 2.2 for each 1°C [89]. Normothermia should be maintained with antipyretics or cooling blankets, but true hypothermia must undergo more investigation before it can be recommended.

Hyperglycemia at the time of stroke admission also appears to correlate with poor outcome [90]. Extraneous glucose can be metabolized to lactic acid, subsequently resulting in acidosis and increased tissue injury. Although the effect of normalizing the level is unknown, rapid control of blood sugars is recommended. Obviously, care must be taken to avoid overshooting into the hypoglycemic range. The administration of parenteral glucose should be minimized in patients with acute stroke.

Treatment of Cerebral Edema

In 10–15% of stroke patients, elevated ICP and compartmental shifts can complicate the clinical course. Pressure is exerted by the expanding zone of infarction and edema, causing both focal and diffuse effects that are typically maximal at 2–5 days [91,92]. The pathophysiology of this phenomenon is poorly understood, but the clinical manifestations are well recognized. In large hemispheric stroke, the malignant MCA syndrome can occur, in which the edematous infarcted tissue causes compression of the anterior and posterior cerebral arteries, resulting in secondary infarctions [91]. Similarly, infarction of the cerebellum can lead to basilar artery compression and brain stem ischemia. Mortality in both conditions approaches 80%. The treatment of elevated ICP caused by stroke is controversial, because each of the available therapeutic maneuvers can theoretically exacerbate the underlying disequilibrium.

Hyperventilation rapidly lowers the ICP by causing cerebral vasoconstriction in response to a low Pco_2. The effect is believed to be brief, however, and may be associated with a rebound increase in ICP when ventilatory status is normalized. Vasoconstriction lowers cerebral blood volume and cerebral blood flow, and can theoretically worsen the ischemic insult to the brain. In the critically ill patient, modest hyperventilation to bring the Pco_2 down to 30–35 mm Hg lowers the ICP by approximately 25% and may be an effective temporizing measure [93].

Mannitol diuresis lowers the ICP by extracting water from the brain and can improve "forward flow" through a bolus effect. Glycerol is also used in some centers, but it has a less potent and less durable effect. The reduction in ICP is rapid and may be longer lasting than that of hyperventilation. In the setting of acute stroke, however, there may be regional variations in the blood-brain barrier that can cause unpredictable effects, including relative expansion of the infarcted region. Moreover, systemic volume shifts can cause either transient dehydration and hypotension or substantial volume overload and congestive heart failure. The role of other diuretics in the treatment of cerebral edema is not well defined.

Steroids are not beneficial in cerebral edema caused by stroke and can exacerbate the situation by causing hyperglycemia and increasing the risk of infection [94,95]. They should be avoided unless they are required for a concomitant medical illness.

Surgical decompression has a potential role for a minority of stroke patients. In acute cerebellar stroke, craniotomy with cerebellar resection is a lifesaving intervention that has become widely accepted [96]. As was noted previously, the major complication of cerebellar infarction is compression of other posterior fossa structures. Surgery removes the mass lesion and alleviates these secondary effects, yet the added morbidity is minimal because only infarcted cerebellar tissue is removed.

The malignant MCA syndrome may be amenable to hemicraniectomy. This seemingly extreme measure has been shown to reduce mortality from 80% to 35% in a few series and may reduce residual infarct volume as well [97,98]. Early decompressive surgery appears to offer the greatest potential benefit of salvaging compromised tissue by improving collateral pial circulation to the ischemic zone. Delayed hemicraniectomy is unlikely to have any effect because the tissue will be irreversibly damaged. Selection criteria for appropriate patients, optimal surgical technique, timing, and the role for adjunctive diagnostic and therapeutic modalities are currently under preliminary investigation in both Europe and the United States.

CONCLUSION

The current management of acute ischemic stroke is only a prelude to stroke treatment in the future. Many options now exist, although the safety and efficacy of most of these remain to be proved. Thrombolysis with t-PA is the only approved treatment for acute stroke, but the time window of 3 hours limits this to a minority of patients. Additions to this armamentarium are expected, with better techniques for improving cerebral blood flow and minimizing neuronal injury. Combined therapies are likely to be particularly beneficial. Moreover, novel imaging modalities may aid in identifying those patients who might respond best to specific treatments. Opportunities to intervene in acute ischemic stroke are emerging, and the prospects for the future are more optimistic than ever before.

ADDENDUM

Since the completion of this chapter, results of the Second European-Australasian Acute Stroke Study (ECASS II) have been published [99]. This was a double-blinded study of 800 acute stroke patients treated within 6 hours of symptom onset with patients randomly assigned to either intravenous t-PA (0.9 mg/kg) or placebo. The protocol was intentionally structured to use tactics and techniques used in the earlier NINDS trial [20]. A favorable outcome, defined as a modified Rankin score ≤ 1 was demonstrated in 40.3% of t-PA–treated patients versus 36.6% of placebo-treated patients ($p = .277$). A less stringent, post-hoc analysis dichotomizing patients into independent versus dependent or dead categories revealed favorable outcomes in 54.3% of t-PA–treated patients compared to 46% of placebo-treated patients ($p = .024$). Symptomatic intracranial hemorrhage occurred in 8.8% of t-PA–treated patients and 3.4% of placebo-treated patients ($p = .001$). The primary efficacy result of ECASS II did not reach statistical significance and therefore does not support the use of t-PA in a 6-hour window. However, the study was not powered to assess the role of t-PA specifically within the first 3 hours. Symptomatic intracranial hemorrhage rates in ECASS II were comparable to those of the NINDS t-PA study, and these data support the safety of t-PA for the treatment of acute ischemic stroke in carefully selected patients. Further research is needed to determine if thrombolysis has any role beyond the first 3 hours after stroke onset.

REFERENCES

1. Hossman K-A. Viability thresholds and the penumbra of focal ischemia. Ann Neurol 1994;36:557.

2. Fisher M, Garcia JH. Evolving stroke and the ischemic penumbra. Neurology 1996;47:884.
3. Minematsu K, Li L, Sotak CH, et al. Reversible focal ischemic injury demonstrated by diffusion-weighted magnetic resonance imaging in rats. Stroke 1992;23:1304.
4. Aronowski J, Strong R, Grotta JC. Treatment of experimental focal ischemia in rats with lubeluzole. Neuropharmacology 1996;35:689.
5. Bratina P, Greenberg L, Pasteur W, Grotta JC. Current emergency department management of stroke in Houston, Texas. Stroke 1995;26:409.
6. Lyden PD, Rapp K, Babcock T, Rothrock J. Ultra-rapid identification, triage, and enrollment of stroke patients into clinical trials. J Stroke Cerebrovasc Dis 1994;4:106.
7. Gomez CR, Malkoff MD, Sauer CM, et al. Code stroke. An attempt to shorten inhospital therapeutic delays. Stroke 1994;25:1920.
8. Adams HP, Bendixen BH, Kappelle LJ, et al., and the TOAST Investigators. Classification of subtype of acute ischemic stroke. Definitions for use in a multicenter clinical trial. Stroke 1993;24:35.
9. Madden KP, Karanjia PN, Adams HP, Clarke WR, and the TOAST Investigators. Accuracy of initial stroke subtype diagnosis in the TOAST study. Neurology 1995;45:1975.
10. Heiss W-D, Herholz K. Assessment of pathophysiology of stroke by positron emission tomography. Eur J Nucl Med 1994;21:455.
11. Marchal G, Beaudouin V, Rioux P, et al. Prolonged persistence of substantial volumes of potentially viable brain tissue after stroke. A correlative PET-CT study with voxel-based data analysis. Stroke 1996;27:599.
12. Alexandrov AV, Grotta JC, Davis SM, Lassen NA. Brain SPECT and thrombolysis in acute ischemic stroke: time for a clinical trial. J Nucl Med 1996;37:1259.
13. Warach S, Dashe JF, Edelman RR. Clinical outcome in ischemic stroke predicted by early diffusion-weighted and perfusion magnetic resonance imaging: a preliminary analysis. J Cereb Blood Flow Metab 1996;16:53.
14. Fisher M, Prichard JW, Warach S. New magnetic resonance techniques for acute ischemic stroke. JAMA 1995;274:908.
15. Minematsu K, Fisher M, Li L, Sotak CH. Diffusion and perfusion magnetic resonance imaging studies to evaluate a noncompetitive N-methyl-D-aspartate antagonist and reperfusion in experimental stroke in rats. Stroke 1993;24:2074.
16. Baron JC, von Kummer R, del Zoppo GJ. Treatment of acute ischemic stroke. Challenging the concept of a rigid and universal time window. Stroke 1995;26:2219.
17. Anderson HV, Willerson JT. Thrombolysis in acute myocardial infarction. N Engl J Med 1993;329:703.
18. Hacke W, Toni D, Steiner T, et al. for the ECASS Study Group. rt-PA in acute ischemic stroke–results from the ECASS three hour cohort (abstract). Stroke 1997;28:272.
19. von Kummer R, Bozzao L, Bastianello S, Manelfe C, for the ECASS Group. Extent of ischemic brain edema and the response to plasminogen activator in acute hemispheric stroke (abstract). Stroke 1997;28:270.
20. National Institute of Neurological Disorders and Stroke rt-PA Stroke Study Group. Tissue plasminogen activator for acute ischemic stroke. N Engl J Med 1995;333:1581.
21. European Cooperative Acute Stroke Study (ECASS). Intravenous thrombolysis with recombinant tissue plasminogen activator for acute hemispheric stroke. JAMA 1995;274:1017–1025.
22. Multicentre Acute Stroke Trial–Italy (MAST-I) Group. Randomised controlled trial of streptokinase, aspirin, and combination of both in treatment of acute ischemic stroke. Lancet 1995;346:1509.
23. Multicentre Acute Stroke Trial–Europe Study Group. Thrombolytic therapy with streptokinase in acute ischemic stroke. N Engl J Med 1996;335:145.
24. Donnan GA, Davis SM, Chambers BR, et al., for the Australian Streptokinase (ASK) Trial Study Group. Streptokinase for acute ischemic stroke with relationship to time of administration. JAMA 1996;276:961.
25. Fieschi C, Argentino C, Lenzi GL, et al. Clinical and instrumental evaluation of patients with ischemic stroke within the first six hours. J Neurol Sci 1989;91:311.
26. Wolpert SM, Bruckmann H, Greenlee R, et al., and the rt-PA Acute Stroke Study Group. Neuroradiologic evaluation of patients with acute stroke treated with recombinant tissue plasminogen activator. AJNR Am J Neuroradiol 1993;14:3.
27. del Zoppo GJ, Higashida RT, Furlan AJ, et al., and the PROACT Investigators. The Prolyse in Acute Cerebral Thromboembolism Trial (PROACT): results of 6 mg dose tier (abstract). Stroke 1996;27:164.
28. Zeumer H, Freitag H-J, Zanella F, et al. Local intra-arterial fibrinolytic therapy in patients with stroke: urokinase versus recombinant tissue plasminogen activator (r-TPA). Neuroradiology 1993;35:159.

29. Barnwell SL, Clark WM, Nguyen TT, et al. Safety and efficacy of delayed intra-arterial urokinase therapy with mechanical clot disruption for thromboembolic stroke. AJNR Am J Neuroradiol 1994;15:1817.
30. Hiramoto M, Yoshimizu N, Satoh K, Takamatsu S. Intra-arterial urokinase therapy in thromboembolic stroke (abstract). Stroke 1994;25:268.
31. Sasaki O, Takeuchi S, Koike T, et al. Fibrinolytic therapy for acute embolic stroke: intravenous, intracarotid, and intra-arterial local approaches. Neurosurgery 1995;36:246.
32. Mori E, Tabuchi M, Yoshida T, Yamadori A. Intracarotid urokinase with thromboembolic occlusion of the middle cerebral artery. Stroke 1988;19:802.
33. Ferguson RDG, Ferguson JG. Cerebral intraarterial fibrinolysis at the crossroads: is a phase III trial advisable at this time? AJNR Am J Neuroradiol 1994;15:1201.
34. del Zoppo GJ, Higashida RT, Furlan AJ. The case for a phase III trial of cerebral intraarterial fibrinolysis. AJNR Am J Neuroradiol 1994;15:1217.
35. Scott PA, Lowell MJ, Longstreth K. Analysis of U.S. population with geographic access to interventional neuroradiology and intra-arterial thrombolysis for acute ischemic stroke (abstract). Stroke 1997;28:266.
36. Emergency Management of Stroke (EMS) Investigators. Combined intra-arterial and intravenous tPA for stroke (abstract). Stroke 1997;28:273.
37. Walters BB, Ojemann RG, Heros RC. Emergency carotid endarterectomy. J Neurosurg 1987;66:817.
38. Beebe HG, Archie JP, Baker WH, et al. Concern about safety of carotid angioplasty. Stroke 1996;27:197.
39. Markus HS, Clifton A, Buckenham T, et al. Improvement in cerebral hemodynamics after carotid angioplasty. Stroke 1996;27:612.
40. Higashida RT, Halbach VV, Cahan LD, et al. Transluminal angioplasty for treatment of intracranial artery vasospasm. J Neurosurg 1989;71:648.
41. Marsh EE, Adams HP, Biller J, et al. Use of antithrombotic drugs in the treatment of acute ischemic stroke: a survey of neurologists in practice in the United States. Neurology 1989;39:1631.
42. International Stroke Trial Collaborative Group. The International Stroke Trial (IST): a randomised trial of aspirin, heparin, both, or neither among 19,435 patients with acute ischaemic stroke. Lancet 1997;349:1569.
43. Cerebral Embolism Study Group. Immediate anticoagulation of embolic stroke: a randomized trial. Stroke 1983;14:668.
44. Cerebral Embolism Study Group. Immediate anticoagulation of embolic stroke: brain hemorrhage and management options. Stroke 1984;15:779.
45. Haley EC, Kassell NF, Torner JC. Failure of heparin to prevent progression in progressing ischemic infarction. Stroke 1988;19:10.
46. Irino T, Watanabe M, Nishide M, et al. Angiographical analysis of acute cerebral infarction followed by "cascade"-like deterioration of minor neurological deficits. What is progressing stroke? Stroke 1983;14:363.
47. Gautier JC. Stroke-in-progression. Stroke 1985;16:729.
48. Baker RN, Broward JA, Fang HC, et al. Anticoagulant therapy in cerebral infarction. Report on cooperative study. Neurology 1962;12:823.
49. Fisher CM. Anticoagulant therapy in cerebral thrombosis and cerebral embolism: a national cooperative study, interim report (part 2). Neurology 1961;11:119.
50. Carter AB. Anticoagulant treatment in progressing stroke. BMJ 1961;2:70.
51. Millikan CH, McDowell FH. Treatment of progressing stroke. Stroke 1981;12:397.
52. Ramirez-Lassepas M, Quinones MR, Nino HH. Treatment of acute ischemic stroke. Open trial with continuous intravenous heparinization. Arch Neurol 1986;43:386.
53. Putnam SF, Adams HP. Usefulness of heparin in initial management of patients with recent transient ischemic attacks. Arch Neurol 1985;42:960.
54. Biller J, Bruno A, Adams HP, et al. A randomized trial of aspirin or heparin in hospitalized patients with recent transient ischemic attacks. A pilot study. Stroke 1989;20:441.
55. Duke RJ, Bloch RF, Turpie AGG, et al. Intravenous heparin for the prevention of stroke progression in acute partial stable stroke: a randomised controlled trial. Ann Intern Med 1986;105:825.
56. Keith DS, Phillips SJ, Whisnant JP, et al. Heparin therapy for recent transient focal cerebral ischemia. Mayo Clin Proc 1987;62:1101.
57. Nehler MR, Moneta GL, McConnell DB, et al. Anticoagulation followed by elective carotid surgery in patients with repetitive transient ischemic attacks and high-grade carotid stenosis. Arch Surg 1993;128:1117.

58. Raschke RA, Reilly BM, Guidry JR, et al. The weight-based heparin dosing nomogram compared with a "standard care" nomogram. Ann Intern Med 1993;119:874.

59. Leizorovicz A, Simonneau G, Decousus H, Boissel JP. Comparison of efficacy and safety of low molecular weight heparins and unfractionated heparin in initial treatment of deep venous thrombosis: a meta-analysis. BMJ 1994;309:299.

60. Hull RD, Raskob GE, Pineo GF, et al. Subcutaneous low-molecular-weight heparin compared with continuous intravenous heparin in the treatment of proximal-vein thrombosis. N Engl J Med 1992;326:975.

61. Kay R, Wong KS, Yu YL, et al. Low-molecular-weight heparin for the treatment of acute ischemic stroke. N Engl J Med 1995;333:1588.

62. Adams HP, Woolson RF, Biller J, Clarke W. Studies of ORG 10172 in patients with acute ischemic stroke. TOAST Study Group. Haemostasis 1992;22:99.

63. CAST (Chinese Acute Stroke Trial) Collaborative Group. CAST: randomised placebo-controlled trial of early aspirin use in 20,000 patients with acute ischemic stroke. Lancet 1997;349:1641.

64. The American Nimodipine Study Group. Clinical trial of nimodipine in acute ischemic stroke. Stroke 1992;23:3.

65. De Ryck M, Keersmaekers R, Clincke G, et al. Lubeluzole, a novel benzothiazole, protects neurologic function after cerebral thrombotic stroke in rats: an apparent stereospecific effect. Soc Neurosci Abstr 1994;20:185.

66. Grotta J. The current status of neuronal protective therapy: why have all neuronal protective drugs worked in animals but none so far in stroke patients? Cerebrovasc Dis 1994;4:115.

67. Olney J, Labruyere J, Wang G, et al. NMDA antagonist neurotoxicity: mechanism and prevention. Science 1991;254:1515.

68. Lipton SA, Rosenberg PA. Excitatory amino acids as a final common pathway for neurologic disorders. N Engl J Med 1994;330:613.

69. Diener HC, Hacke W, Hennerici M, et al., for the Lubeluzole International Study Group. Lubeluzole in acute ischemic stroke. A double-blind, placebo-controlled phase II trial. Stroke 1996;27:76.

70. Grotta J, Hantson L, Wessel T, for the LUB-INT-9 Lubeluzole Study Group. The efficacy and safety of lubeluzole in patients with acute ischemic stroke (abstract). Stroke 1997;28:271.

71. Diener HC, Kaste M, Hacke W, et al, for the LUB-INT-5 Lubeluzole Study Group. Lubeluzole in acute ischemic stroke (abstract). Stroke 1997;28:271.

72. Muir KW, Grosset DG, Gamzu E, Lees KR. Pharmacological effects of the non-competitive NMDA antagonist CNS 1102 in normal volunteers. Br J Clin Pharmacol 1994;38:33.

73. Bowes MP, Rothlein R, Fagan SC, Zivin JA. Monoclonal antibodies preventing leukocyte activation reduce experimental neurologic injury and enhance efficacy of thrombolytic therapy. Neurology 1995;45:815.

74. Enlimomab Acute Stroke Trial Investigators. The Enlimomab Acute Stroke Trial: final results (abstract). Neurology 1997;48(suppl 2):A270.

75. Schabitz WR, Weber J, Takano K, et al. The effects of prolonged treatment with citicoline in temporary experimental focal ischemia. J Neurol Sci 1996;138:21.

76. D'Orlando KJ, Sandage BW. Citicoline (CDP-choline): mechanisms of action and effects in ischemic brain injury. Neurol Res 1995;17:281.

77. Pettigrew LC, Clark WM, Warach S, Sabounjian LA, for the Citicoline Stroke Study Group. Effect of citicoline on cognitive function in acute stroke (abstract). Stroke 1997;28:271.

78. Warach S, Sabounjian LA. Effects of citicoline on the evolution of lesion volume as measured by diffusion-weighted imaging (abstract). Stroke 1997;28:233.

79. Grotta JC, Pasteur W, Khwaja G, et al. Elective intubation for neurologic deterioration after stroke. Neurology 1995;45:640.

80. Vender RL. Respiratory management after stroke: what to do, what to avoid. J Crit Illness 1992;7:1895.

81. Lisk DR, Grotta JC, Lamki LM, et al. Should hypertension be treated after acute stroke? A randomized controlled trial using single photon emission computed tomography. Arch Neurol 1993;50:855.

82. Grotta JC, Pettigrew LC, Allen S, et al. Baseline hemodilution state and response to hemodilution in patients with acute cerebral ischemia. Stroke 1985;16:790.

83. Lee SH, Heros RC, Mullan JC, Korosue K. Optimum degree of hemodilution for brain protection in a canine model of focal cerebral ischemia. J Neurosurg 1994;80:469.

84. Koller M, Haenny P, Hess K, et al. Adjusted hypervolemic hemodilution in acute ischemic stroke. Stroke 1990;21:1429.

85. Strand T, Asplund K, Eriksson S, et al. A randomized controlled trial of hemodilution therapy in acute ischemic stroke. Stroke 1984;15:980.
86. Italian Acute Stroke Study Group. Hemodilution in acute stroke: results of the Italian haemodilution trial. Lancet 1988;1:318.
87. Maher J, Hachinski V. Hypothermia as a potential treatment of cerebral ischemia. Cerebrovasc Brain Metab Rev 1993;5:277.
88. Azzimondi G, Bassein L, Nonino F, et al. Fever in acute stroke worsens prognosis: a prospective study. Stroke 1995;26:2040.
89. Reith J, Jorgensen S, Pedersen PM, et al. Body temperature in acute stroke: relation to stroke severity, infarct size, mortality, and outcome. Lancet 1996;347:422.
90. Pulsinelli WA, Levy DE, Sigsbee B, et al. Increased damage after ischemic stroke in patients with hyperglycemia with or without established diabetes mellitus. Am J Med 1983;74:540.
91. Hacke W, Schwab S, Horn M, et al. The "malignant" middle cerebral artery territory infarction: clinical course and prognostic signs. Arch Neurol 1996;53:309.
92. Frank JI. Large hemispheric infarction, deterioration, and intracranial pressure. Neurology 1995;45:1286.
93. James HE, Langfitt TW, Kumar VS, Ghostine SY. Treatment of intracranial hypertension. Analysis of 105 consecutive, continuous recordings of intracranial pressure. Acta Neurochir 1977;36:189.
94. Norris JW, Hachinski VC. High dose steroid treatment in cerebral infarction. BMJ 1986;292:21.
95. Norris JW. Steroid therapy in acute cerebral infarction. Arch Neurol 1976;33:69.
96. Rieke K, Krieger D, Adams HP, et al. Therapeutic strategies in space-occupying cerebellar infarction based on clinical, neuroradiological and neurophysiological data. Cerebrovasc Dis 1993;3:45.
97. Rieke K, Schwab S, Krieger D, et al. Decompressive surgery in space-occupying hemispheric infarction: results of an open, prospective trial. Crit Care Med 1995;23:1576.
98. Steiner T, Krieger D, Jauss M, et al. Hemicraniectomy for massive cerebral infarction: presurgical prognostic factors (abstract). Stroke 1995;26:172.
99. Hacke W, Kaste M, Fieschi C, et al., for the Second European-Australasian Acute Stroke Study Investigators. Randomised double-blind placebo-controlled trial of thrombolytic therapy with intravenous alteplase in acute ischaemic stroke (ECASS II). Lancet 1998;352:1245.

8
Thrombosis of the Cerebral Veins and Sinuses

R. W. Ross Russell

Thrombosis of the cerebral veins or sinuses is a relatively neglected aspect of vascular disease. It differs from arterial thrombosis in a number of respects: It affects a much younger age group, has a much wider variety of causes, and has distinctive though varied symptoms. Most important, patients can make a remarkable recovery if the correct treatment is given promptly. This treatment must not only be directed at thrombosis but also at the underlying cause. The initial symptoms of venous thrombosis, consisting of headache, seizures, focal deficit, and altered consciousness, may be sudden and severe, and patients are often admitted to an intensive care unit. The attending physician should be familiar with the clinical symptoms, the most appropriate investigations, and the general management and complications of the disease as well as with emergency treatment.

This chapter briefly outlines the venous anatomy of the brain and the consequences of venous occlusion both in the brain and in the blood vessels. This is followed by an account of the causes of thrombosis of veins and sinuses and of the clinical symptoms and signs. The final sections deal with management, investigation, and treatment, with an emphasis on acute cases and on the major advances that have occurred since 1990, notably the crucial role of early and effective antithrombotic therapy.

STRUCTURE AND FUNCTION OF CEREBRAL VEINS

The venous drainage of the forebrain takes place through a system of surface veins draining the superficial 2 cm of each hemisphere and a system of internal (galenic) veins draining much of the interior of the hemispheres, including the basal nuclei. The blood then passes directly or indirectly into one of the dural sinuses and then to the internal jugular veins.

The superficial veins of each hemisphere comprise a superior group draining the superior surface upward into the superior sagittal sinus (SSS); a middle group draining the remainder of the cortex over the convexity of the brain into the cavernous sinus; and an inferior group draining the undersurface of the brain into the cavernous, superior petrosal, and lateral (transverse) sinuses (LSs). The internal veins drain much of the deep cerebral white matter, the basal nuclei, the hypothalamus and choroid plexus via the basal and internal cerebral veins that converge on the unpaired great vein of Galen, and then the straight sinus and torcular (confluence of the sinuses).

Small veins communicate freely on the surface of the brain; in addition, there are two larger anastomotic channels, the superior anastomotic vein (Trolard's vein), which links the SSS with the middle cerebral vein, and the inferior anastomotic vein (Labbé's vein), which links the middle cerebral vein with the transverse sinus. Within the cerebral substance, the veins run perpendicularly to the surface in a similar manner to arteries, each draining a cylindrical core of tissue; few vein-to-vein anastomoses are found within the brain.

The veins of the cerebellum and brain stem are situated on the surface and drain directly into adjacent sinuses: occipital, transverse, and straight sinuses.

The venous sinuses are relatively thick-walled structures enclosed by folds of dura. In addition to receiving the cerebral veins, they also drain the diploic vein of the skull and communicate with the scalp veins by a series of transcranial emissary veins. The SSS has a number of lateral expansions (venous lakes) within the dura.

Blood from the SSS flows mainly into the right transverse sinus, whereas the straight sinus drains mainly to the left side (Figure 8.1). The extent to which the two sides communicate at the torcular is very variable. As well as being a major route of venous drainage, the SSS has an important role in the circulation of cerebrospinal fluid (CSF). The arachnoid granulations project into the sinus or the lateral lacunae and act as minute valves that allow the passage of CSF from the subarachnoid space into the venous system.

The structure of the sinuses, which are enveloped by folds of dura, ensures that they do not collapse but remain open at all times, even with a negative transmural pressure. Cerebral veins do not have this rigid structure but they, too, remain open because the intraluminal pressure is always higher than the pressure in the surrounding CSF. Cerebral arteries show autoregulation, changing caliber in response to changes in blood pressure or CSF pressure but venous caliber remains relatively constant. The veins are also much less sensitive than arteries to the effects of changes in pH or potassium concentration in the perivascular fluid.

CONSEQUENCES OF VENOUS OCCLUSION

The consequences of venous occlusion depend partly on the rate of occlusion but more importantly on its extent. If a superficial vein is occluded at a single point, blood can be rerouted via existing channels and no damage ensues. If the blockage is more extensive and involves anastomotic vessels, venous pressure may rise, with venous distention and localized edema. Finally, if pressure rises still further,

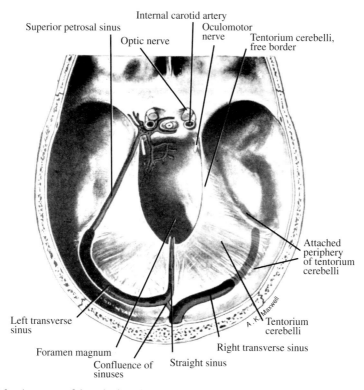

Figure 8.1   Anatomy of the principal dural venous sinuses. (Reprinted with permission from PL Williams. Gray's Anatomy. New York: Churchill Livingstone, 1995.)

perfusion pressure may be inadequate to sustain cerebral blood flow, and cerebral infarction, often hemorrhagic, results. Should venous occlusion occur slowly, allowing anastomotic channels to develop, the brain may escape damage.

If the SSS or LS is involved, the rise in venous pressure can impede absorption of CSF or the arachnoid granulations can become blocked by thrombus. In either case, the result is a rise in intracranial pressure

Venous thrombi have a different composition from those formed in arteries. Although initiated by platelet adhesion and aggregation, they are composed mainly of a fibrin meshwork that contains clumps of red cells and are formed under conditions of slow or stagnant flow. As in the systemic veins, cerebral venous thrombi tend to extend and propagate forward and backward. Thrombi beginning in surface veins can spread to the venous sinuses, and thrombi formed initially in the dural sinuses can extend retrogradely to the surface or anastomotic veins.

The naturally occurring fibrinolytic system is capable of completely removing freshly formed thrombus and restoring normal venous patency. If lysis does not occur, the thrombus may undergo organization and become adherent to the vessel wall. Recanalization of the organized thrombus may follow with partial or complete restoration of the lumen. Before the thrombus becomes adherent, there

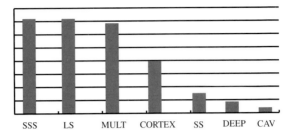

SSS	LS	MULT	CORTEX	SS	DEEP	CAV

Figure 8.2   Location of sinovenous thrombosis and relative frequency of thrombosis at various sites. (SSS = superior sagittal sinus; LS = lateral sinus; MULT = multiple sites; CAV = cavernous sinus; SS = straight sinus.) (Adapted from A Ameri, MG Bousser. Cerebral venous thrombosis. Neurol Clin 1993;10:87.)

is a risk of embolism to the heart and lungs; this is especially the case when the sigmoid sinus or internal jugular veins are involved.

The location of sinus thrombosis varies with the underlying cause (Figure 8.2). In noninfective thrombosis, the SSS is most often involved, whereas in infective thrombosis, the LS is most involved because of its proximity to the temporal bone and mastoid. Cavernous sinus thrombosis, now rare, is almost always infective. In thrombosis that results from prothrombotic disorders or from dehydration, it is not uncommon to have multiple sites of thrombosis, usually including the SSS (Table 8.1).

Table 8.1   Varieties of cerebral sinovenous thrombosis

Site	Prevalence (%)	Causes	Clinical features
SSS	72	Idiopathic, puerperal; pro-thrombotic states; obstruction by tumor; trauma	Raised intracranial pressure; spread to cortical veins
LS	72	Otitic infection; prothrombotic states	Spread to SSS; raised intracranial pressure; spread to cortical veins; temporal venous infarction
Straight sinus	15	Dehydration; prothrombotic states	Bilateral thalamic infarction
Cavernous sinus	3	Infection of face, mouth; dural arteriovenous fistula	Cavernous sinus syndrome; proptosis, bilateral spread
Cortical veins	40	Spread from SSS, LS; puerperal	Seizures; focal deficit
Deep veins	8	Dehydration; prothrombotic states	Bilateral signs; alteration of consciousness
Combined	68	Dehydration; prothrombotic states	Encephalitic syndrome

SSS = superior sagittal sinus; LS = lateral sinus.

CLINICAL FEATURES

Onset

The clinical features of sinovenous thrombosis are set out in Table 8.2. In contrast to arterial thrombosis, there is great variation in the rate of onset; in one-third of cases, it is acute (less than 48 hours to presentation), and the main features are seizures and focal deficit. This type is characteristic of puerperal cases. A subacute onset (2–30 days to presentation) occurs in approximately 40% of patients and a chronic onset (more than 30 days) in the remainder. A subacute or chronic onset is the rule in inflammatory or idiopathic cases [1].

Headache

Headache is rarely absent but can be of any grades of severity. In acute cases, it is caused by brain swelling and by the leakage of small quantities of blood from distended veins on the surface of the brain. It can be sudden and severe. In more chronic cases with thrombosis of the SSS or LS, the headache may be intermittent and milder and often has the characteristics of raised intracranial pressure. It is usually accompanied by bilateral papilledema and sometimes by vomiting, visual obscurations, and diplopia from sixth nerve palsy.

Focal Deficit

A focal deficit is present at some time in approximately 60% of patients and indicates cerebral venous infarction, which can be ischemic or hemorrhagic. The most common variety is a unilateral hemiparesis with cortical sensory loss, often predominating in the patient's leg. Spread of thrombosis to both sides can result

Table 8.2   Neurologic signs and symptoms in 110 patients with cerebral venous thrombosis

Signs and symptoms	No. of patients (%)
Headache	83 (75)
Papilledema	54 (49)
Seizures	41 (37)
Motor or sensory deficit	38 (34)
Drowsiness, mental changes, confusion, or coma	33 (30)
Dysphasia	13 (12)
Multiple cranial nerve palsies	13 (12)
Cerebellar incoordination	3 (3)
Bilateral or alternating cortical signs	3 (3)
Nystagmus	2 (2)
Hearing loss	2 (2)

Source: Reprinted with permission from A Ameri, MG Bousser. Cerebral venous thrombosis. Neurol Clin 1993;10:88.

in a cerebral paraparesis. In other cases, the hemiparesis is mainly brachio-facial with or without dysphasia. Isolated homonymous hemianopia is relatively uncommon but a partial hemianopia with visual disorientation and a defect in visually guided movement, indicating a parieto-occipital location, may be found on one or both sides. Cerebellar venous infarction is not often described but can produce an ipsilateral dysmetria and tremor with ataxia, nystagmus, and dysarthria.

Cranial Nerve Palsies

Cranial nerve palsies are a feature of venous thrombosis at specific sites in the venous sinuses. Cavernous sinus thrombosis produces ophthalmoplegia from combined third, fourth, and sixth nerve lesions, sometimes bilateral and with signs of orbital venous congestion and proptosis. Combined fifth and sixth nerve involvement points to thrombosis of the superior petrosal sinus, and combined ninth and tenth cranial nerve palsies indicate thrombosis of the internal jugular vein.

Seizures

Seizures are much more common in venous than in arterial thrombosis and are found in approximately 40% of patients. They indicate an irritative cortical lesion, usually a hemorrhagic venous infarct that can be located in any site, although they most commonly occur anterior to the central sulcus. The seizures can be partial, generalized, or combined and are often followed by aggravation of focal signs. Seizures are often difficult to control, and focal or generalized status epilepticus is common.

Consciousness Level

Impairment of consciousness is not usually a presenting feature of venous thrombosis but is present at some time during the course of the disease in approximately one-half of patients. In its usual form, it consists of drowsiness, lack of concentration, and irritability frequently accompanied by headache and is caused in most cases by raised intracranial pressure. Deep unconsciousness can occur during or after a seizure or in thrombosis involving the galenic system, particularly bilateral thalamic infarction.

Subacute Encephalopathy

Widespread venous thrombosis, especially in the very young or very old and in patients who are terminally ill from malignant disease, cardiac failure, malnutrition, or dehydration, may present as a subacute encephalopathic illness without focal signs and with varying degrees of drowsiness, confusion, headache, and seizures. Often, no signs of raised intracranial pressure are present. The cause is generalized brain swelling, and pathologic examination shows laminar cortical necrosis.

Figure 8.3   Causes of cerebral venous thrombosis.

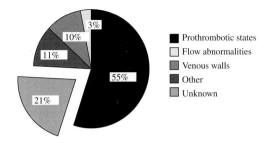

Prothrombotic states
Flow abnormalities
Venous walls
Other
Unknown

PATHOGENESIS

The known causes of cerebral venous thrombosis can be grouped under the three headings originally suggested by Virchow: those arising (1) from an increased thrombotic tendency in the blood, (2) from a defect in the vessel wall causing mural thrombosis, and (3) from a disturbance in blood flow, either local or generalized (Figure 8.3). However, in spite of the many known diseases and abnormalities that have been recorded in association with cerebral venous thrombosis (now more than 100), the cause remains unknown, even after full investigation, in approximately 20% of patients (Table 8.3; see Figure 8.3).

An increased thrombotic tendency may be congenital, acquired, or physiologic (as in pregnancy) and may arise from an abnormality in the coagulation or fibrinolytic systems, in the platelets, or in the vascular endothelium. In contrast to arterial thrombosis, in venous thrombosis abnormalities of coagulation leading to impaired generation of fibrin are of greater importance than are platelet disorders. In the cerebral veins, as in the systemic venous system, thrombi tend to form under conditions of stasis or slow flow and tend to be composed mainly of a fibrin meshwork and red cells.

Prothrombotic States

See Figure 8.4 for a breakdown of the causes of prothrombotic states.

Pregnancy

Pregnancy can be regarded as a physiologic prothrombotic state in which minor changes upset the delicate equilibrium between coagulation, platelet, or fibrinolytic factors. Thrombosis tends to develop in patients with any underlying inherited coagulation defect at this time. Pregnancy is the most commonly identified cause of cerebral venous thrombosis, occurring in approximately 20% of cases, with higher percentages in underdeveloped countries [2] (see Figure 8.4). Many factors contribute to this tendency; in the third trimester the concentrations of procoagulant proteins such as factor II, factor VII, and factor X are increased. Fibrin generation is also increased while the concentration of natural anticoagulant factors, such as protein S, diminishes [3]. Protein C concentration is usually

Table 8.3   Causes of cerebral sinovenous thrombosis

Abnormalities of the blood
  Prothrombotic states
    Physiologic
      Pregnancy
    Blood disease
      Polycythemia (all types)
      Sickle cell disease
      Hemolytic anemia
      Iron deficiency anemia
      Myeloproliferative disease
      Thrombocytosis
      Leukemia
      Paroxysmal nocturnal hemoglobinuria
      Protein C and protein S deficiency
      Antithrombin III deficiency
      Prothrombin gene (20210A) mutation
      Antiphospholipid syndrome
      Cryofibrinogenemia
    Systemic disease
      Carcinomatosis
      Inflammatory bowel disease
      Nephrotic syndrome
      Systemic lupus erythematosus
      Carcinoid syndrome
      Septicemia, human immunodeficiency virus infection
    Iatrogenic
      Steroid therapy
      Other drugs
      Intravenous cannulas
Abnormalities of vessel wall
  Local sepsis
  Trauma, surgery
  Wegener's granuloma
  Sarcoidosis
  Lymphoma, leukemic infiltration
  Behçet's disease
Abnormalities of flow
  Dehydration
  Congenital heart disease
  Congestive heart failure
  Arterial occlusion
  Compression by tumor
  Arteriovenous malformation

unchanged. Other rheologic factors that may play a part are the increased venous distensibility and capacity associated with pregnancy and the venous stasis that occurs with prolonged bed rest, instrumental delivery, and multiparity (Table 8.4).

Thrombosis can occur at any site but is most often in the unpaired dural sinuses, such as the SSS, and can spread to involve cortical veins, producing venous infarction, most often in the posterior parietal or posterior temporal

Figure 8.4   Causes of prothrombotic
states.

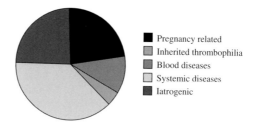

Pregnancy related
Inherited thrombophilia
Blood diseases
Systemic diseases
Iatrogenic

region on one or both sides. The peak prevalence of the illness is 10 days post-partum, but it can occur at any time in the third trimester and, exceptionally, earlier. The onset is usually acute, with severe headache and focal signs such as hemiparesis, which is usually unilateral but may be bilateral or alternating. Seizures are frequent and may be focal or generalized. Signs of raised intracranial pressure, such as papilledema and drowsiness, can develop.

Inherited Prothrombotic States

Congenital absence or reduction in the concentration of naturally occurring anticoagulant proteins can result in venous thrombosis, usually with onset early in life (Table 8.5). Protein C is a serine protease synthesized by the liver and acts as an anticoagulant by virtue of its ability to inactivate factors V and VIII. Protein C is activated by thrombin, and protein S is a cofactor in this reaction. Antithrombin III binds irreversibly to the active site of thrombin and other serine protease coagulation factors, thus inactivating them. Approximately 20% of patients younger than age 45 years who have venous thrombosis are said to be deficient in protein C, protein S, or antithrombin III. Another prothrombotic congenital disorder has been described in which there is a mutation in the gene responsible for factor V, rendering it resistant to the action of protein C (Leiden mutation). This

Table 8.4   Venous thrombosis in pregnancy and puerperium

Prevalence
    4 per 1,000 (systemic)
    1 per 3,000 (cerebral)
Possible factors
    Inherited prothrombotic states
    Protein C, protein S, and antithrombin III deficiency
    Factor V resistant to protein C (Leiden mutation)
Coagulation system changes induced by pregnancy
    Increase in factor II, VII, X
    Reduction in protein S
Flow changes induced by pregnancy
    Venous stasis from bed rest, surgery, age, multiparity
    Increase in venous distensibility and capacity
Other factors
    Sepsis, hemorrhage, instrumental delivery

Table 8.5   Inherited prothrombotic disorders

Disease	Suggested mechanism
Protein C deficiency	Decrease in inhibition of factor V
Protein S deficiency	Decreased cofactor for protein C
Factor Va resistance	Factor Va resistant to action of protein C (Leiden mutation)
Antithrombin III deficiency	Decreased inactivation of thrombin
Familial plasminogen defect	Decreased fibrinolysis
Homocystinuria	Vascular endothelial injury; increased platelet deposition
Prothrombin gene (20210A) mutation	Increased prothrombin concentration

abnormality appears to account for approximately one-half of the previously idiopathic cases of venous thrombosis in young subjects and may prove to be the most important cause of inherited thrombophilia [4]. All of these conditions are inherited in a mendelian-dominant fashion; affected patients are usually heterozygotes and present in the second or third decade with venous thrombosis, most often in their legs and commonly provoked by other factors such as pregnancy, surgery, or oral contraceptive use. When thrombosis affects the cerebral venous system, it is frequently subacute or chronic in onset and may present as intracranial hypertension without focal signs caused by occlusion of the SSS.

Other Inherited Prothrombotic Conditions

Rarely, inherited thrombophilia is caused by a quantitative or qualitative defect in plasminogen, leading to defective fibrinolysis. Widespread cerebral venous thrombosis has been reported [5]. Homocystinuria is a recessively inherited condition in which there is a deficiency in cystathione B synthase, the enzyme responsible for normal cross linkages in collagen. A strong tendency to premature cardiovascular disease exists, both arterial and venous, and the risk of thrombosis is proportional to the plasma concentration of homocysteine. Thrombosis is thought to be initiated by platelet deposition on abnormal vascular endothelium.

Other abnormalities that may predispose to thrombosis include heparin cofactor 11 deficiency or a mutation at position 20210A of the prothrombic gene, leading to increased plasma concentrations of prothrombin. It is at present uncertain if these mutations are causal [6].

Acquired Thrombotic States Secondary to Blood Diseases

A tendency to thrombosis is a common feature in a number of blood disorders (Table 8.6), and in many cases there may be more than one underlying abnormality. These may include defects of platelets and of coagulation as well as physical factors such as slowing of blood flow or changes in viscosity. The myeloproliferative disorders include primary proliferative polycythemia, essential thrombocythemia, chronic myeloid leukemia, and myelofibrosis. Not only are

Table 8.6 Prothrombotic blood disorders

Disease	Suggested mechanism
Polycythemia vera	Increased blood viscosity, slowed flow; increased platelet numbers; abnormal platelet behavior
Primary thrombocythemia	Increased platelet numbers; abnormal platelet behavior
Leukemias	Increased viscosity; meningeal infiltration; effects of treatment (asparaginase)
Sickle cell disease	Increased viscosity; venous endothelial damage
Hemolytic anemias, paroxysmal nocturnal hemoglobinuria	Excess hemolysis; increased thromboplastin release

there increased numbers of red cells, white cells, and platelets, but, in addition, the platelets are often qualitatively abnormal. Patients with these disorders have an increased thrombotic tendency that affects both arteries and veins and occurs in usual and unusual sites, including portal hepatic and mesenteric veins and in the cerebral sinuses.

Primary Proliferative Polycythemia

In proliferative polycythemia, in which there is increased viscosity and slowed blood flow from raised hematocrit as well as an increase in cells and platelets, thrombosis of cerebral arteries or veins is five times more common than in the general population, and documented events include hemispheric venous infarction, raised intracranial pressure from SSS obstruction, and nonseptic cavernous sinus thrombosis. An increased thrombotic tendency in secondary polycythemia and many recorded cases in children with cyanotic heart disease also exist. Altitude polycythemia also causes cerebral sinovenous thrombosis on rare occasions [7].

In primary thrombocythemia, there is hyperplasia of megakaryocytes with a consequent increase in platelet numbers, usually greater than $600 \times 10^9 l^{-1}$ and sometimes as high as $2,500 \times 10^9 l^{-1}$. The platelets are also qualitatively abnormal and may show spontaneous aggregation in the microcirculation. Often, a poor correlation between platelet numbers and thrombosis exists. Cerebral venous thrombosis in this condition is often benign and of slow onset with raised intracranial pressure. The occurrence of thrombosis can be provoked by secondary factors such as pregnancy [8].

Leukemia

Very high white blood cell counts in acute leukemia can increase blood viscosity with stasis and impaction of cellular masses in the microcirculation. Infiltration of meninges and vascular walls by leukemic deposits may also occur.

Thrombosis of cerebral veins or sinuses has been reported mainly in children with acute lymphoblastic leukemia and may present either as venous infarction

Table 8.7   Prothrombotic states secondary to systemic disease

Disease	Suggested mechanism
Malignant disease	Increased thromboplastin (secreted by monocytes, macrophages); tumor proteases (raised factor Xa); increased fibrinogen; increased factors V, VIII, IX, XI; decreased AT III; effects of treatment
Inflammatory bowel disease	Raised thromboplastin; increased platelet numbers; raised factors III, V, VIII; lowered AT III; effects of treatment
Nephrotic syndrome	Increased platelets; increased factors V, VIII; decreased AT III, protein C, plasminogen
Systemic lupus erythematosus	Raised lupus anticoagulant, varied antiphospholipid antibodies; low protein C, protein S, and AT III; decreased fibrinolysis; increased fibrinogen; platelets abnormal

AT III = antithrombin III.

or raised intracranial pressure without focal signs. Treatment with asparaginase, which produces deficiency in antithrombin III, may be an additional causative factor here [9].

Paroxysmal Nocturnal Hemoglobinuria

In paroxysmal nocturnal hemoglobinuria, an unusual acquired genetic disorder caused by a mutation of primitive precursor cells in the bone marrow, chronic hemolytic anemia begins in the third or fourth decade. The risk of venous thrombosis, especially cerebral, appears to be high. This is attributed to excessive release of thromboplastin during hemolysis. Clinical presentation may be either as venous infarction or as intracranial hypertension [10].

Other Types of Anemia

The older literature contains a number of reports of cerebral sinovenous thrombosis in patients with iron deficiency anemia, mainly young women with chronic blood loss. Patients with hemolytic anemias, such as sickle cell disease, are also at increased risk, partly from the sludging effect of deformed erythrocytes in the microcirculation and partly from increased release of thromboplastin. Paraproteinemia does not seem to predispose to cerebral venous thrombosis, but in cryofibrinogenemia extensive thrombosis may occur on exposure to cold. This mainly affects the legs but can extend to other organs, including the brain [11].

Cerebral Venous Thrombosis as a Complication of Systemic Disease or Therapy

Many patients with malignant disease develop thrombosis (Tables 8.7 and 8.8), mainly in the pelvic or leg veins. Up to 50% of patients with pancreatic or mucin-

Table 8.8 Drug-induced cerebral venous thrombosis

Drug	Suggested mechanism
Oral contraceptives	Increased fibrinogen, factors II, VII, VIII, IX, X; decreased antithrombin III; decreased fibrinolysis
Corticosteroids	Increased factor VIII, IX
Epsilon-aminocaproic acid	Decreased plasmin activity
L-Asparaginase	Low plasma proteins, including protein C, protein S, and antithrombin III

secreting carcinoma may be affected. Possible causative factors are an increase in thromboplastin-like substances secreted by macrophages under the influence of tumor antigens. Secretion of proteases by the tumor can also activate coagulation factors and decrease natural anticoagulants. Paradoxically there may also be increased fibrinolytic activity, leading to a hemorrhagic tendency in some patients. Many examples of cerebral venous thrombosis in patients with malignant disease in the absence of local pathology have been reported [12]. The clinical presentation is often as multiple regions of hemorrhagic venous infarction producing seizures and focal signs, and the distinction from metastatic disease may be difficult [13].

Inflammatory Bowel Disease

Venous thrombosis is a common event in ulcerative colitis and may be present in as many as 40% of patients coming to autopsy. Multiple sites are involved, mainly abdominal or thoracic, and cerebral venous thrombosis has frequently been reported [14]. Again, no shortage of possible causes exists, including accelerated thromboplastin generation; thrombocytosis; increased fibrinogen and coagulation factors III, V, and VIII; decreased antithrombin III; and the effects of steroid treatment. Many cases have a fatal outcome from extensive thrombosis of multiple venous sinuses, causing generalized brain edema.

Other types of inflammatory bowel disease, notably regional enteritis (Crohn's disease) and malabsorption states, such as celiac disease, may also occur in association with cerebral venous thrombosis.

Nephrotic Syndrome

An increased risk of either arterial or venous thrombosis is a recognized feature of children with nephrotic syndrome. Possible causative influences include elevated concentrations of coagulation factors V and VIII, increased platelet numbers, and excess loss of natural anticoagulant proteins and plasminogen as a consequence of the heavy proteinuria [15]. Most cases occur in children and can be of any grade of severity, from fatal, generalized brain swelling to chronic, intracranial hypertension with full recovery.

Systemic Lupus Erythematosus

Cerebral venous thrombosis in systemic lupus erythematosus is well documented [16], usually as a complication of well-established disease. The most common presenting features are stroke-like episodes with focal deficit caused by venous infarction. Seizures and headache are also frequent and signs of raised intracranial pressure may be seen. The SSS is the sinus that is most often involved.

Drug-Induced Thrombosis

Oral contraceptive drugs with a high estrogen content were associated early with an increased risk of venous thrombosis in the legs and arterial thrombosis in the brain (see Table 8.8). The mode of action is complex and includes a rise in fibrinogen and coagulation factors II, VII, VIII, IX, and X with a decrease in antithrombin III and fibrinolytic activity.

   Cases of intracranial venous thrombosis usually have involvement of the large venous sinuses, often in more than one site, rather than the cortical veins [17]. Raised intracranial pressure occurring within a short time of starting the drug is the most common presentation.

Other Thrombogenic Drugs

Thrombosis of cerebral venous sinuses has been described in many patients who are receiving corticosteroids and also in patients with Cushing's disease, suggesting that steroids rather than any underlying disease are responsible. Androgenic steroids may carry a similar risk [18]. L-Asparaginase, an inhibitor of protein synthesis used in combination chemotherapy, can cause hemorrhages or thrombosis from a disturbance in the balance between pro- and anticoagulant naturally occurring proteins. Many cases of sinovenous thrombosis have been reported [19].

Venous Cannulas

The increasing use of long-term cannulas placed in the brachial, subclavian, or superior vena cava for parenteral feeding, drug therapy, or fluid replacement has undoubtedly been responsible for the large number of reported cases of cerebral sinus thrombosis, from intracranial spread of infected or bland thrombus. The usual presentation is as raised intracranial pressure [20].

Disturbance of Flow

Disturbance of flow is an important factor when venous thrombosis occurs in infancy [21] or in terminal states of cachexia and dehydration [22]. Underlying causes include fluid and electrolyte loss from gastroenteritis, dysphagia, and inadequate hydration in unconscious patients, especially in diabetic coma. The

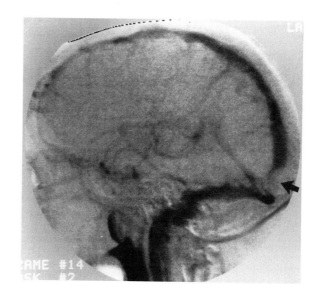

Figure 8.5 Intravenous digital subtraction angiogram shows partial obstruction of the superior sagittal sinus by a plasmacytoma (*arrow*). (Courtesy of Dr. Gordon Plant, London.)

midportion of the SSS is the favored site for thrombosis, and involvement of multiple veins, both intracranial and extracranial, is common. The diagnosis can be difficult, and the most common presenting features are seizures, confusion, and altered consciousness. Signs of raised intracranial pressure may be absent. Slowing of the circulation secondary to arterial thrombosis or cardiac failure can also predispose to venous thrombosis, and, in many such cases, cerebral thrombosis is clinically silent and discovered only at autopsy [23].

Obstruction or thrombosis of cerebral veins or sinuses from neoplastic or traumatic lesions is also included in this category. Tumors are usually meningiomas or sarcomas that arise in the skull or dura in the parasagittal area and slowly obstruct the SSS. Metastatic tumors can also occur, with the breast and cervix the most common primary sites [24].

Hematogenous deposits that occur in lymphoma or acute lymphocytic leukemia can also narrow or obstruct the sinuses (Figure 8.5). Glomus tumors that arise in the temporal bone adjacent to the jugular foramen are especially prone to cause jugular vein thrombosis on one or both sides [25].

Traumatic thrombosis may, on rare occasions, result from tangential bullet wounds to the skull vertex but in peacetime is more often seen as a consequence of depressed skull fractures. Raised intracranial pressure has been recorded in patients in whom the SSS has been compressed but not thrombosed. The pressure returns to normal after elevation of the fracture [24].

Arteriovenous Malformations

The association of arteriovenous malformations and venous thrombosis has been recognized only since 1990. The malformations can be dural or intracerebral, usually the former, and generally are situated at the base of the brain near a major venous sinus. The causative mechanism is often difficult to determine, and it is uncertain whether malformations antedate the thrombosis or whether they are the result of venous collateral development after obstruction of the vessel. Patients usually present in middle life with intracranial hypertension, pulsatile tinnitus, or focal venous infarction from obstruction of the sagittal, transverse, or cavernous sinuses [26].

Meningeal Infection or Infiltration

In the days before antibiotics, infection was by far the most common cause of sinovenous thrombosis, predominantly affecting the LS by contiguous spread from the mastoid region and middle ear. The infecting organism was most often a beta-hemolytic *Streptococcus*; however, this has now been replaced by *Proteus*, *Escherichia coli*, or anaerobes. Clinically, onset of sinus thrombosis was signaled by worsening of fever and the appearance of severe headache, vomiting, and convulsions [27]. A chronic variety, with minimal signs of infection, caused raised intracranial pressure by interference with drainage of CSF and was named *otitic hydrocephalus* by Symonds [28].

Cavernous sinus thrombosis is almost always infective in origin, with the infection originating in pyogenic lesions of the face, mouth, sinuses, or orbit and reaching the sinus via the pterygoid veins. In the past, the predominant infecting organisms were *Staphylococcus aureus*, *Streptococcus pneumoniae*, and *Haemophilus influenzae*, but these have now been replaced by unusual or resistant organisms such as *Aspergillus* or *Mucor*, and the affected patients may be immunocompromised, diabetic, or receiving steroid therapy. The mortality of septic cavernous sinus thrombosis used to be close to 100%, and even with modern antibiotic treatment it is still approximately 30% [29].

Behçet's Syndrome

The first descriptions of Behçet's syndrome were of chronic relapsing orogenital ulceration and uveitis. More recently, a number of other features have been added, including arthritis, erythema nodosum, and venous occlusion. Neurologic involvement in the form of relapsing meningitis or focal necrotic lesions, usually in the brain stem or spinal cord, may also exist. The cause is unknown, but it is thought to be an immunologic abnormality. Circulating immune complexes can be detected in 40–60% of patients.

Thrombophlebitis occurs in approximately 25% of patients; it can affect veins at any site, including the venae cavae, but has a predilection for the cerebral venous sinuses. In some parts of the world, notably Japan and the Middle East, Behçet's disease is the most common cause of cerebral venous thrombosis (Figures 8.6 and 8.7) [30].

Affected patients are usually young men, and the most common mode of presentation is as intracranial hypertension. Most patients are treated with corticosteroids, immunosuppressive or immunopotentiating treatment, or colchicine. Anticoagulants have been recommended for patients with cerebral venous thrombosis, but the presence of pulmonary artery aneurysms has limited this form of treatment.

Figure 8.6   Enhanced magnetic resonance imaging shows extensive pachymeningitis and thrombosis of the superior sagittal sinus (*arrow*) in the course of Behçet's disease. (A = anterior; P = posterior.) (Courtesy of Dr. J. Arruga, Barcelona, Spain.)

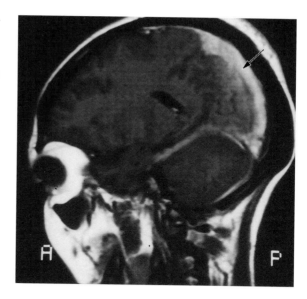

Wegener's Granulomatosis

In Wegener's granulomatosis, granulomatous vasculitis mainly affects the respiratory tract and the kidneys. Cerebral lesions are rare, but sinus thrombosis can occur as a complication of meningeal granulomatosis [31].

Sarcoidosis is another chronic systemic disease that can involve the meninges, and there are a number of reports of dural venous sinus thrombosis, mainly at the base of the brain. Marked meningeal enhancement on computed tomographic (CT) scanning is a helpful diagnostic pointer, and there is a marked lymphocytic cellular reaction in the CSF [32].

Figure 8.7   Magnetic resonance imaging shows thrombosis of the cavernous sinus (*arrow*) in Behçet's disease (same patient as in Figure 8.6). (R = right; L = left; M = medial.) (Courtesy of Dr. J. Arruga, Barcelona, Spain.)

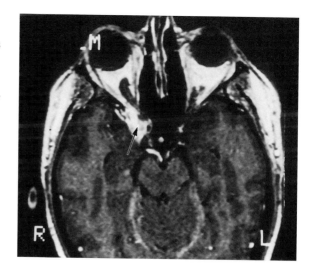

Non-Hodgkin's lymphoma can infiltrate the walls of cerebral veins and sinuses as part of generalized meningeal spread. It may present clinically as venous infarction or intracranial hypertension [33].

DIFFERENTIAL DIAGNOSIS

Cerebral venous thrombosis should be considered as a possible diagnosis (1) in any acute cerebral event in late pregnancy or the puerperium; (2) in any stroke-like illness in a young patient, especially if associated with severe headache or seizures; and (3) in patients who present with headache that is suggestive of raised intracranial pressure without signs of a cerebral mass lesion.

Headache

In taking the clinical history, particular attention should be paid to the character of the headache, the circumstances of onset, and the presence or absence of associated features, such as vomiting and focal symptoms, especially visual. In venous thrombosis, headache can be of any grade of severity, including sudden intense "thunderclap" headache that simulates subarachnoid hemorrhage.

Although the headache of venous thrombosis is usually generalized and seldom accompanied by a visual aura, it is sometimes difficult to distinguish cerebral venous thrombosis from migraine. A history of similar attacks is a valuable indication of migraine.

Seizures

If seizures have occurred, it is relevant to inquire whether the patient has had them in the past, whether they were focal or generalized, and whether a seizure was followed by postictal paralysis, a common event in venous thrombosis.

If a stroke-like event has occurred, it is important to record its character, whether motor, sensory, or visual; whether it was of sudden or gradual onset and evolution; and whether it varied from minute to minute or changed in location or laterality. Fluctuating signs of this kind are prone to occur in venous thrombosis.

History

Other important points in the history include any unexplained venous thrombosis in any site, either occurring spontaneously or after events such as pregnancy, prolonged bed rest, or surgery. A history of inflammation, either recent or remote, that involved ears, paranasal sinuses, face, or mouth may suggest a septic sinus thrombosis. Finally, it is relevant to inquire after a history of systemic illness, especially hematologic disease, inflammatory bowel disease, or nephritis. A family history of venous thrombosis may also be an indication of a congenital pro-thrombotic state.

CLINICAL EXAMINATION

Clinical examination should begin with assessment of the patient's general state: Does he or she have any evidence of infection, especially of ears or sinuses? Is fever or neck stiffness present? Does he or she show signs of dehydration, weight loss, or cachexia, suggesting systemic or malignant disease?

In the neurologic examination, is the patient fully alert or obtunded; does his or her speech show evidence of dysphasia? It is important to look repeatedly for raised intracranial pressure, shown by papilledema, headache, and vomiting with or without sixth nerve palsy. Papilledema may take some days to develop.

Local hemispheric signs normally take the form of unilateral hemiparesis and cortical sensory loss, sometimes more marked in the patient's leg than in his or her arm. Bilateral or alternating signs are rare but characteristic of venous disease. Homonymous hemianopia is also an unusual feature of venous infarction, but defects of visual orientation and attention indicative of damage to the parieto-occipital regions on one or both sides may be present, and the most reliable clinical sign is a localized defect in visually directed reaching.

Altered Consciousness

Patients whose principal feature is an alteration in consciousness present the most difficulty in diagnosis. They are often either very young or very old and are frequently dehydrated and seriously ill from other causes. They are often unable to give an adequate history. The classic triad of headache, seizures, and focal cerebral deficit may be absent or obscured. Depression of consciousness may vary from mild confusion to deep coma. Although the main pathologic process is generalized cerebral swelling, signs of raised intracranial pressure are often absent. The clinical features are those of a meningoencephalitis or cerebral abscess, but fever is slight and inconstant, and there is little meningeal inflammatory reaction in the CSF. Clinical diagnosis may be impossible without the help of brain imaging.

Drug Abuse

Drug abuse is a diagnosis that often must be considered in a young patient who presents with an acute or subacute cerebral event with seizures and depressed consciousness but no focal signs and no systemic features of an infectious illness. Diagnostic pointers in favor of intoxication are early brain stem signs such as loss of respiratory, cardiovascular, or temperature control and abnormal pupil reactions. A diagnostic screening test for commonly used drugs of abuse should be part of the routine investigation in cases of doubt.

Intracranial Hypertension

Patients with sagittal or LS thrombosis who have raised intracranial pressure without focal signs or epilepsy often experience a long delay before the correct diagnosis is reached. Headache may not be severe but usually has the characteristics of raised intracranial pressure, presence on waking from sleep, and aggravation by coughing or recumbency. Other features, such as vomiting, drowsiness, and visual obscurations, may or may not be present. The main physical sign is papilledema; contraction of the visual fields and consecutive optic atrophy are present in advanced cases.

Isolated intracranial hypertension in a young patient at once raises the possibility of a cerebral tumor causing obstructive hydrocephalus, a low-grade tumor in a silent area, or a subdural hematoma. These are easily recognized on a CT scan. Patients with a negative scan may have benign intracranial hypertension or sinus thrombosis, and it is here that the greatest diagnostic difficulty arises, because the two conditions may be clinically indistinguishable.

In favor of benign intracranial hypertension is an overweight female patient in the second or third decade, often with a history of menstrual irregularity. In favor of sinus thrombosis is a past or family history of venous thrombosis in any site or any underlying disease or medication that is known to predispose to thrombosis. In both conditions, measurement of CSF pressure shows a marked elevation, 300–600 mm; the composition of the spinal fluid is normal. CT scanning shows the cerebral ventricles to be normal or small, and usually no diagnostic signs of sinus thrombosis are present. Direct confirmation of sinus obstruction is provided by angiography; an intravenous digital subtraction study is usually adequate. Advances in magnetic resonance angiography make this the method of choice for the demonstration of major sinus obstruction.

INVESTIGATIONS

The purpose of investigations in cerebral venous thrombosis is to confirm the clinical diagnosis of sinovenous thrombosis and to detect any underlying abnormality (Table 8.9). The routine screening tests listed in Table 8.9 may point to a systemic disorder but are frequently negative. The diagnosis of venous thrombosis relies heavily on imaging.

Imaging

A CT scan is normally the first rapidly available method of imaging and should be performed as soon as the diagnosis is suspected. Unenhanced CT scan is very suitable for the detection of recent intracerebral hemorrhage and hemorrhagic infarction. It can also give an indication that the infarction is venous from the location of the infarct, particularly if it is bilateral and parasagittal. Occasionally, a recently thrombosed large cortical vein is visible as a hyperdense cord on the unenhanced scan. Patients with very recent infarcts may show deterioration after injection of contrast, and enhancement is not recommended as a routine investigation. However, it can give valuable additional information in patients who present with a subacute or chronic onset or those without focal signs. The empty delta sign is an inconstant finding, with thrombosis showing as a filling defect in the SSS on the enhanced CT scan (Figure 8.8). Excessive enhancement of the meninges can also be shown by this technique and gives an indication of

Table 8.9   Routine investigations in suspected cerebral venous thrombosis

Test	Purpose
Computed tomographic scan	Detects hemorrhage, infarction, brain swelling
Full blood cell count, including platelets, erythrocyte sedimentation rate, C-reactive protein	Detects primary blood disorders, underlying inflammatory and malignant disease
Thrombosis screen	Detects prothrombotic states, primary or secondary
Fibrinogen, protein C, protein S	
Antithrombin III, factor V resistance	
Prothrombin gene (20210A) mutation	
Lupus anticoagulant	
Antiphospholipid antibody	
Lumbar puncture	Only if computed tomographic scan normal; not if on anticoagulants
	Detects intracranial hypertension, meningeal inflammation, infiltration
Magnetic resonance imaging	Detects infarction, sinus thrombus, intra-vascular thrombus
Contrast angiography or magnetic resonance angiography	Detects venous nonfilling defects, filling defects, collaterals

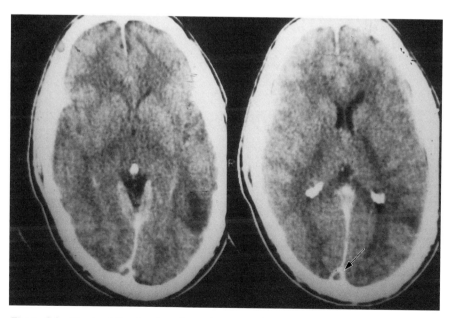

Figure 8.8   Empty delta sign in enhanced computed tomographic scan in a patient with superior sagittal sinus thrombosis (*arrow*).

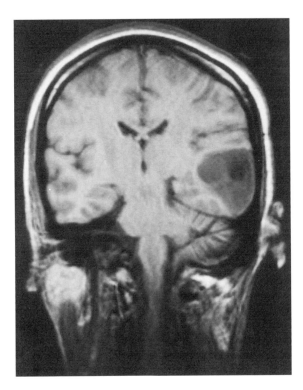

Figure 8.9 Magnetic resonance imaging shows hemorrhagic infarction of the temporal lobe in a patient with thrombosis of the lateral sinus and inferior anastomotic vein.

meningeal inflammation or infiltration, which may have led to sinus thrombosis. Computed tomography can also detect evidence of infection in the temporal bone and in the paranasal sinuses.

Magnetic resonance imaging is undoubtedly the investigation of choice and is capable of providing information not only on cerebral lesions but also on the venous sinuses. It is more sensitive than CT scan for the detection of ischemic cerebral infarction and edema and can also visualize thrombus as a filling defect within the large midline sinuses (Figures 8.9 and 8.10). Magnetic resonance imaging can detect hemorrhage as well and give some estimate of its age. Fresh thrombus is also hyperdense on T1-weighted images and contrasts with the flow void that is present in uninvolved veins (Figure 8.11).

Angiography

For many years, angiography was the definitive investigation; if performed by the intra-arterial route with subtraction technique, it provides excellent views of the surface and deep veins and of the sinuses. Thrombosis is inferred from a failure of filling of veins or by a filling defect within a sinus. Collateral veins that develop after occlusion are also shown by this technique, either on the surface or within the brain (Figure 8.12). Intravenous digital subtraction angiography can

Figure 8.10   Magnetic resonance imaging shows thrombus within the superior sagittal sinus (*arrows*) in a patient with essential thrombocythemia.

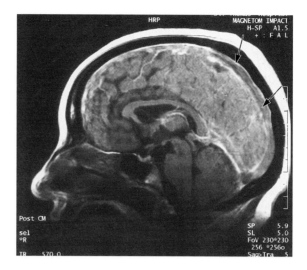

Figure 8.11   Magnetic resonance imaging shows thrombus within the lateral sinus (high signal) (*arrow*) in a patient with antithrombin III deficiency.

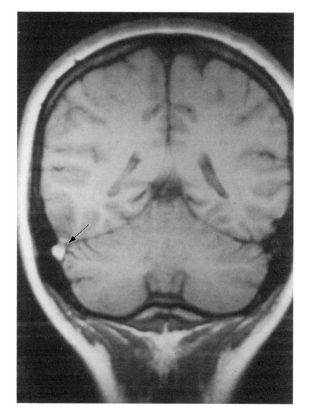

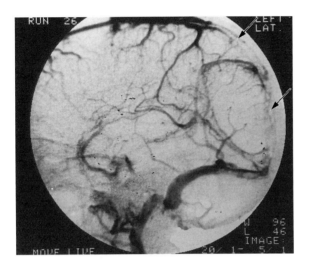

Figure 8.12   Intra-arterial digital subtraction angiogram (venous phase) shows partial thrombosis of the superior sagittal sinus (*arrows*).

be used as well; this has the advantage of low morbidity but reliably demonstrates only the sinuses (Figure 8.13).

Magnetic resonance angiography is becoming the method of choice for show-ing thrombosis, especially of the SSS, usually using a two-dimensional time-of-flight technique (Figure 8.14). It is sometimes difficult to distinguish intravenous thrombus from a region of slow flow, but it may be possible to overcome this by using a phase contrast technique that is sensitive to different flow rates.

All angiographic methods may fail to separate hypoplasia (commonly found in the anterior part of the SSS) from partial thrombosis or a recanalized vessel. Magnetic resonance angiography does not often demonstrate the cavernous sinus clearly.

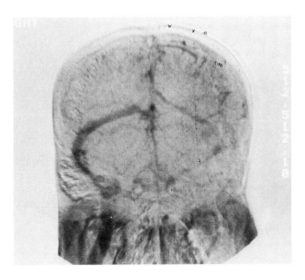

Figure 8.13   Intravenous digital subtraction angi-ography shows failure of filling of the right lateral and superior sagittal sinuses.

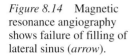

Figure 8.14 Magnetic resonance angiography shows failure of filling of lateral sinus (*arrow*).

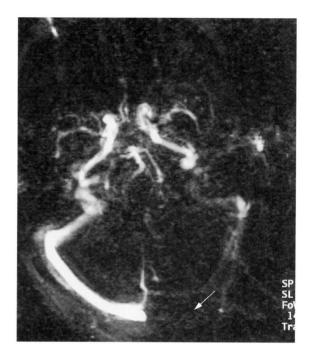

MANAGEMENT

The principles of early treatment of cerebral venous disease are (1) to limit the spread of thrombosis, (2) to combat brain swelling if necessary, (3) to treat any infection or underlying cause, (4) to treat and prevent seizures, and (5) to relieve headache and raised intracranial pressure.

Thrombosis

In venous thrombosis, there is a disturbance in the delicate balance between procoagulant forces and the natural anticoagulant and fibrinolytic properties of the blood. Thrombi are formed of friable masses of fibrin and red cells; they tend to grow slowly and extend along veins in both directions, especially when flow is slow or stagnant. Anticoagulant treatment aims to limit the spread and embolization of thrombus and to allow the balance of forces to alter in favor of thrombolysis and organization (Table 8.10).

The attitude toward anticoagulant treatment in cerebral venous thrombosis has changed considerably. At one time, both heparin and warfarin were considered to be contraindicated because of the risk of cerebral hemorrhage [23], and there were reports of patients receiving heparin whose conditions deteriorated [34]. Since 1988, however, many series of patients have been treated with heparin without clinical worsening and with a good outcome [1,35,36]. Even patients who show evidence of hemorrhage on CT scan have been treated without deterioration, with remarkable improvement in some cases. Anticoagulation also has the advantage

Table 8.10   Treatment of cerebral venous thrombosis

Type	Drug, dosage	Comments
Antithrombotic	Heparin IV, 3,000 IU, followed by 25,000–50,000 IU/day IV infusion to keep the partial thromboplastin time at 80–100 secs	Except neonates; controversial in severe hemorrhage, paroxysmal nocturnal hemoglobinuria
	Warfarin, international normalized ratio 2.0–2.5	Not in pregnancy
Antibiotic	Penicillin (co-amoxiclav IV, 1 g q8h); cefotaxime IV, 1 g q8h	Treat source of infection
	? Metronidazole IV, 500 mg q8h	? Surgery; caution in pregnancy
Anticonvulsant	Benzodiazapine, 10–20 mg slow IV, or chlormethiazole, 0.8% IV, 10 ml/min up to 100 ml	Established seizures
	Phenytoin, 300–400 mg/day	Preventive
Antiedema	Mannitol IV 20%, 500–1,000 ml/24 hrs	Contraindicated in cardiac failure, pulmonary edema
	Acetazolamide, 0.25–1.00 g/day, IV or oral	Contraindicated in pregnancy

of preventing venous thrombosis in other areas, such as the patient's legs, and in lessening the risk of pulmonary embolism.

Although these reports are encouraging, only a single randomized controlled study of heparin treatment has been published [37]. This was planned to include 60 patients but was stopped after an interim analysis when only 20 patients had been treated, at which time a significant difference had been found in favor of the heparin over the control group (Table 8.11). This trial has been criticized on the basis of a nonvalidated severity scale, and a further trial comparing low–molecular-weight heparin with placebo is currently in progress [38].

Most authorities now agree that the dangers of anticoagulation have been overestimated in the past and that heparin should be given to all patients except those who show large confluent amounts of cerebral hemorrhage on CT scan. Treatment should begin as early as possible after diagnosis, with an initial intravenous bolus of 3,000 IU followed by 25,000–50,000 IU daily by continuous

Table 8.11   Randomized controlled trial of heparin treatment in cerebral venous thrombosis

Result*	Treated group (n = 10)	Control group (n = 10)
Complete recovery	8	1
Residual deficit	2	6
Died	0	3

*Results at 3 months.

Source: Reprinted with permission from KM Einhaupl, A Villringer, W Meister, et al. Heparin treatment in sinus venous thrombosis. Lancet 1991;338:598.

intravenous infusion, adjusted to keep the partial thromboplastin time at 80–100 seconds. Daily blood cell counts are indicated because of the risk of heparin-induced thrombocytopenia. If the clinical condition of the patient deteriorates, a repeat CT scan is performed.

In patients with severe protein C or antithrombin III deficiency, heparin alone may be relatively ineffective, and concentrates of protein C or antithrombin III are available for emergency treatment or during periods of high risk as in pregnancy or after surgery.

After approximately a week or when the patient's condition has stabilized, anticoagulation should be continued with warfarin in a dose adjusted to achieve an international normalized ratio of ×2–3. In idiopathic or puerperal cases, warfarin is continued for 3 months and then discontinued over a 2-week period.

Patients with an underlying thrombotic tendency, either congenital or acquired, may need to stay on warfarin indefinitely. During pregnancy or when the possibility of pregnancy exists, warfarin cannot be used because of its teratogenic effects. Low-molecular-weight heparin or low-dose heparin can be used instead and is continued throughout pregnancy.

In patients with congenital protein C or S deficiency, anticoagulation must be started with heparin for a few days before a change to warfarin; this is because warfarin, which acts by depressing prothrombin formation in the liver, can also lower still further the levels of proteins C and S.

Brain Swelling

Cerebral venous infarction, when extensive, is commonly associated with intra-cerebral hemorrhage and a variable amount of surrounding edema. This is probably caused by ischemia and is similar in type to the edema that may accompany arterial infarction; it is partly cytotoxic and partly vasogenic and responds poorly to corticosteroids. The combination of hemispheric swelling and hemorrhage can lead to displacement of midline structures, uncal herniation, and secondary distortion of the brain stem. Hydrocephalus can occur from blockage of the CSF pathways, especially in children. A similar sequence of events may follow cerebellar infarction. Ischemic edema takes some time to develop and is maximal 4 days after infarction; this contrasts with the effects of hemorrhage, which appear within minutes or hours.

Brain displacement and swelling from either infarction or hemorrhage should be suspected clinically by deterioration in the patient's level of consciousness; with worsening of the focal deficit; by the appearance of brain stem signs, such as pupillary enlargement and loss of light reaction beginning on the side ipsilateral to the lesion; with respiratory irregularity; and with bradycardia. They are confirmed by CT scan or magnetic resonance imaging showing displacement and swelling in one hemisphere, usually with signal change, suggesting increased water content in white matter.

Generalized brain swelling without much displacement can occur with thrombosis of the deep venous system or when extensive thrombosis involves a number of sinuses. In such cases, which most often affect the very old or very young, no focal signs may be present, and the patient may present only with a progressive decline in the level of consciousness. When an individual with cerebral venous thrombosis shows clinical deterioration and changes on scanning that are compatible with edema, the most appropriate treatment is mannitol.

Infection

Fulminating septic thrombosis of the cavernous sinus or LS spreading from facial or otitic infection is now a rarity in the developed world, but low-grade infection of the adjacent bone is still an important cause of thrombosis of the LS and one that may be difficult to diagnose. Septic thrombosis still occurs in steroid-treated, diabetic, or immunocompromised patients or in the presence of atypical infecting organisms. In septic cerebral sinus thrombosis, there are often a bacteremia and the attendant dangers of dissemination of infection throughout the body, especially septic embolism to the lungs. Identification of the infecting organism by blood culture is of primary importance, and the microbiologist may indicate the most appropriate antibiotic. Treatment with intravenous antibiotics should not, however, await the results of culture and should be started at once using an intravenous penicillinase-resistant penicillin such as co-amoxiclav, 1 g every 8 hours, combined with a third-generation cephalosporin (cefotaxime, 1 g intravenously every 8 hours) with or without metronidazole (500 mg every 8 hours). If the source of infection can be identified, as in the mastoid area, surgical treatment may be necessary even in the early stages to remove infected bone adjacent to the sinus. Surgical ligation of the jugular vein to prevent septic embolism to the lungs is sometimes recommended, but surgical thrombectomy is no longer performed.

Treatment of Other Underlying Conditions

If cerebral venous thrombosis is secondary to a systemic disease or to a meningeal lymphoma or granuloma, such as sarcoidosis or Wegener's granulomatosis, these require treatment that may often include corticosteroids. In patients with the nephrotic syndrome or ulcerative colitis, in whom natural anticoagulants protein C, protein S, or antithrombin III may be depleted, emergency treatment may include fresh frozen plasma or intravenous concentrated preparations.

Retardation of blood flow secondary to dehydration is an important contributory cause of cerebral venous thrombosis, particularly in infants and in the aged. Prompt replacement of fluid and electrolytes is mandatory. Cardiac failure or severe systemic hypotension can also lead to slowing of the cerebral circulation and should be corrected

Venous sinus thrombosis secondary to obstruction by tumor or by a depressed skull fracture may require neurosurgical treatment. Surgical excision or embolization may also be required for arteriovenous malformations that cause venous thrombosis.

Seizures

Seizures are a common and sometimes a presenting feature of cerebral venous thrombosis and (except in children) usually indicate venous infarction in the cerebral hemispheres. They can be focal or generalized and are often difficult to control. At the first sign of seizure activity, immediate treatment with intravenous diazepam, 10 mg in 2 ml, should be given over 5 minutes. An immediate bolus injection carries some risk of respiratory depression. Intravenous diazepam can be repeated on one or two occasions at 15-minute intervals if seizures are not controlled. Chlormethiazole or lorazepam is an alternative if diazepam is ineffective. For longer term prevention of recurrent seizures, phenytoin sodium is suitable. Because seizures can aggravate brain swelling, raise intracranial pressure, and increase the risk of intracerebral venous bleeding, many recommend anticonvulsant treatment as a precautionary measure even if no fits have occurred [35] or if electroencephalography shows epileptic activity [39].

It is unusual for epileptic attacks to continue after recovery from cerebral venous thrombosis. Anticonvulsants are continued for at least a year in patients who have had seizures in the acute phase and for 3 months in those who have not [40].

Isolated Intracranial Hypertension

Raised intracranial pressure without cerebral infarction is a feature of thrombosis of the SSS or LS and is caused by interference with the drainage of CSF from the arachnoid villi. The clinical features are similar to those of "benign intracranial hypertension"; headache may not be a prominent symptom but there is a risk of permanent damage to the optic nerves if pressure remains high. Slight, generalized cerebral swelling may be shown by scanning, but it is not clinically significant and requires no treatment.

Once the diagnosis has been made, it is advisable to check the CSF pressure and to remove 25–50 ml of fluid to restore the pressure to normal. This can be repeated at weekly intervals. The pressure may return to normal spontaneously as venous drainage improves on anticoagulant treatment. Acetazolamide, 250–500 mg by mouth or intravenously, is also recommended to reduce both the secretion of CSF and intracranial pressure. It is not suitable for use in pregnancy.

Careful monitoring of the visual fields and acuity is necessary in patients with intracranial hypertension, as well as repeated photography of the optic disks to assess the degree of papilledema and disk pallor. If there is evidence that progressive optic nerve damage is occurring in spite of medical treatment, ventriculo-atrial shunting or fenestration of the optic nerve sheaths should be undertaken. These appear to be more effective ways of protecting the optic nerves than the alternative procedure of lumboperitoneal shunting.

Headache is a prominent symptom in some patients and is caused at least in part by raised intracranial pressure. It may improve after lumbar puncture and acetazolamide but, if not, it can be treated with paracetamol or codeine by mouth. Aspirin is best avoided because it carries an increased risk of bleeding.

PROGNOSIS

Before the introduction of modern imaging, cerebral venous thrombosis was a diagnosis that was usually made at autopsy, and the disease was thought to carry a high initial mortality of approximately 30–50% [2]. In more recent series of patients, the mortality has been nearer to 10% [1]. The change is only partly explained by improved diagnosis and reflects a genuine advance in treatment, both of the thrombotic tendency and the underlying cause, especially in cases that are secondary to infection and to dehydration. Some of the early mortality was caused by massive hemorrhagic infarction and brain swelling, but many deaths also occurred from complications such as septicemia, seizures, and pulmonary embolism.

Patients who survive cerebral venous infarction may be left with a severe motor, sensory, or cognitive deficit, especially after thrombosis of the deep venous system, but in general the degree of recovery is much better than in arterial thrombosis. Here again, the site of thrombosis is relevant: LS thrombosis carries the best prognosis and deep venous thrombosis the worst. In general, individuals with cranial nerve palsies recover well as do patients with isolated intracranial hypertension from SSS thrombosis. Unfavorable prognostic factors include age (either very young or very old), a rapid onset, deep coma, bilateral signs, and generalized seizures. The underlying cause also exerts a great influence on the outcome; patients with thrombosis caused by sepsis, malignancies, or blood diseases (especially paroxysmal nocturnal hemoglobinuria) tend to do badly compared with those who have idiopathic or postpartum causes. Of those patients with seizures during the acute stage, 10% may continue to have them after recovery. It is rare for seizures to occur for the first time after recovery from venous infarction.

REFERENCES

1. Ameri A, Bousser MG. Cerebral venous thrombosis. Neurol Clin 1993;10:87.
2. Krayenbuhl HA. Cerebral venous and sinus thrombosis. Clin Neurosurg 1967;14:1.
3. Conard J, Horellou MH, Van Dreden P, Samama M. Pregnancy and congenital deficiency of antithrombin III or protein C (abstract). Thromb Haemost 1987;58:39.
4. Martinelli I, Landi G, Merati G, et al. Factor V gene mutation is a risk factor for cerebral venous thrombosis. Thromb Haemost 1996;75:393.
5. Schutta HS, Williams EC, Baranski BG, Sutula TP. Cerebral venous thrombosis with plasminogen deficiency. Stroke 1991;22:401.
6. Kellett MW, Martin PJ, Enevoldson TP, et al. Cerebral venous sinus thrombosis associated with 20210A mutation of the prothrombin gene [letter]. J Neurol Neurosurg Psychiatry 1998;65:611.
7. Melamed E, Rachmilewicz EA, Reches A, Lavy S. Aseptic cavernous sinus thrombosis after internal carotid artery occlusion in polycythaemia vera. J Neurol Neurosurg Psychiatry 1976;39:320.
8. Haan J, Caekebeke JFV, van der Meer FJM, Wintzen AR. Cerebral venous thrombosis as a presenting sign of myeloproliferative disorders. J Neurol Neurosurg Psychiatry 1988;51:1219.
9. David RB, Hadfield MG, Vines FS. Dural sinus occlusion in leukemia. Pediatrics 1975;56:793.
10. Al Hakim M, Katirji MB, Osorio I, Weisman R. Cerebral venous thrombosis in paroxysmal nocturnal hemoglobinuria: report of two cases. Neurology 1993;43:742.
11. Dunsker SB, Torres Reyes E, Peden JC. Pseudotumor cerebri associated with idiopathic cryofibrinogenemia. Arch Neurol 1970;23:120.
12. Averback P. Primary cerebral venous thrombosis in young adults: the diverse manifestations of an underrecognized disease. Ann Neurol 1978;3:81.

13. Sigsbee B, Deck MDF, Posner JB. Non-metastatic superior sagittal sinus thrombosis complicating systemic cancer. Neurology 1979;29:139.
14. Das R, Vasishta RK, Banerjee AK. Aseptic cerebral venous thrombosis associated with idiopathic ulcerative colitis: a report of two cases. Clin Neurol Neurosurg 1996;98:179.
15. Freycon MT, Richard O, Allard D, et al. Thrombose des sinus veineux intracraniens au cours d'un syndrome nephrotique. Pediatrie 1992;47:513.
16 Vidailet M, Piette JC, Weschler B, et al. Cerebral venous thrombosis in systemic lupus erythematosus. Stroke 1990;21:1226.
17. Estanol B, Rodriguez A, Conte A, et al. Intracranial venous thrombosis in young women. Stroke 1979;10:680.
18. Hamed LM, Glaser JS, Schatz NJ, Perez FH. Pseudotumor cerebri induced by danazol. Am J Ophthalmol 1989;107:105.
19. Steinherz PG, Miller LP, Ghavimi F, et al. Dural sinus thrombosis in children with acute lymphoblastic leukemia. JAMA 1981;246:2837.
20. Souter RG, Mitchell A. Spreading cortical venous thrombosis due to infusion of hyperosmolar solutions into the internal jugular vein. BMJ 1982;285:935.
21. Banker BQ. Cerebral vascular disease in infancy and childhood. 1. Occlusive vascular disease. J Neuropathol Exp Neurol 1961;20:127.
22. Byers RK, Hass GM. Thrombosis of dural venous sinuses in infancy and childhood. Am J Dis Child 1933;45:1161.
23. Barnett HJM, Hyland HH. Non-infective intracranial venous thrombosis. Brain 1953;76:36.
24. Plant GT, Donald JJ, Jackowski A, et al. Partial non-thrombotic superior sagittal sinus occlusion due to occipital skull tumours. J Neurol Neurosurg Psychiatry 1991;54:520.
25. Enevoldson TP, Ross Russell RW. Cerebral venous thrombosis: new causes for an old syndrome. QJM 1990;77:1255.
26. Houser OW, Campbell JK, Campbell RJ, et al. Arteriovenous malformation affecting the transverse venous sinus: an acquired lesion. Mayo Clin Proc 1979;54:651.
27. Reading PV, Schurr P. Thrombosis of the sigmoid sinus. Lancet 1956;2:473.
28. Symonds CP. Hydrocephalic and focal cerebral symptoms in relation to thrombophlebitis of the dural sinuses and cerebral veins. Brain 1937;60:531.
29. DiNubile MJ, Boom WH, Southwick FS. Septic cortical thrombophlebitis. J Infect Dis 1990;161:1216.
30. Daif A, Awada A, Al-Rejeh, et al. Cerebral venous thrombosis in adults. A study of 40 cases from Saudi Arabia. Stroke 1995;26:1193.
31. Mickle JP, McLennan JE, Chi JG, Lidden CW. Cortical vein thrombosis in Wegener's granulomatosis. J Neurosurg 1977;46:248.
32. Akora YA, Kansu T, Dumas S. Pseudotumor cerebri secondary to dural sinus thrombosis in neurosarcoidosis. J Clin Neurol Ophthalmol 1993;l13:188.
33. Meininger V, James JM, Rio B, Zittoun R. Occlusions des sinus veineux de la dure-mere au cours des hemopathies. Rev Neurol 1985;141:228.
34. Gettelfinger DM, Kokman E. Superior sagittal sinus thrombosis. Arch Neurol 1977;34:2.
35. Einhaupl KM, Masuhr F. Cerebral venous and sinus thrombosi; an update. Eur J Neurol 1994;1:109.
36. Villringer A, Mehraein S, Einhaupl KM. Treatment of sinus venous thrombosis—beyond the recommendation of anticoagulation. J Neuroradiol 1994;21:72.
37. Einhaupl KM, Villringer A, Meister W, et al. Heparin treatment in sinus venous thrombosis. Lancet 1991;338:597.
38. Stam J. Treatment of cerebral venous thrombosis. Cerebrovasc Dis 1993;3:329.
39. Chopra JS, Banerjee AK. Primary Intracranial Sinovenous Thrombosis in Youth and Pregnancy. In JF Toole (ed), Handbook of Clinical Neurology (Pt 11, Vol 10). Amsterdam: Elsevier, 1989;425–452.
40. Preter M, Tzourio CH, Ameri A, Bousser MG. Long-term prognosis in cerebral venous thrombosis. Stroke 1996;27:243.

9
Thrombotic and Vasculitic Disorders That Affect the Central Nervous System

David P. D'Cruz

The practicing neurologist and intensive care physician are often called on to assess patients with autoimmune connective tissue diseases complicated by critical central nervous system involvement. These patients may present as neurologic emergencies, and their morbidity and mortality are significant. A working knowledge of these disorders would help physicians who manage these patients, and the purpose of this chapter is to outline the variety of these diseases and their assessment in terms of clinical features, relevant investigations, and therapy. The main conditions described here include systemic lupus erythematosus (SLE); the antiphospholipid syndrome; the primary systemic vasculitides, including isolated angiitis of the nervous system; and cerebral vasculitis associated with other rheumatologic disorders, infections, and drugs.

SYSTEMIC LUPUS ERYTHEMATOSUS

Once thought to be a rare disease, SLE, a multisystem connective tissue disorder, is one of the great mimics in clinical medicine. It has a prevalence of approximately 1 in 2,000 individuals, and in some countries (e.g., in the Far East) it is more common than rheumatoid arthritis. The usual presenting features include photosensitive rashes, arthritis, oral and genital ulceration, renal disease, and serositis.

The spectrum of central neurologic involvement is enormous and ranges from minor psychological disturbances to memory loss, cognitive impairment, psychoses, chorea, organic brain syndromes, transverse myelopathy, demyelinating polyneuropathy, cranial nerve lesions, major cerebral infarctions, convulsions, coma, and death. If careful neurologic and psychometric assessments are used, the prevalence of neuropsychiatric abnormalities may be as high as 75% [1]. Central nervous system disease is usually seen in the context of active, established lupus, most often within the first year, but in one study, 10% of lupus patients with neuropsychiatric manifestations presented before lupus was diagnosed [2]. These authors showed a close correlation between the presence of vasculitis, both mucocutaneous and visceral, and neuropsychiatric disease. Pathologic studies suggest that true cerebral vasculitis in lupus is rare [3,4], although vascular hyalinization and perivascular inflammation can occur. The most striking aspect of these pathologic studies is the relatively normal macroscopic appearance of the brain despite significant neuropsychiatric dysfunction before death.

Organic brain syndromes may be due to causes other than the direct effects of lupus. For example, patients with severe glomerulonephritis who are uremic may be obtunded. Aseptic meningitis has been observed in lupus patients treated with nonsteroidal anti-inflammatory agents, in particular ibuprofen [5] and, more rarely, azathioprine [6]. The clinical features of meningitis occur within hours of drug ingestion and can be dramatic but resolve rapidly on stopping the drug; the etiology is almost certainly a hypersensitivity reaction [7].

Transverse myelitis is an uncommon neurologic complication of lupus. Presentation can be rapid with paraparesis or even quadriparesis when involvement of the high cervical cord exists, requiring mechanical ventilation.

Clinical Assessment

The diagnosis of severe neuropsychiatric disease is usually readily made in a patient known to have SLE in whom new central nervous system symptoms develop. Exclusion of other conditions, notably sepsis, is essential because patients frequently require immunosuppressive therapy. A prospective study highlighted the difference between primary cerebral lupus and other conditions that can give rise to a similar clinical picture in patients with lupus [8]. These included acute and chronic bacterial (*Staphylococcus* and tuberculosis), fungal (*Aspergillus*, *Cryptococcus*, *Nocardia*, or *Candida*), or viral (hepatitis or cytomegalovirus) infections. When these infections occur in patients with SLE, patients can also present with major behavioral changes, confusion, seizures, hallucinations, and altered levels of consciousness. One patient had a hypertensive encephalopathy and two others had steroid-associated psychoses, a relatively rare occurrence in most series [8].

Most patients undergo scanning, either computed tomographic (CT) scans or preferably magnetic resonance imaging (MRI), followed by cerebrospinal fluid (CSF) examination. No specific tests that unequivocally define neuropsychiatric lupus are available, however, and the diagnosis is fundamentally based on clinical grounds and exclusion. The CSF may be abnormal in one-third of patients, with nonspecific findings such as elevated protein levels and, occasionally, pleocytosis, for which there may be a higher risk of death in patients with abnormal CSF findings [2].

Investigations, such as electroencephalograms, are frequently nonspecifically abnormal (up to 71% in Feinglass and associates' study) with either diffuse slow-wave activity or focal changes associated with epilepsy [2]. CT scans are often normal but may show cerebral atrophy. MRI frequently shows periventricular or discrete white matter lesions. The nature of these lesions remains unknown, and they are certainly not specific for neuropsychiatric lupus as they are commonly seen in lupus patients without any evidence of neurologic dysfunction [9,10]. Gadolinium-enhancing lesions on MRI may improve with immunosuppressive therapy in a small number of patients [11]. Other forms of imaging, such as single-photon emission CT scans, frequently show areas of reduced cerebral blood flow (up to 82% in one study) but, again, these defects were also seen in asymptomatic lupus patients [12,13]. More recently, it has been found that positron emission tomography (PET), including [18]fluoro (F)-labeled 2-F-2-deoxyglucose–PET, may be more useful, particularly in showing reversible deficits [14]. Glucose metabolism may be a better measure of brain activity than cerebral blood flow measured, for example, by xenon-133 [15]. Cognitive impairment correlated with 2-F-2-deoxyglucose uptake on PET scanning in three patients with the antiphospholipid syndrome and highlights the potential usefulness of this technique [1].

Serologically, antinuclear and anti–DNA antibodies are frequently present, and complement levels, especially complement factors C3 and C4, are often low in active lupus, although this is not always the case. Anti–DNA antibodies may also be found in the CSF, but this finding does not necessarily correlate with neuropsychiatric lupus. Cytokine levels in the CSF may also correlate with neuropsychiatric lupus, and, in particular, elevated interleukin-6 levels have been noted [16]. More recently, antiribosomal P antibodies have been correlated with neuropsychiatric lupus, particularly with psychosis and depression [17]. Antibodies to a wide variety of antigens in the nervous system have been described in association with neuropsychiatric lupus, but few have been used clinically on a regular basis. These include antibodies directed against lymphocytes that cross-react with brain antigens and neuroblastoma cells, myelin-associated glycoprotein, mycobacterial glycosphingolipids, and galactocerebrosides (reviewed in reference 18).

Probably the most helpful, simple laboratory investigations in the context of acute cerebral lupus are the C-reactive protein (CRP) and erythrocyte sedimentation rate (ESR). The classic finding is that of a high ESR with a normal CRP in active SLE. When elevated, however, CRP is a good pointer toward sepsis, particularly if markedly elevated, and should caution the physician against immunosuppressive therapy until sepsis has been firmly excluded [8].

Management

Having excluded sepsis, immunosuppressive therapy with corticosteroids, such as pulse intravenous methylprednisolone and intravenous pulse cyclophosphamide, is the most effective treatment. My colleagues and I have noted excellent responses to low-dose weekly or fortnightly pulse intravenous cyclophosphamide in a series of patients with neuropsychiatric lupus [19,20]. Patients with transverse myelitis on the whole have a better outcome when treated with intravenous cyclophosphamide [21]. Once a good response has been obtained with intravenous cyclophosphamide or methylprednisolone, or both, azathioprine is a useful agent for the maintenance of remission [21].

ANTIPHOSPHOLIPID SYNDROME

SLE may be complicated by acute neurologic events, such as strokes, which may be catastrophic in terms of morbidity and mortality. Antiphospholipid syndrome

Table 9.1   Clinical features of antiphospholipid syndrome

Thrombosis
Heart valve disease
Recurrent fetal losses
Transverse myelopathy
Thrombocytopenia
Pulmonary hypertension
Livedo reticularis
Adrenal infarction
Labile hypertension
Skin necrosis
Epilepsy
Ocular ischemia
Accelerated atherosclerosis
Chorea

is a striking clinical constellation of widespread arterial and venous thromboses, recurrent fetal losses, and thrombocytopenia. In 1983–1986, this clinical constellation was associated with antibodies directed against phospholipids [22]. Since its original description, the clinical spectrum of this syndrome has broadened considerably [23] to include features such as livedo reticularis, pulmonary hypertension, valvular heart disease, transient ischemic attacks, epilepsy, and transverse myelopathy (Table 9.1). Although originally described in association with SLE, the syndrome may be seen in the absence of a connective tissue disease—the so-called primary antiphospholipid syndrome.

Clinical Features

Thrombosis, both venous and arterial, remains the hallmark of antiphospholipid syndrome. Vessels of all sizes have been involved, ranging from small vessels in the skin to the aortic arch. Neurologic features include recurrent migraine; transient ischemic attacks with visual disturbances or dysarthria, or both; and a previous history of chorea. Cerebral ischemia ranging from transient ischemia to infarction is commonly seen, and, in some untreated patients, recurrent cerebral infarcts have led to multi-infarct dementia. Epilepsy [24], chorea, and movement disorders [23] have been associated with antiphospholipid antibodies, and a reasonable hypothesis would include small vessel thromboses or emboli resulting in these clinical features. Of great interest is the clinical observation that some patients with epilepsy and chorea improve strikingly after anticoagulation [23]. Transverse myelitis is an uncommon manifestation of SLE that is frequently associated with the presence of antiphospholipid antibodies [25]. Studies of unselected stroke populations have shown a relatively low prevalence of antiphospholipid antibodies, but in young stroke patients this rises to 18% [26] compared to a prevalence of approximately 30% in patients with SLE.

    Asherson and associates [27] have proposed the term *catastrophic antiphospholipid syndrome* to describe a condition in which patients with antiphospholipid antibodies rapidly develop widespread multiorgan failure associated with a mortality of 58%. Adult respiratory distress syndrome was the predominating feature in 6 of the 31 patients described, and severe neurologic involvement was also seen [27].

The epidemiology of the antiphospholipid syndrome is still being investigated, and it is unclear whether other risk factors, such as oral contraceptives, smoking, or dietary intake, can add to the risk of thrombosis in these patients. Certainly, thrombosis-prone families exist, and human leukocyte antigen studies have suggested an association between antiphospholipid antibodies and an increased prevalence of one or more of the major histocompatibility complex class II alleles HLA-DR4, -DR53, and -DQ7 (DQB1*0301) (reviewed in reference 28).

Mechanisms of Thrombosis

Antibodies against phospholipids are heterogenous, and negatively charged phospholipids are the predominant antigens. Monoclonal antibodies, both human and animal, have suggested that antibodies react predominantly to phospholipids in their hexagonal but not their lamellar phase.

Very wide disturbances of function have been described in endothelial cells, platelet membranes, and the clotting cascade, particularly with components such as protein C and protein S, although this area of research has been complex with conflicting results. In 1990, a cofactor beta$_2$-glycoprotein 1 was found to be an absolute requirement for binding of both the anticardiolipin antibodies and the lupus anticoagulant in plasma from thrombotic patients. Furthermore, domain V is a crucial area of the cofactor molecule and contains a phospholipid binding site between residues 281 and 288 [29]. Antibodies to beta$_2$-glycoprotein 1 have been closely correlated with thrombosis, and, in the future, these antibodies may become the specific marker for this syndrome [30,31].

Management

Very few prospective controlled trials of therapy in patients with the antiphospholipid syndrome exist, mainly owing to the small number of patients seen at any single center and the need for very long-term follow-up. However, a retrospective study of a cohort of 147 patients with antiphospholipid antibodies and a history of thrombosis who were followed for 10 years clearly showed that those who received warfarin with a maintenance international normalized ratio (INR) of 3.0 or greater had the lowest risk of further thrombosis [32]. The other important point to emerge from this study was that patients in whom anticoagulation was stopped all had a further thrombosis. Obviously, anticoagulation with INRs of 3.0 or greater has its risks, and in this study 29 bleeding episodes occurred, seven of which were severe but not fatal. A prospective study of patients with venous thrombosis alone and no other features of the antiphospholipid syndrome suggests that this more straightforward condition can be managed with INRs of 2.0–3.0, which would perhaps lower the risk of bleeding [33].

One of the features of antiphospholipid syndrome is that many patients are relatively resistant to warfarin, requiring up to 25 mg per day to maintain adequate anticoagulation; this is particularly true of patients who are also taking azathioprine to control their SLE. Azathioprine interacts with warfarin, reducing its efficacy, possibly by hepatic enzyme induction. Conversely, patients receiving warfarin who stop azathioprine may be at risk of bleeding and should be monitored carefully [34].

Immunosuppressive therapy alone is unlikely to reduce the risk of further thrombosis in the antiphospholipid syndrome [34]. Fibrinolytic therapy has been successfully administered in a small number of patients, and prostacyclin analogues, such as iloprost, have also been used to manage small-vessel digital thromboses.

Management of catastrophic antiphospholipid syndrome remains unsatisfactory, although it appears that anticoagulation alone is probably insufficient. Measures such as plasma exchange, high-dose corticosteroids, and immunosuppressives have all been used anecdotally in these severely ill patients [27].

SYSTEMIC VASCULITIS

Although relatively uncommon, the systemic vasculitides comprise a group of multisystem connective tissue diseases that are often severe and may be life-threatening. Neurologists may be called on to assess these patients, because they frequently have peripheral neurologic disease. However, central nervous system involvement is certainly seen in these patients and is associated with high morbidity and mortality. Nevertheless, early assessment and therapy can be gratifying.

Vasculitis is characterized by inflammation and necrosis of vessel walls, resulting in compromise of vascular blood flow and ischemia. Because vasculitis can affect any organ in the body, the presenting clinical features may be extremely diverse and confusing. Several vasculitic syndromes are known and have characteristic clinical features, although the classification of these systemic vasculitides has been very difficult. One of the better-known classifications is that described by the American College of Rheumatology [35], which classifies seven conditions: Wegener's granulomatosis, polyarteritis nodosa, Churg-Strauss syndrome, hypersensitivity vasculitis, Takayasu's arteritis, giant-cell arteritis, and Henoch-Schönlein purpura (Table 9.2). This is by no means an ideal system, but it does have the merit of being validated and relatively easy to use and uses fairly characteristic features, although it does omit the use of antineutrophil cytoplasmic autoantibodies (ANCAs), which are specific for vasculitides such as Wegener's granulomatosis.

Primary angiitis of the central nervous system (PACNS), also known as *granulomatous angiitis of the nervous system*, has been extensively described in the literature [36]. It is a very rare vasculitic condition that presents with exclusively neurologic features without other organ involvement and in the absence of other connective tissue diseases. Calabrese and associates [37] classified the disease into true PACNS, benign angiitis of the nervous system, and other varieties, including cerebral amyloid angiopathy and postpartum angiopathy.

Clinical Features

Moore and Fauci [38] found central nervous system involvement in 40% of 25 patients with systemic vasculitides, a surprisingly high proportion. Development

Table 9.2   American College of Rheumatology criteria for the classification of vasculitis

Disease	Criteria	Number required	Sensitivity (%)	Specificity (%)
Wegener's granulomatosis	Nasal/oral inflammation; abnormal chest radiograph (nodules, infiltrates, or cavities); abnormal urine sediment; biopsy: granulomatous, inflammation	≥2	88.2	92.0
Churg-Strauss syndrome	Asthma; eosinophilia >10%; neuropathy; pulmonary infiltrates (nonfixed); paranasal sinus abnormality; extravascular eosinophils	≥4	85.0	99.7
Polyarteritis nodosa	Weight loss; livedo reticularis; testicular tenderness; myalgia or weakness; mono-/poly-neuropathy; diastolic blood pressure ≥90 mm Hg; elevated urea or creatinine; hepatitis B virus; arteriographic abnormality; biopsy of small/medium artery containing granulocytes	≥3	82.2	86.6
Giant-cell/ temporal arteritis	Age at onset ≥50 yrs; new headache; temporal artery tenderness or decreased pulsation; erythrocyte sedimentation rate ≥50; biopsy: mononuclear cell infiltrates or granulomatous inflammation	≥3	93.5	91.2
Takayasu's arteritis	Age at onset ≤40 yrs; claudication of extremities; decreased brachial artery pulse; blood pressure difference ≥10 mm Hg between arms; subclavian or aortic bruit; arteriographic narrowing or occlusion of aorta or its main branches	≥3	90.5	97.8
Hypersensitivity vasculitis	Age >16 yrs at onset; palpable purpura; maculopapular rash; extravascular or perivascular granulocytes	≥3	71.0	83.9
Henoch-Schönlein purpura	Palpable purpura; age <20 yrs at onset; bowel angina; biopsy: vessel wall granulocytes	≥2	87.8	87.7

of central nervous system disease is often late in the disease course, usually 2–3 years after diagnosis of the systemic vasculitis. Onset of these symptoms is likely to be insidious and nonspecific. For example, memory loss, irritability, lethargy, and mild impairment of intellectual activity are easy to overlook in a patient with active vasculitic disease. Major organ involvement may itself account for some of these symptoms (e.g., by resulting in uremia or hypoxia).

Two patterns of central nervous system disease are seen in the systemic vasculitides: diffuse and focal or multifocal [38,39]. Diffuse disease was seen in 5 of the 10 patients with central nervous system involvement in Moore and Fauci's study [38]. This was characterized by an encephalopathy in four patients with generalized or focal seizures and occasional minor focal features such as limb paresis and visual hallucinations. CT scanning and CSF examination were unremarkable apart from elevated protein levels in two patients. The other five patients had clinical evidence of focal disease in the cerebrum, cerebellum, or brain stem. One patient also had progressive dementia and another had seizures. On the whole, seizures were seen acutely and were not a long-term consequence of cortical damage from cerebral vasculitis. Psychosis was not seen in this series, possibly owing to relatively low corticosteroid doses. Of the 10 patients, 4 were hypertensive and in 9 of the 10 patients with central nervous system involvement, the neurologic features appeared despite the fact that the patients were taking oral corticosteroids.

Specific diseases may differ in the pattern of neurologic disease. In polyarteritis nodosa, for example, central nervous system disease can be seen in 23–53% of patients, particularly when aneurysms are also found on celiac axis angiography [36]. In one series, central nervous system disease was second only to renal disease as a cause of death [40]. Neurologic deafness, sometimes bilateral, has occasionally been noted in polyarteritis nodosa. In Wegener's granulomatosis, central nervous system involvement can be mediated by granulomatous nasal and sinus lesions invading the brain or orbits, isolated granulomatous lesions within the brain, or, more rarely, necrotizing cerebral vasculitis. The eye is often involved in the systemic vasculitides and can produce visual impairment from retinal vasculitis, corneal melts, and uveitis. Blindness caused by direct pressure on the optic nerve from a granulomatous lesion and deafness, mostly owing to otitis media but also from eighth nerve involvement, have been documented [41]. Ophthalmoplegia can also occur.

The presentation of PACNS is acute in up to 88% of patients with a heterogenous clinical picture, including headaches, transient ischemic attacks, paresis, neurocognitive deficits, altered consciousness, seizures, and vision loss in young to middle-aged patients [42]. Laboratory findings are often nonspecific with a leukocytosis in 80%, but a raised ESR is uncommon. CSF examination often shows an elevated protein and a mononuclear pleocytosis. CT and MRI scans may show cerebral hemorrhages, infarcts, and atrophy, or punctate gadolinium-enhancing lesions. Some patients show beading or alternating ectasia, or both, and stenosis on angiography; these abnormalities involve the smaller secondary and tertiary branches distal to the termination of the internal carotid arteries [42]. In one study, treatment with corticosteroids and oral cyclophosphamide was associated with remission in 88% of patients and repeat angiograms in three patients returned to normal; however, permanent disease-related neurologic deficit was also common (between 15% and 67% of patients) [42].

Clinical Assessment

When faced with a patient suspected of having cerebral vasculitis, the neurologist should carefully evaluate the patient clinically before considering further investigations. As with cerebral lupus, sepsis should always be excluded before immunosuppressive therapy is considered. Most patients undergo CT scan or preferably MRI before CSF examination, although the appearances are often nonspecific. CT scan is most useful in patients with Wegener's granulomatosis to document sinus and orbital disease, which can erode bony structures [41]. Electroencephalograms may show diffuse or bitemporal slowing or nonspecific abnormalities. Cerebral angiography is advocated by some clinicians, but this has its own morbidity and can sometimes be normal in a patient with cerebral vasculitis. Magnetic resonance angiography is at present relatively insensitive at visualizing small cerebral vessels, but the techniques may improve in time. CSF examination in the absence of sepsis is often unremarkable apart from occasional increases in CSF protein levels, with or without mild to moderate pleocytosis. Elevated CSF interleukin-6 levels have been reported in three patients with cerebral vasculitis in whom levels correlated with clinical and serologic evidence of active disease [43].

Serologic investigations may be useful, although CRP levels are not as helpful in vasculitis as they are in lupus in considering sepsis because they are usually elevated in active vasculitis. Hepatitis B and C status may be relevant in polyarteritis nodosa and cryoglobulinemic vasculitis. Antibodies directed against neutrophil cytoplasmic components (ANCA) may be particularly helpful in the diagnosis of systemic vasculitis. Two main patterns of immunofluorescence are known with distinct antigenic and disease specificities, and the test is readily available in most immunology laboratories (Table 9.3).

Table 9.3 Clinical significance and binding specificities of antineutrophil cytoplasmic autoantibodies

Pattern (target antigens)	Major associations	Other associations
cANCA (proteinase 3, BPI)	Wegener's granulomatosis	Minority of PAN, Churg-Strauss syndrome, Kawasaki's disease
pANCA (myeloperoxidase, elastase, cathepsin G, lactoferrin, lysozyme)	Microscopic PAN; rapidly progressive glomerulo-nephritis	Churg-Strauss syndrome; rheumatoid arthritis, Felty's, Still's disease; systemic lupus erythematosus, Sjögren's disease; Takayasu's arteritis; inflammatory bowel disease; drugs: hydralazine
xANCA (lactoferrin, lysozyme, cathepsin G, beta-glucuronidase)	Inflammatory bowel disease; autoimmune hepatitis	—

BPI = bactericidal permeability increasing protein; PAN = polyarteritis nodosa; cANCA = cytoplasmic staining antineutrophil cytoplasmic antibody; pANCA = perinuclear staining antineutrophil cytoplasmic antibody; xANCA = atypical/cross-staining antineutrophil cytoplasmic antibody.

Source: Adapted from WL Gross, WH Schmitt, E Csernok. ANCA and associated diseases: immunodiagnostic and pathogenetic aspects. Clin Exp Immunol 1993;91:1.

Some clinicians suggest that monitoring ANCA titers may be a good guide to disease activity and predicting disease flares, but this has not lived up to its initial promise in many patients [44]. Although ANCAs remain most useful in the acute situation in assisting diagnosis, every effort should be made to obtain histologic confirmation of vasculitis because many conditions (e.g., some malignancies) can mimic vasculitis. Cerebral biopsy is advocated by several authors [36] but this is probably only really necessary in patients who are suspected of having an isolated PACNS. In patients with an established systemic vasculitis with typical clinical features, cerebral biopsy is only indicated if another condition, such as a malignancy, is being considered. Histology may reveal arterial and arteriolar abnormalities involving various stages of vascular infiltration, necrosis, thrombosis, fibrosis, occlusion, and scarring [38]. These are found either diffusely or in patches throughout the meninges, cranial nerves, cerebrum and cerebellum, brain stem, and spinal cord but are most commonly located in the cerebral hemispheres.

Treatment

Many of the early descriptions of systemic vasculitis were autopsy studies, and this underscored the extremely poor prognosis of these patients before the advent of modern immunosuppressive therapies. Although the use of prednisolone was encouraging, its adverse effects and the high incidence of relapses on dose reduction led to a search for other therapies. Novak and Pearson [45] first used oral cyclophosphamide in the treatment of Wegener's granulomatosis and achieved dramatic improvements in prognosis. Combination therapy with cyclophosphamide and corticosteroids is now the treatment of choice for the systemic vasculitides and has resulted in dramatic improvements in life expectancy of Wegener's granulomatosis [46].

Cyclophosphamide is an oxazaphosphorine alkylating agent that acts on the "S" and other phases of the cell cycle. It has profound effects on T- and B-cell function and numbers that are dose- and time-dependent. Certainly, the suppression of autoantibody production by B cells and impairment of T-cell function are accompanied by clinical improvement in most patients with systemic vasculitis, although this is by no means always true.

It is useful to approach the treatment of a patient with severe life-threatening systemic vasculitis in two phases: induction and maintenance of remission. A variety of regimens exist for the initial treatment of acute necrotizing systemic vasculitis. Intravenous pulse cyclophosphamide therapy has been widely adopted and is relatively safe, well tolerated, and rapidly effective [19]. Mesna can be incorporated to reduce the risk of hemorrhagic cystitis. The rationale for intravenous bolus doses is that oral cyclophosphamide does not begin to exert an effect for at least 2 weeks and there is evidence that an immunosuppressive effect is seen much earlier with pulse therapy [47]. However, the long-term results in Wegener's granulomatosis in terms of disease relapse have not been as encouraging as in lupus nephritis [20,48]. Plasma exchange can also be used in the induction phase, particularly in severe disease with rapidly progressive glomerulonephritis.

Consensus on the best maintenance therapy has not been reached. Some groups continue monthly pulses of cyclophosphamide whereas others use oral cyclophosphamide, azathioprine, or methotrexate. Therapy continues for a minimum of 1 year and usually extends to 18–24 months with gradual withdrawal of therapy. Whatever regimen is used, it is clear that very frequent close monitoring of the patient is required to assess both response and adverse effects of therapy.

Adverse effects of corticosteroids and cyclophosphamide are legion and have been well documented. Long-term use of oral cyclophosphamide is associated with a high risk of infections, hemorrhagic cystitis, bladder malignancies, gonadal failure, solid tumors such as lymphomas, and a high incidence of marrow suppression [47]. Thus, although it is an extremely effective and often life-saving agent, the risk-benefit ratio of prolonged oral use is poor. Debate over the dose, duration, and route of administration of cyclophosphamide continues, and prospective studies are in progress in Europe to address some of these issues.

Azathioprine is safer than cyclophosphamide but is not effective in the initial treatment of severe necrotizing systemic vasculitis. It does, however, have a useful role in patients who have responded well to intensive induction therapy and can be used in the maintenance therapy of polyarteritis nodosa or Churg-Strauss syndrome in which the risk of a major relapse after successful initial therapy is not high. The main adverse effects include marrow suppression and hepatitis. Occasional rashes have been reported, and, rarely, pancreatitis and sterility are seen.

Methotrexate has been used in moderately high doses (20–25 mg/week) for the treatment of Wegener's granulomatosis. Although initially encouraging, studies showed a significant risk of *Pneumocystis carinii* infections together with abnormalities of liver and lung function [49].

A number of other therapies have been tried in systemic vasculitis with varying degrees of success. Cotrimoxazole has received attention [50] in the treatment of Wegener's granulomatosis. Although reports have been mainly anecdotal, larger studies in progress are modestly encouraging.

Etoposide is a well-established agent in the treatment of lung and testicular tumors. It has been used successfully to induce and maintain remission in a patient with Wegener's granulomatosis that did not respond to intensive standard therapies [51], and two additional patients have also had positive results with monthly courses of etoposide, 75–100 mg per day for 1 week each month. Its main adverse effects are a transient neutropenia that occurs at day 15 and some hair loss, although these problems have been mild in these patients.

Other experimental therapies include the successful use of intravenous immunoglobulin in the treatment of seven patients with ANCA-positive vasculitis that did not respond to conventional therapies [52]. Monoclonal antibodies have also been used successfully in a patient with Wegener's granulomatosis. A combination of anti-CD4 and an anti-CDw52 (Campath-1H) monoclonal antibody was used to profoundly reduce circulating lymphocyte numbers and was associated with a prolonged remission [53].

The improvement of central nervous system manifestations of vasculitis with treatment can be rapid. This speed of recovery in diffuse cerebral disease suggests that functional rather than structural abnormalities may be responsible for the clinical features and may be mirrored by improvements in electroencephalographic changes [38]. Although many patients achieve some improvement, this is not always the case, and cerebral vasculitis can develop as a new manifestation despite cyclophosphamide therapy [54].

OTHER DISORDERS ASSOCIATED WITH CEREBRAL VASCULITIS

Cerebral vasculitis can complicate adult and juvenile rheumatoid arthritis, but this is notable by its rarity [36]. In primary Sjögren's syndrome, true cerebral disease is uncommon, but cranial nerve lesions, especially trigeminal neuropathy, are well described [55]. Peripheral neuropathy is common in Sjögren's syndrome; other cerebral features include aseptic meningoencephalitis, necrotizing spinal arteritis and hemorrhage, focal and multifocal cerebral disease (reviewed in reference 36), and diffuse cerebral vasculitis [56,57]. Trigeminal neuropathy, often bilateral, has been described in 4% of patients with progressive systemic sclerosis and may predate other features of the disease [58]. Other cranial nerve lesions may be seen, although true cerebral vasculitis is very rare in systemic sclerosis (reviewed in reference 36). Mixed connective tissue disease, which overlaps clinically with lupus, scleroderma, and the inflammatory myopathies, may also be complicated by central nervous system features, especially trigeminal neuropathy, in up to 10% of cases [59].

Giant-cell arteritis can be diagnosed easily because of its characteristic clinical features. In addition to the well-known risk of blindness, it has been associated with meningoencephalitis, seizures, hemiplegia, dysarthria, and dysphagia. Giant-cell arteritis may even be a presenting feature of Wegener's granulomatosis [60].

Behçet's disease is commonly associated with central neurologic disease, usually as a late manifestation, and is seen in up to 29% of patients (reviewed in reference 36). Clinical features include ocular disease, strokes, hemi- and quadriparesis, pseudobulbar palsy, cranial neuropathy, cerebellar disease, and dysarthria. Cerebrospinal fluid examination shows a lymphocytic pleocytosis and MRI is often useful in detecting lesions, which often preferentially involve the brain stem, basal ganglia, and internal capsules. True angiitis is rare, although perivascular lymphocytic infiltrates with demyelination, axonal degeneration, and necrotic lesions may be seen (reviewed in reference 36).

Lyme disease that results from infection with *Borrelia burgdorferi* classically causes a distinctive rash (erythema chronicum migrans), arthritis, carditis, and, in up to 20% of patients, neurologic disease. Among the most common features is fluctuating meningoencephalitis with superimposed cranial or radicular neuropathies; slow resolution occurs with high-dose penicillin [61].

Sarcoidosis is complicated by central nervous system disease in 3–5% of patients and may be a presenting clinical feature. Clinical features include cranial nerve palsies, hypothalamic dysfunction, hydrocephalus, encephalopathy, seizures, optic neuropathy, myelopathy, and retinal vasculitis. Histologically, a granulomatous angiitis has been described coexisting with a granulomatous leptomeningitis. Nearly all patients with neurosarcoidosis have some evidence of systemic disease that helps in diagnosis (reviewed in reference 36).

Other diseases that can either cause or mimic cerebral vasculitis include thrombotic thrombocytopenic purpura, left atrial myxoma, multiple cholesterol emboli, mitral valve prolapse, and some migraine syndromes (reviewed in reference 36). Celiac disease has been complicated by cutaneous, renal, and cerebral vasculitis (reviewed in reference 62). Many infections can be associated with cerebral vasculitis, including herpes zoster, which can result in delayed contralateral hemiplegia and human immunodeficiency virus disease.

Drugs and chemicals occasionally cause or mimic cerebral vasculitis. These include poisons, such as carbon monoxide and arsenic, ergotamine, and intravenous drug abuse, especially with amphetamines (reviewed in reference 63).

CONCLUSIONS

Although some of the conditions described here are uncommon, careful evaluation of the patient at the bedside and with appropriate laboratory and imaging investigations can lead to a diagnosis that yields satisfying clinical results from therapy. Since the 1980s, laboratory assays, such as antiphospholipid antibodies and ANCA, together with improvements in imaging, including MRI, have transformed the investigation of patients with inflammatory and thrombotic vascular central nervous system disease. Further refinements in noninvasive techniques to aid diagnosis are just around the corner, but as in any branch of clinical medicine, there is no substitute for clinical skills, knowledge, and experience of these diseases when assessing these complex diagnostic problems.

REFERENCES

1. Carbotte RM, Denburg SD, Denburg JA, et al. Fluctuating cognitive abnormalities and cerebral glucose metabolism in neuropsychiatric systemic lupus erythematosus. J Neurol Neurosurg Psychiatry 1992;55:1054.
2. Feinglass EJ, Arnett FC, Dorsch CA, et al. Neuropsychiatric manifestations of systemic lupus erythematosus: diagnosis, clinical spectrum and relationship to other features of the disease. Medicine (Baltimore) 1976;55:323.
3. Johnson RT, Richardson EP. The neurological manifestations of systemic lupus erythematosus: a clinical pathological study of 24 cases and review of the literature. Medicine 1968;47:337.
4. Devinsky O, Pettito CK, Alonso DR. Clinical and neuropathological findings in systemic lupus erythematosus: the role of vasculitis, heart emboli and thrombotic thrombocytopenic purpura. Ann Neurol 1988;23:380.
5. Widener HL, Littman BH. Ibuprofen-induced meningitis in systemic lupus erythematosus. JAMA 1978;239:1062.
6. Sergent JS, Lockshin M. Azathioprine-induced meningitis in systemic lupus erythematosus. JAMA 1978;240:529.
7. Reik L. Disorders that mimic CNS infections. Neurol Clin 1986;4:223.
8. Wong KL, Woo EKW, Yu YL, Wong RWS. Neurological manifestations of systemic lupus erythematosus: a prospective study. QJM 1991;81:857.
9. Cauli A, Montaldo C, Peltz MT, et al. Abnormalities of magnetic resonance imaging of the central nervous system in patients with systemic lupus erythematosus correlate with disease severity. Clin Rheumatol 1994;13:615.
10. Gonzalez-Crespo MR, Blanco FJ, Ramos A, et al. Magnetic resonance imaging of the brain in systemic lupus erythematosus. Br J Rheumatol 1995;34:1055.

11. Miller DH, Buchanan N, Barker G, et al. Gadolinium-enhanced magnetic resonance imaging of the central nervous system in systemic lupus erythematosus. J Neurol 1992;239:460.
12. Emmi L, Bramati M, De Cristofaro MT, et al. MRI and SPECT investigations of the CNS in SLE patients. Clin Exp Rheumatol 1993;11:13.
13. Kodama K, Okada S, Hino T, et al. Single photon emission computed tomography in systemic lupus erythematosus with psychiatric symptoms. J Neurol Neurosurg Psychiatry 1995;58:307.
14. Stoppe E, Wildhagen MD, Seidel MD, et al. Positron emission tomography in neuropsychiatric lupus erythematosus. Neurology 1990;40:304.
15. Awada HH, Mamo HL, Luft AG, et al. Cerebral blood flow in systemic lupus erythematosus with and without central nervous system involvement. J Neurol Neurosurg Psychiatry 1987;50:1597.
16. Hirohata S, Miyamoto T. Elevated levels of interleukin-6 in cerebrospinal fluid from patients with systemic lupus erythematosus and central nervous system involvement. Arthritis Rheum 1990;33:644.
17. Teh LS, Hay EM, Amos N, et al. Anti-P antibodies are associated with psychiatric and focal cerebral disorders in patients with systemic lupus erythematosus. Br J Rheumatol 1993;32:287.
18. Asherson RA, Denburg SD, Denburg JA, et al. Current concepts of neuropsychiatric systemic lupus erythematosus (NP-SLE). Postgrad Med J 1993;69:602.
19. Haga HJ, D'Cruz D, Asherson RA, Hughes GRV. The short-term effect of pulse cyclophosphamide in the treatment of connective tissue diseases. Ann Rheum Dis 1992;51:885.
20. Martin-Suarez M, D'Cruz D, Mansoor M, et al. Immunosuppressive therapy in severe connective tissue diseases: effects of low dose intravenous cyclophosphamide. Ann Rheum Dis 1997;56:1.
21. Lopez Dupla M, Khamashta MA, Sanchez A, et al. Transverse myelitis as a first manifestation of systemic lupus erythematosus: a case report. Lupus 1995;4:239.
22. Hughes GRV, Harris EN, Gharavi AE. The anticardiolipin syndrome. J Rheumatol. 1986;13:486.
23. Hughes GRV. The antiphospholipid syndrome: ten years on. Lancet 1993;342:341.
24. Herranz MT, Rivier G, Khamashta MA, et al. Association between antiphospholipid antibodies and epilepsy in patients with systemic lupus erythematosus. Arthritis Rheum 1994;37:568.
25. Alarcon-Segovia D, Deleze M, Oria CV, et al. Antiphospholipid antibodies and the antiphospholipid syndrome in systemic lupus erythematosus: a prospective analysis of 500 consecutive patients. Medicine (Baltimore) 1989;68:353.
26. Nencini P, Baruffi MC, Abbati R, et al. Lupus anticoagulant and anti-cardiolipin antibodies in young adults with cerebral ischemia. Stroke 1992;23:189.
27. Asherson RA, Piette J-C. The catastrophic antiphospholipid syndrome 1996: acute multi-organ failure associated with antiphospholipid antibodies: a review of 31 patients. Lupus 1996;5:414.
28. Wilson WA, Gharavi AE. Genetic risk factors for aPL syndrome. Lupus 1996;5:398.
29. Hunt JE, Krilis SA. The fifth domain of 2 glycoprotein I contains a phospholipid binding site (Cys 281–Cys 288) and a region recognized by anticardiolipin antibodies. J Immunol 1994;152:653.
30. Cabiedes J, Cabral AR, Alarcon-Segovia D. Clinical manifestations of the antiphospholipid syndrome in patients with systemic lupus erythematosus associate more strongly with anti-2-glycoprotein-1 than with antiphospholipid antibodies. J Rheumatol 1995;22:1899.
31. Amengual O, Atsumi T, Khamashta MA. Specificity of ELISA for antibody to β_2-glycoprotein 1 in patients with antiphospholipid syndrome. Br J Rheumatol 1996;35:1239.
32. Khamashta MA, Cuadrado MJ, Mujic F, et al. The management of thrombosis in the antiphospholipid-antibody syndrome. N Engl J Med 1995;332:993.
33. Ginsberg JS, Wells PS, Brill-Edwards P, et al. Antiphospholipid antibodies and venous thromboembolism. Blood 1995;86:3685.
34. Khamashta MA. Management of thrombosis in the antiphospholipid syndrome. Lupus 1996;5:463.
35. Hunder GG, Arend WP, Bloch DA, et al. The American College of Rheumatology 1990 criteria for the classification of vasculitis. Arthritis Rheum 1990;33:1065.
36. Sigal LH. The neurologic presentation of vasculitis and rheumatologic syndromes. Medicine (Baltimore) 1987;66:157.
37. Calabrese LH, Furlan AJ, Gragg LA, Popos TJ. Primary angiitis of the central nervous system: diagnostic criteria and clinical approach. Cleve Clin J Med 1992;59:293.
38. Moore PM, Fauci AS. Neurologic manifestations of systemic vasculitis. A retrospective and prospective study of the clinicopathologic features and responses to therapy in 25 patients. Am J Med 1981;71:517.
39. Kissel JT. Neurologic manifestations of systemic disease. Neurol Clin 1989;7:655.
40. Travers RL, Allison DJ, Brettle RP, Hughes GRV. Polyarteritis nodosa: a clinical and angiographic analysis of 17 cases. Semin Arthritis Rheum 1979;8:184.
41. D'Cruz DP, Baguley E, Asherson RA, Hughes GRV. Ear, nose and throat symptoms in sub-acute Wegener's granulomatosis. BMJ 1989;299:419.

42. Abu-Shakra M, Khraishi M, Grosman H, et al. Primary angiitis of the CNS diagnosed by angiography. QJM 1994;87:351.
43. Hirohata S, Tanimoto K, Ito K. Elevation of cerebrospinal fluid interleukin-6 activity in patients with vasculitides and central nervous system involvement. Clin Immunol Immunopathol 1993;66:225.
44. Kerr GS, Fleisher TA, Hallahan CW, et al. Limited prognostic value of antineutrophil cytoplasmic antibody titer in patients with Wegener's granulomatosis. Arthritis Rheum 1993;36:365.
45. Novak SN, Pearson CM. Cyclophosphamide therapy in Wegener's granulomatosis. N Engl J Med 1971;284:938.
46. Hoffman GS, Kerr GS, Leavitt RY, et al. Wegener's granulomatosis: an analysis of 158 patients. Ann Intern Med 1992;116:488.
47. De Vita S, Neri R, Bombardieri S. Cyclophosphamide pulses in the treatment of rheumatic diseases: an update. Clin Exp Rheumatol 1991;9:179.
48. Hoffman GS, Leavitt RY, Fleisher TA, et al. Treatment of Wegener's granulomatosis with intermittent high dose intravenous cyclophosphamide. Am J Med 1990;89:403.
49. Hoffman GS, Leavitt RY, Kerr GS, Fauci AS. The treatment of Wegener's granulomatosis with glucocorticoids and methotrexate. Arthritis Rheum 1992;35:1322.
50. DeRemee RA. The treatment of Wegener's granulomatosis with trimethoprim/sulfamethoxazole: illusion or vision? Arthritis Rheum 1988;31:1068.
51. D'Cruz D, Payne H, Timothy A, Hughes GRV. Response of cyclophosphamide resistant Wegener's granulomatosis to etoposide. Lancet 1992;340:425.
52. Jayne DRW, Davies MJ, Fox CJV, et al. Treatment of systemic vasculitis with pooled intravenous immunoglobulin. Lancet 1991;337:1137.
53. Mathieson PW, Cobbold SP, Hale G, et al. Monoclonal-antibody therapy in systemic vasculitis. N Engl J Med 1990;323:250.
54. Kroneman OC III, Pevzner M. Failure of cyclophosphamide to prevent cerebritis in Wegener's granulomatosis. Am J Med 1986;80:526.
55. Kaltreider HB, Talal N. The neuropathy of Sjögren syndrome: trigeminal nerve involvement. Ann Intern Med 1969;70:751.
56. Ferreiro JE, Robalino BD, Saldana MJ. Primary Sjögren's syndrome with diffuse cerebral vasculitis and lymphocytic interstitial pneumonitis [letter]. Am J Med 1987;82:1227.
57. Calabrese CH. "Possible" primary Sjögren's syndrome with diffuse cerebrovasculitis and lymphocytic interstitial pneumonitis [letter]. Am J Med 1987;83:1175.
58. Farrell DA, Medsger TA Jr. Trigeminal neuropathy in progressive systemic sclerosis. Am J Med 1982;73:57.
59. Sharp GC. Mixed connective tissue disease. Bull Rheum Dis 1975;25:828.
60. Howe L, D'Cruz D, Chopdar A, Hughes G. Anterior ischaemic optic neuropathy in Wegener's granulomatosis. Eur J Ophthalmol 1995;5:277.
61. Steere AC, Pachner AR, Malawista SE. Neurologic abnormalities of lyme disease: successful treatment with high-dose intravenous penicillin. Ann Intern Med 1983;99:767.
62. Rush PJ, Inman R, Bernstein M, et al. Isolated vasculitis of the central nervous system in a patient with celiac disease. Am J Med 1986;81:1092.
63. Ferris EJ, Levine HL. Cerebral arteritis: classification. Radiology 1973;109:32.

10
Subarachnoid Hemorrhage

Gary L. Bernardini, Stephan A. Mayer,
and Robert A. Solomon

Subarachnoid hemorrhage (SAH) represents 5% of all strokes and is unique in that the risk of recurrence can be effectively eliminated by treatment. Saccular (or berry) aneurysms on vessels at the base of the brain cause 80% of all cases of SAH. Other nonaneurysmal causes are listed in Table 10.1. Despite remarkable advances in medical and surgical treatment since the early 1980s, SAH remains a devastating neurologic disease in which up to 25% of patients die within the first 24 hours. Of those who survive, more than half are left with significant neurologic deficits as a direct result of the hemorrhage or from delayed complications [1]. This review discusses the clinical presentation and pathogenesis of SAH and provides an update on current diagnostic procedures and clinical management.

INCIDENCE AND NATURAL HISTORY
OF SUBARACHNOID HEMORRHAGE

Aneurysmal SAH is a major clinical problem in the United States, with an annual incidence of 6–16 per 100,000 people [2,3]. Based on this rate, it is estimated that approximately 28,000 Americans will experience a ruptured intracranial aneurysm each year. The prevalence of unruptured intracranial aneurysms in the general population is probably between 0.5% and 1.0%, or approximately 2 million individuals in the United States [4]. Aneurysms are found in up to 4% of routine adult autopsies but are rare in children [5]. Although the incidence of other types of stroke (e.g., cerebral infarction and intracerebral hemorrhage) has substantially decreased since the 1960s, the incidence of aneurysmal SAH has remained unchanged [6,7].

SAH occurs more frequently in women than in men, with a ratio of 3 to 2, but before the age of 40 years it tends to predominate in men [8]. Aneurysms are rare in childhood; the incidence of aneurysmal rupture increases with age and is highest in the fifth to sixth decades. In patients who harbor a previously unrup-

Table 10.1   Nonaneurysmal causes of subarachnoid hemorrhage

Trauma
Arterial dissection
Mycotic aneurysm
Arteriovenous malformation
Cocaine and amphetamine use
Moyamoya disease
Central nervous system vasculitis
Idiopathic perimesencephalic subarachnoid hemorrhage

tured aneurysm, the risk of bleeding is approximately 1–2% per year, with greater risk for aneurysms of 7 mm or more in size [9].

ANATOMY AND PATHOGENESIS OF ANEURYSMAL RUPTURE

Approximately 85% of intracranial aneurysms occur in the anterior circulation. The most common sites are the junction of the internal carotid and the posterior communicating arteries, the anterior communicating–anterior cerebral arteries, or the trifurcation of the middle cerebral artery (Figure 10.1). Aneurysms of the posterior circulation are most commonly located at the bifurcation of the basilar artery or the junction of a vertebral artery and the posterior inferior cerebellar artery [10,11]. Multiple intracranial aneurysms are found in 15–20% of patients and are commonly seen as "mirror" aneurysms—that is, located on the same artery on the contralateral side [12–14]. Intracranial aneurysms are occasionally found at the origin of the ophthalmic artery, or in the cavernous sinus, where rupture can cause a carotid-cavernous fistula rather than SAH [5,15]. In addition, approximately 7% of patients with an arteriovenous malformation have an aneurysm on a feeding artery [16].

Microscopically, saccular or berry aneurysms characteristically have a very thin tunica media or none at all, and the internal elastic lamina is either absent or severely fragmented [12,17]. Growth and subsequent rupture of aneurysms are thought to result from increased hydrostatic pressure and turbulence at bifurcations of the major arteries at the base of the brain. Most ruptures occur through the dome of the aneurysm, which may be as thin as 0.3 mm [18]. With rupture, a jet of blood under high pressure can cause local tissue damage and an abrupt increase in intracranial pressure, which can approximate mean arterial pressure and lead to loss of consciousness. The probability of occurrence of aneurysmal rupture is related to size; aneurysms smaller than 7 mm in diameter have a very low rate of rupture [9].

RISK FACTORS FOR SUBARACHNOID HEMORRHAGE

Although the exact cause of aneurysm formation remains obscure, both congenital and environmental factors appear to play a role. Association of aneurysms

Figure 10.1 **A.** Computed tomographic scan demonstrates a large left temporo-parietal hemorrhage with surrounding edema and effacement of the lateral ventricle; also note mild subfalcine herniation. **B.** Four-vessel cerebral angiogram reveals a 1-cm left middle cerebral artery–trifurcation aneurysm *(long arrow)* with a small lobulated component that may represent a "tit"—that is, the site of rupture *(arrowhead)*.

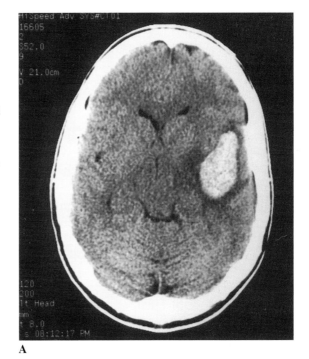

A

B

with diseases such as fibromuscular dysplasia, Marfan's syndrome, pseudoxanthoma elasticum, Ehlers-Danlos syndrome, polycystic kidney disease, and coarctation of the aorta suggests that heritable connective tissue disorders can predispose to aneurysm formation [19]. The preponderance of SAH in women suggests that hormonal factors may play a role in aneurysm formation. Subarachnoid hemorrhage is more common in women after menopause, and use of low-dose oral contraceptives in postmenopausal women has been associated with a reduced risk of SAH [20].

Among modifiable risk factors for SAH, cigarette smoking, excessive alcohol use, and hypertension are associated with aneurysmal rupture [21]. The number of cigarettes smoked per day and duration of smoking are closely associated with the risk of SAH [22,23]. Pathologically, smoking leads to increased amounts of proteolytic enzymes released into the systemic circulation [24] and decreased effectiveness of alpha$_1$-antitrypsin, an inhibitor of proteolytic enzymes. These enzymes can contribute to arterial wall degradation and subsequent aneurysm formation [25]. Heavy alcohol use and binge drinking increase the risk of SAH [23]. This association can be mediated by transient hypertension, which occurs with intoxication or withdrawal [26,27], as well as alcohol-induced platelet dysfunction and coagulopathy. Hypertension and cocaine use are risk factors for both SAH and intracerebral hemorrhage.

CLINICAL PRESENTATION
OF SUBARACHNOID HEMORRHAGE

SAH classically presents with an explosive headache of sudden onset, followed by brief loss of consciousness and neck stiffness [28]. Although this characteristic presentation occurs in more than 50% of cases, up to 25% of patients with SAH are initially misdiagnosed, which can lead to delays in treatment and increased morbidity and mortality [29,30]. In most cases, the location of the headache is generalized but may refer to the site of aneurysmal rupture—that is, the occipital region with posterior circulation aneurysms or the periorbital region with ophthalmic artery aneurysms. Rupture of an intracranial aneurysm can lead to intraventricular, intracerebral, or subdural hemorrhage, as well as SAH (Figure 10.2).

Associated symptoms of aneurysmal rupture include neck stiffness, nausea and vomiting, back or leg pain, lethargy, and photophobia [28]. The presence of neck pain or nuchal rigidity owing to meningeal irritation in SAH is caused by the breakdown of blood products circulating within the subarachnoid space. If the blood settles into the thoracic or lumbar subarachnoid space, back pain can overshadow the more characteristic complaints of occipital or neck pain. Ophthalmologic examination may reveal unilateral or bilateral subhyaloid hemorrhages in one-fourth of patients with SAH [31]. Although aneurysmal rupture often takes place during periods of exercise or physical stress, SAH can occur at any time [32].

Patients often present with a history of a recent but less severe headache days to weeks before the onset of aneurysmal rupture. These sentinel or "warning leak" headaches are believed to result from minor leaking of blood into the subarachnoid space and may be misdiagnosed as migraine headache, systemic viral infection, hypertensive encephalopathy, sinusitis, or malingering [33].

Figure 10.2 **A.** Computed tomographic scan demonstrates extensive subarachnoid hemorrhage with thick clot in the anterior interhemispheric fissure, along with intracerebral hemorrhage and surrounding edema in the right frontal region. **B.** Note also dilatated temporal horns and lateral ventricles consistent with acute hydrocephalus. This 43-year-old man presented with acute onset of a bifrontal headache followed by brief loss of consciousness.

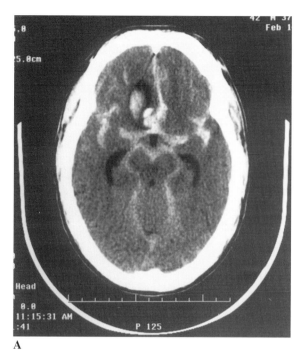

A

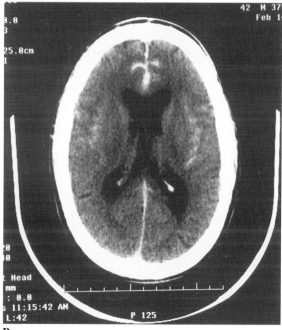

B

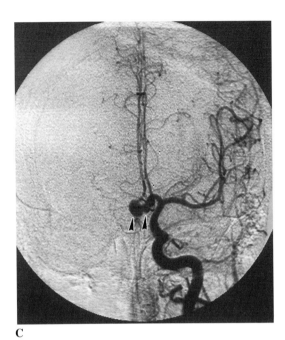

Figure 10.2 (continued)   **C.** Four-vessel cerebral angiogram reveals a bilobed anterior communicating aneurysm *(arrowheads)* that was successfully clipped.

C

An expanding, unruptured aneurysm can present with a visual field deficit; oculomotor palsy; or eye, face, or local head pain. In rare cases, cerebral ischemia in the vascular territory distal to an aneurysm is the presenting clinical manifestation of an unruptured intracranial aneurysm [34,35]. Ischemic events from unruptured aneurysms are thought to result from thrombus within the aneurysm, which serves as a nidus for embolization [34].

The syndrome of "perimesencephalic" nonaneurysmal SAH, as seen on computed tomographic (CT) scans, has a relatively benign course (Figure 10.3). The clinical presentation of these patients is similar to that of patients with aneurysmal SAH, with sudden headache, meningismus, and nausea. Changes in level of consciousness and sentinel headaches do not occur; their presence should raise suspicion for an aneurysmal source of bleeding. Compared to patients with aneurysmal SAH, those with perimesencephalic SAH tend to be younger and are more often men. Although significant hydrocephalus can develop in up to 5% of patients, vasospasm and rebleeding never occur after perimesencephalic SAH [36,37]. The pathogenesis of perimesencephalic SAH is unknown, but the origin is thought to be venous or capillary rather than arterial. Repeat angiography is usually unnecessary in patients with uncomplicated perimesencephalic SAH when the initial angiogram is negative [36].

Patients may have global or focal neurologic abnormalities depending on the location and severity of the SAH. The modified Hunt and Hess grading serves as a means for risk stratification of acute SAH based on the initial neurologic examination [38]. This five-point scale (Table 10.2) categorizes level of consciousness and presence of cranial nerve or focal neurologic deficits. Patients who present with grade I or II SAH have a relatively good prognosis; grade III carries an intermediate prognosis, and grades IV and V carry a poor prognosis. Radiographi-

Figure 10.3 Computed tomographic scan demonstrates typical perimesencephalic subarachnoid hemorrhage in a 44-year-old man. An angiogram was negative for aneurysm. (R = right.)

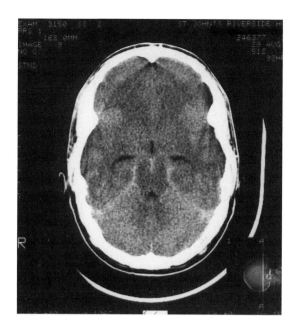

cally, the Fisher scale is used to grade the amount of subarachnoid blood on the initial CT scan (Table 10.3); thick clot in the basal cisterns (grades 3 and 4) indicates a high risk for delayed ischemia from vasospasm.

DIAGNOSTIC STUDIES

Detection of Subarachnoid Blood

A noncontrast CT scan remains the diagnostic study of choice for evaluating suspected SAH (see Figure 10.3). The sensitivity of computed tomography is highest within the first 24 hours after the hemorrhage (90–95%) but declines to 80%

Table 10.2   Modified Hunt and Hess scale

Grade	Description	Mortality (%)
I	Asymptomatic or mild headache with normal neurologic examination	2
II	Moderate to severe headache with normal neurologic examination or oculomotor palsy	5
III	Lethargy, confusion, or mild focal neurologic signs	15–20
IV	Stupor	30–40
V	Coma	50–80

Table 10.3   Fisher grade*

Grade	Description
1	No or minimal subarachnoid blood
2	Diffuse, thin subarachnoid blood
3	Thick (>1 mm) subarachnoid blood
4	Focal intracerebral or intraventricular hemorrhage

*For quantification of subarachnoid blood on the initial computed tomographic scan.

by the third day and 50% by the end of the first week [11,39]. When the initial CT scan is negative but there is a reasonable suspicion of an SAH, a lumbar puncture should be performed. Subarachnoid hemorrhage can be differentiated from a traumatic tap by the presence of xanthochromia of the cerebrospinal fluid (CSF) supernatant after centrifugation. Caused by blood breakdown products circulating within the CSF, xanthochromia can take up to 12 hours to appear; thus, a lumbar puncture done very recently after an SAH may fail to reveal xanthochromia [40].

The usefulness of magnetic resonance imaging (MRI) in the initial evaluation of patients with SAH is limited by the fact that hyperacute blood appears isodense on both T1- and T2-weighted images and by the need for patient cooperation and the length of time necessary to complete the test. The use of T2-weighted spin echo MRI images has been suggested to have a high sensitivity in demonstrating subtle evidence of acute SAH that is not visible on CT scan [41]. At present, however, computed tomography is generally considered to be superior to standard MRI for diagnosing acute SAH.

Diagnosis of Intracranial Aneurysms

Cerebral four-vessel angiography is the method of choice for detecting intracranial aneurysms and determining their precise anatomic location and size. If SAH is demonstrated on CT scan or by lumbar puncture, an angiogram should be performed as soon as possible. In 15–20% of patients with SAH, the initial cerebral angiogram is negative [42–44]. A repeat angiogram should be performed in these individuals 1–2 weeks after the initial study, because at least 5% of patients with an initially negative angiogram have an aneurysm detected on follow-up [45]. The exception to this rule is in patients with perimesencephalic SAH [36]. False-negative angiograms after SAH can result from aneurysm obliterated by clot, local vasospasm, or inadequate technique [44,46].

An MRI scan can reveal an occult vascular malformation, rupture of a small penetrating arteriole or venule, or a thrombosed aneurysm in patients with SAH [47]. Magnetic resonance angiography (MRA) can detect intracranial aneurysms as small as 2–3 mm, but in most studies the level of detection is approximately 5 mm [48]. Thus, smaller aneurysms can be missed with this technique. Helical CT angiography (CTA) is a newer, noninvasive method for detecting aneurysms [49]. A particular advantage of CTA is that images can be rotated on the screen to mimic the operative approach. Although aneurysms located near the base of the skull are more difficult to visualize with CTA, improved bone-removal algorithms may make this less of a problem in the future. Because of their limited sensitivity, however, with present technology CTA or MRA should not be used as a substitute for conventional angiography in the initial evaluation of acute SAH.

Screening for Asymptomatic Aneurysms

Screening for unruptured aneurysms is generally indicated in two settings: (1) in individuals with two or more first-degree family members with a history of intracranial aneurysm and (2) in family members of patients with autosomal-dominant polycystic kidney disease [50,51]. In one study, asymptomatic aneurysms were detected in almost 9% (38 of 438) of asymptomatic, first-degree relatives of patients with a ruptured intracranial aneurysm [52]. Approximately 5–10% of asymptomatic relatives of SAH patients with polycystic kidney disease are found to have an intracranial aneurysm [53,54]. Because of its low risk, MRA is the best imaging modality available for screening asymptomatic relatives of patients with SAH.

TREATMENT OF ACUTE SUBARACHNOID HEMORRHAGE

Initial Medical Management

All patients with SAH should be closely monitored in an intensive care unit, where frequent neurologic examinations can be performed. Blood pressure should be measured with an automated cuff, or an arterial line if active treatment is required. Patients with the more severe SAH (Hunt and Hess grades III–V) may require intubation to protect the airway. Intubation-induced hypertension can pose a significant risk of rebleeding; therefore, appropriate premedication with lidocaine or a short-acting barbiturate should be used before placement of an endotracheal tube. Admission electrocardiogram, chest x-ray, serum electrolytes, cardiac enzymes, hematologic and coagulation profiles, and a blood sample for type and cross should be obtained (Table 10.4). Patients should be kept at strict bed rest and given adequate sedation when necessary to prevent excessive elevations in blood pressure that might precipitate rebleeding. Agents such as propofol and fentanyl are useful for providing short-acting and reversible sedation in intubated, poor-grade patients.

The optimal blood pressure at which SAH patients should be maintained before surgical clipping is not entirely clear; a reasonable approach is to avoid elevations higher than 150 mm Hg systolic or greater than 10% of baseline premorbid levels. The appropriate choice for an intravenous antihypertensive agent in this setting is one with a short half-life that can be easily titrated. Labetalol, a mixed alpha$_1$ and nonselective beta blocker, and the calcium channel blocker nicardipine both possess these properties and do not increase intracranial pressure [55]. Both nitroprusside and nitroglycerin should be avoided because their use can lead to cerebral vasodilation, increased intracranial blood volume, and elevated intracranial pressure [56].

Table 10.4   Management protocol for acute subarachnoid hemorrhage (SAH)

Parameter	Treatment
Blood pressure	Treat persistently elevated blood pressure (systolic blood pressure >150 mm Hg) to prevent rebleeding during preoperative phase
Intravenous hydration	Aggressively hydrate with isotonic crystalloid (with or without colloid) to induce mild hypervolemia; use a central venous or pulmonary artery catheter to guide fluid administration in high-risk patients
Laboratory testing	Periodically check complete blood cell count and maintain hematocrit at 30%; monitor electrolytes to detect hyponatremia; obtain three serial electrocardiograms and check admission CK-MB to evaluate for neurogenic cardiac injury
Seizure prophylaxis	Fosphenytoin intravenous load (15–20 mg/kg); discontinue phenytoin on postoperative day 2
Vasospasm prophylaxis	Nimodipine, 60 mg orally q4h for 21 days
Vasospasm diagnosis	Transcranial Doppler sonography every 1–2 days through SAH day 8
Gastrointestinal prophylaxis	H_2 blockers (e.g., ranitidine) or sucralfate (Carafate)
Deep vein thrombosis prophylaxis	Heparin, 5,000 units subcutaneously q12h, and/or pneumatic compression boots

CK-MB = isoenzyme of creatine kinase with muscle and brain subunits.

Patients with SAH should be given nimodipine, 60 mg orally every 4 hours, as tolerated by blood pressure, for 21 consecutive days [57,58]. A loading dose of an intravenous anticonvulsant such as fosphenytoin (15–20 mg/kg) should be given to prevent rebleeding related to seizures. Anticonvulsants can routinely be discontinued on postoperative day 2 or 3 if the patient has not had a seizure [59]. The use of dexamethasone in acute SAH is controversial; it is frequently used in the perioperative period for brain relaxation without specific evidence to suggest that it is beneficial. Serum glucose and bedside fingerstick monitoring should be followed closely in patients given steroids. Prophylaxis against deep vein thrombosis in immobilized patients can be achieved with pneumatic boots or administration of heparin, 5,000 units subcutaneously twice a day.

Surgical Management

The goal of surgical treatment is to exclude the aneurysmal sac from the intracranial circulation by placement of a clip across the neck of the aneurysm while preserving the parent artery and its branches. Neurosurgical techniques have improved dramatically since the 1970s with the introduction of the operating microscope and microsurgical techniques [60–63]. As a result, the operative mortality of aneurysm surgery has fallen from more than 50% in the 1950s to less than 5% in the 1990s. These dramatic improvements in surgical results have been complemented by advances in neuroanesthesia and neurologic intensive care.

In some instances, owing to size, location, or configuration, aneurysms that are not amenable to safe clipping with standard techniques may require parent artery occlusion with vascular bypass grafting, or surgery under hypothermic circulatory arrest [60–63]. Clipping of large, complex basilar artery aneurysms under hypothermic circulatory arrest has a reported mortality of 10%, compared to 50% using standard neurosurgical techniques [64].

The optimal timing of surgery for repair of ruptured intracranial aneurysm has been an area of continuing controversy. Early surgery can be difficult owing to intraoperative rerupture of the aneurysm, swollen brain, or tenacious clot surrounding the aneurysm [65]. For decades, surgeons routinely operated days to weeks after SAH in an attempt to reduce perioperative morbidity and mortality. A majority of these patients deteriorated or died from rebleeding or delayed cerebral ischemia and never made it to surgery [66]. By the late 1980s, a number of neurosurgical series suggested that early surgery effectively reduces the risk of rebleeding with acceptable operative morbidity and mortality [67,68]. In 1990, the International Cooperative Study on the Timing of Aneurysm Surgery reported on the surgical and medical management of 3,521 patients followed in a prospective, nonrandomized, observational survey [69]. No difference was found in mortality between early surgery (0–3 days post-SAH) and late surgery (11–14 days post-SAH). Outcome was worse in patients operated on 7–10 days after SAH, however, the peak interval for symptomatic vasospasm. Regardless of the timing of surgery, patients with good Hunt and Hess grades consistently had the best outcomes.

Current evidence supports the recommendation that patients in good clinical condition at the time of hospital admission (Hunt and Hess grades I–III) undergo early surgery (within 3 days of SAH). Patients in worse condition (Hunt and Hess grades IV and V) may also benefit from early surgery, but this remains dependent on the experience of the individual surgical team. Endovascular treatment of acutely ruptured aneurysms provides a less invasive method for "protecting" against rebleeding in high-risk patients who are not considered candidates for early operation [70].

Surgical management of patients with unruptured intracranial aneurysms remains controversial. In one series of more than 200 aneurysm operations performed by a single neurosurgeon, the key predictor of risk for surgical morbidity in these patients was the size, not the location, of the aneurysm [71]. The exceptions to this finding were giant basilar aneurysms. Excellent or good outcome was achieved in 100% of patients with aneurysms less than 10 mm in diameter, 95% with aneurysms of 11–25 mm, and 79% with aneurysms larger than 25 mm. These data may be useful when discussing with patients the risk-benefit ratio of choosing between conservative management, endovascular embolization, or microsurgical clipping on discovery of an asymptomatic intracranial aneurysm.

Endovascular Therapy

Endovascular therapy represents a promising alternative to surgical clipping of intracranial aneurysms in selected cases that are not amenable to surgical repair. Early endovascular attempts to treat aneurysms involved parent artery occlusion and packing with balloons [72–74]. Newer methods using thrombogenic coils

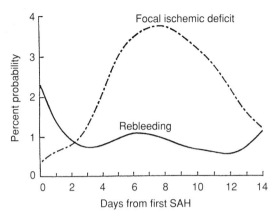

Figure 10.4   Graph depicting the daily percent probability of developing symptomatic vasospasm or rebleeding after subarachnoid hemorrhage (SAH). Day 0 denotes day of onset of SAH. (Reprinted with permission from NF Kassell, T Sasaki, ART Colohan, et al. Cerebral vasospasm following aneurysmal subarachnoid hemorrhage. Stroke 1985;16:563.)

have demonstrated good occlusion rates and low procedure-related complications [75–77]. The most common indication for endovascular rather than surgical treatment of aneurysms is high surgical risk related to anatomy (e.g., giant, posterior circulation, and cavernous sinus aneurysms), poor Hunt and Hess grade, vasospasm, or medical instability.

The current technique of endovascular embolization with detachable platinum coils involves positioning of a microcatheter into the aneurysmal neck, followed by electrolytic detachment of soft metallic coils into the lumen of the aneurysm. A process of electrothrombosis induces local clot formation around the coils within the aneurysm [78]. The most important factor for complete obliteration is the ratio of the neck to the fundus of the aneurysm; complete obliteration can be achieved in 80–90% of small-necked aneurysms [76,79].

The main disadvantage of endovascular treatment is the potential for delayed rebleeding owing to regrowth at the neck of the aneurysm. The short-term risk of rebleeding from aneurysms that are completely occluded with coils appears to be small [77,80]. Even in partially occluded aneurysms, a low risk of rebleeding has been reported within 3 years of Guglielmi detachable coiling [81]. However, efficacy in long-term outcome studies has yet to be demonstrated.

NEUROLOGIC COMPLICATIONS OF SUBARACHNOID HEMORRHAGE

Rebleeding

Aneurysmal rebleeding is a devastating complication of SAH. The risk of rebleeding peaks within the first 24 hours after the initial aneurysmal rupture and remains a significant risk over the ensuing 14 days post-SAH (Figure 10.4). Studies on the natural history of SAH indicate that rebleeding occurs in 20% of patients with unclipped aneurysms during the 2 weeks after the initial SAH and in 40% within 6 months; the risk of rebleeding is approximately 3% per year thereafter [11,82]. The prognosis for patients who rebleed is poor; approximately

50% die immediately, while another 30% die from further complications after the rebleed. Only 20% of patients are surviving at 3 months, and many are left with severe brain damage.

The pathogenesis of rebleeding is not completely understood. It has been suggested that fluctuations in arterial blood pressure can precipitate a rebleed. However, studies of rebleeding after SAH have not found a relationship with either systolic or diastolic blood pressure fluctuations before the event [83]. Endogenous fibrinolysis of the clot around the aneurysm may be an important mechanism underlying rebleeding. CSF has been shown to have enhanced fibrinolytic activity during the first week after SAH with potential for lysis of the blood clot surrounding the aneurysm [84]. The dura mater and pia mater also possess considerable fibrinolytic activity that may be significant. It is thought that subarachnoid blood stimulates the irritated meninges to convert plasminogen to plasmin. The plasmin formed can cause early lysis of the clot that seals the ruptured aneurysm [84].

Antifibrinolytic treatment with agents such as epsilon-aminocaproic acid have been used to prevent rebleeding based on the hypothesis that rebleeding is caused by premature lysis of the blood clot surrounding the ruptured aneurysm. In an analysis of patients undergoing delayed surgery, the International Cooperative Study demonstrated that antifibrinolytic drugs caused a reduction in rebleeding rate of 50%, but this result was offset by an associated increased risk of cerebral ischemic complications, hydrocephalus requiring shunt placement, deep vein thrombosis, and pulmonary embolism [85]. Overall, the effects canceled each other, and equal morbidity and mortality occurred in both groups. A randomized, double-blind, placebo-controlled trial of tranexamic acid also showed no difference in outcome between the drug and placebo groups [86].

At present, early surgical clipping of the aneurysm is the most effective measure to prevent rebleeding. Endovascular aneurysm occlusion with Guglielmi detachable coils is the next best alternative in patients who are not candidates for early operation.

Vasospasm

Delayed cerebral ischemia from vasospasm accounts for up to 30% of the morbidity and mortality that occurs after SAH [87]. A clear relationship exists between the amount of blood seen in the basal cisterns on CT scan and the development of clinically symptomatic vasospasm [88]. The severity of postoperative angiographic spasm, timing of surgery, and pre-existing hypertension have also been implicated as risk factors for delayed cerebral ischemia [89]. Although thick subarachnoid blood is the principal precipitating factor, the precise cause of arterial narrowing after SAH is poorly understood. The prevailing view is that substances released from the blood clot interact with the vessel wall to cause inflammatory arterial spasm [90]. Possible mediators of cerebral vasospasm include oxyhemoglobin, with its intrinsic vasoconstrictive properties, hydroperoxides and leukotrienes, free radicals, prostaglandins, thromboxane A_2, and serotonin [91,92]. Vasospasm is not simply caused by vascular smooth muscle contraction; arteriopathic changes are seen in the vessel wall and consist of subintimal edema and infiltration of leukocytes, lymphocytes, and macrophages [93].

Table 10.5   Criteria for detection of vasospasm by transcranial Doppler ultrasonography

Artery	Mean flow velocity
Middle cerebral	≥140 cm/sec
Anterior cerebral	≥120 cm/sec
Basilar	≥80 cm/sec
Vertebral	≥60 cm/sec

Source: Adapted from L Lennihan, GW Petty, ME Fink, et al. Transcranial Doppler detection of anterior cerebral artery vasospasm. J Neurol Neurosurg Psychiatry 1993;56:906; and MA Sloan, CM Burch, MA Wozniak, et al. Transcranial Doppler detection of vertebrobasilar vasospasm following subarachnoid hemorrhage. Stroke 1994;25:2187.

Delayed cerebral ischemia usually presents as a change in level of consciousness, focal neurologic deficit, or both. Angiographic vasospasm generally begins 3–5 days after the hemorrhage, with maximal narrowing at 5–14 days and gradual resolution over 2–4 weeks. Angiographic evidence of arterial narrowing develops in approximately 70% of patients after SAH [94], but delayed neurologic ischemic deficits develop in 20–30% of patients [90]. Neurologic deficits associated with symptomatic vasospasm usually appear shortly after the onset of angiographic vasospasm and can resolve or progress to cerebral infarction [87]. In some cases, focal CT hypodensities that occur after SAH are reversible, suggesting that areas of potentially reversible ischemia can be rescued with aggressive use of hypervolemic-hypertensive therapy [95].

Transcranial Doppler (TCD) ultrasonography is widely used to diagnose vasospasm of the larger cerebral arteries after SAH (Table 10.5). It has a sensitivity of 90% for detecting angiographic narrowing of the middle cerebral artery but a sensitivity of only less than 20% for detecting anterior cerebral artery spasm [96]. TCD is similarly specific (>80%) but not sensitive (approximately 50%) for detecting spasm of the vertebral and basilar arteries [97]. The ability of TCD to predict which patients will develop neurologic symptoms from cerebral vasospasm is poor. In one study, maximal mean TCD velocity had no predictive value whatsoever, whereas a 50-cm-per-second increase in flow velocity had a positive predictive value of only 53%, compared to a 37% frequency of symptomatic vasospasm in the study population overall [98].

Acetazolamide-activated single-photon emission computed tomography (SPECT) is a newer technique that may be useful for detecting presymptomatic ischemia from vasospasm after SAH [99]. In one preliminary study, a territorial or severe watershed flow deficit identified by acetazolamide-activated SPECT 4–7 days after SAH had a 100% sensitivity for symptomatic vasospasm [100]. Further study is required to directly compare the predictive value of TCD and SPECT for identifying patients at risk for delayed ischemia.

Prevention of vasospasm has been attempted by intraoperative removal of subarachnoid clot with intrathecal administration of recombinant tissue plasminogen activator (t-PA) and has shown encouraging results in small, uncontrolled trials in humans. Administration of t-PA was by a single intracisternal bolus [101,102] or via multiple intrathecal injections through a ventricular catheter [103,104]. However, one study [105] of intracisternal t-PA failed to show prevention of vasospasm in a subset of patients who either had massive

SAH, pre-existing poor collateral flow, or prior SAH. Larger, multicenter, placebo-controlled studies are needed to demonstrate a definitive effect of intrathecal t-PA on outcome after SAH.

Efficacy of the calcium channel blocker nimodipine for preventing delayed cerebral ischemia after SAH is well established. In the British Aneurysm Nimodipine Trial in 1989, oral nimodipine given to patients with SAH significantly reduced the occurrence of a poor outcome by 40% and the incidence of cerebral infarction by 34%, with the improvement in disability and death attributed to a reduction in cerebral ischemia [58]. Nimodipine does not reduce vasospasm as detected by angiography or TCD [58,106,107]. The anti-ischemic effects of nimodipine pretreatment after SAH may be mediated by an effect on cerebral pial vessels to increase collateral flow or blockade of calcium entry into ischemic neurons.

Tirilazad, a nonglucocorticoid 21-aminosteroid free-radical scavenger, has been shown to reduce cerebral vasospasm, improve cerebral blood flow, and reduce infarct size in animal models of SAH [108,109]. However, results from the randomized, double-blind cooperative study in North America of use of tirilazad mesylate in 897 patients demonstrated no statistically significant benefit on mortality, functional outcome, or ischemic symptoms from vasospasm [110]. This negative result may have resulted in part from concurrent use of phenytoin, which accelerates the metabolism of tirilazad.

Treatment of acute symptomatic vasospasm relies on increasing blood pressure and cardiac output in an attempt to improve cerebral blood flow. Hypertensive-hypervolemic-hemodilution ("triple-H therapy") is currently an accepted treatment for symptomatic vasospasm after SAH. Crystalloid or colloid solutions can be given to maintain pulmonary artery diastolic pressure at 14 mm Hg or higher or central venous pressure at 8 mm Hg or higher, and pressors such as dopamine and phenylephrine can be used to elevate systolic blood pressure to levels as high as 180–220 mm Hg (Table 10.6). Kassell and associates [111] reported clinical improvement in 75% of patients treated with triple-H therapy who experienced progressive neurologic deterioration from angiographically confirmed vasospasm. In one-third of the treated patients, transient lowering of the blood pressure brought on the return of neurologic symptoms, which resolved with reinstitution of triple-H therapy.

Triple-H therapy is associated with risks, including myocardial infarction, cardiac arrhythmias, pulmonary edema, rebleeding, and neurologic deterioration, in patients with large, established infarcts. Individuals who receive this therapy should be in an intensive care unit setting with a pulmonary artery or central venous catheter and an arterial line for blood pressure monitoring. Volume given to maintain a pulmonary artery diastolic pressure of 14 mm Hg has been shown to correlate with optimal cardiac output after SAH; volume expansion beyond this level is probably unnecessary [112].

Patients with symptomatic vasospasm that is unresponsive to medical therapy have been treated with transluminal angioplasty. Higashida and associates [113] treated 28 patients and achieved improved luminal diameter in all treated vessels, with clinical improvement in 60% of cases. Other series have reported similar results, with improvement in 60–80% of patients and serious complications in approximately 5% of patients [114,115]. Controlled clinical trials are required to further define the role of angioplasty in the management of refractory vasospasm.

Table 10.6 Fluid management protocols for subarachnoid hemorrhage
at Columbia–Presbyterian Medical Center

Pre- and postoperative volume status	*Protocol*
Preoperative	Normal (0.9%) saline at 80–100 ml/hr
Postoperative normovolemia	Normal (0.9%) saline at 80–100 ml/hr; 250 ml of 5% albumin IV q2h for PADP of ≤7 mm Hg or central venous pressure of ≤5 mm Hg
Postoperative hypervolemia	Normal (0.9%) saline at 80–100 ml/hr; 250 ml of 5% albumin IV q2h for PADP of ≤14 mm Hg or central venous pressure of ≤8 mm Hg
Symptomatic vasospasm	500 ml of 5% albumin IV over 20 mins
	If no response: raise systolic blood pressure with IV pressors until deficit resolves (to maximum of 220 mm Hg); postoperative hypervolemia protocol

PADP = pulmonary artery diastolic pressure.

Source: Adapted from SA Mayer. Fluid management in subarachnoid hemorrhage. Neurologist 1995;1:71.

Hydrocephalus

Acute hydrocephalus occurs in 15–20% of patients with SAH and is primarily related to the volume of intraventricular and subarachnoid blood (see Figure 10.2). Hydrocephalus causes increased intracranial pressure and clinically presents as impaired level of consciousness or abulia. Impairment of consciousness in patients with acute hydrocephalus may be caused by mechanical pressure from the ventricles, impairing conduction of white matter tracts, globally decreased cerebral perfusion, or both [116]. Up to one-third of patients with hydrocephalus on CT scan after SAH have a normal level of consciousness [117]. In more severe cases, in addition to depressed level of consciousness, examination may reveal limitation of upward gaze, sixth cranial nerve palsies, and lower-extremity hyperreflexia.

Treatment for acute hydrocephalus that leads to stupor or coma requires placement of an external ventricular drain by insertion of a catheter through a burr hole in the cranium. Clinical improvement after ventricular drainage can be dramatic or can take 1–3 days. Complications include ventriculitis, bleeding along the catheter tract, or cerebral infarction. The risk of ventriculitis, which occurs in approximately 15% of patients, increases sharply after a catheter has been in place for 5 days [118]; however, it remains controversial as to whether routine replacement of ventricular drains every 5 days can reduce this risk [119]. Use of prophylactic antibiotics or long subcutaneous tunneling of the catheter is frequently practiced to decrease the risk of infection, although the efficacy of these techniques remains to be demonstrated. In patients with mildly depressed level of consciousness, serial drainage of CSF by lumbar puncture may be a safer alternative to ventricular drainage for treating hydrocephalus [120].

Delayed hydrocephalus can develop anywhere from 3 to 21 days after SAH. Any change in the clinical status during this period may be difficult to differentiate from symptomatic vasospasm. Hydrocephalus that occurs 10 days or more after SAH may be indistinguishable from that of normal pressure hydrocephalus, with insidious onset of dementia, gait disturbance, and urinary incontinence [121]. The clinical response to ventriculoperitoneal shunting is usually excellent. Overall, 20% of patients with SAH require shunting for chronic hydrocephalus [122].

Seizures

The overall incidence of seizures after SAH is relatively low, ranging from 5% to 10%; two-thirds of seizures occur within the first month [123]. Baker and associates [59] retrospectively studied the frequency of occurrence of postoperative seizures in aneurysmal SAH patients given anticonvulsants postoperatively for an average of 3 days. The seizure rate in the study group was 5.4% over an average follow-up of 2.4 years, and none of these patients went on to develop epilepsy. Only volume of SAH and rebleeding are risk factors for seizures after SAH [123]. These data support the notion that anticonvulsant medication should be restricted to the immediate perioperative period for most patients with aneurysms.

MEDICAL COMPLICATIONS OF SUBARACHNOID HEMORRHAGE

Fluid and Electrolyte Disturbances

Proper fluid management after SAH is based on maintenance of normal or increased volume status using isotonic fluids and strict avoidance of hypotonic fluids such as 0.45% saline or 5% dextrose in water. This goal can be achieved during both the pre- and postoperative periods, as well as during periods of symptomatic vasospasm, by the administration of crystalloid or colloid solutions, or both (see Table 10.6).

Hyponatremia and intravascular volume contraction occur frequently after SAH and reflect homeostatic derangements that favor excessive free water retention and sodium loss. Hyponatremia, defined as a serum sodium concentration of less than 135 mEq/liter, has been reported in 10–30% of patients with SAH [124,125]. Hypovolemia or extracellular fluid volume contraction, defined as greater than a 10% reduction of plasma volume from baseline, has been described in 30–50% of SAH patients during the first week of hospitalization [124]. Hyponatremia after SAH is related to inappropriate secretion of antidiuretic hormone and retention of free water. This process can be further exacerbated by the excessive natriuresis that occurs after SAH (cerebral salt wasting), because untreated intravascular volume contraction can act as a further stimulus for antidiuretic hormone secretion. Excessive renal sodium excretion after SAH has been related to elevations of atrial natriuretic factor and increased glomerular filtration rate [126].

The frequency and severity of hyponatremia and hypovolemia after SAH generally depend on the volume and composition of intravenous fluid given. Diringer and associates [127] found that a reduction of blood volume does not occur in patients who are given large volumes of isotonic crystalloid. Although hypervolemic therapy does not prevent hyponatremia in all patients, its severity can be greatly minimized by avoiding intravenous solutions that contain excess free water (e.g., 0.45% saline or 5% dextrose in water).

Whereas hyponatremia after SAH is usually asymptomatic, volume contraction after SAH can adversely affect outcome in many patients by increasing the risk of delayed ischemia from vasospasm. Wijdicks and associates [124] reported a significant increase in frequency of cerebral infarction from vasospasm in SAH patients treated with fluid restriction. The authors concluded that, regardless of the mechanism of hyponatremia, fluid restriction that leads to hypovolemia and intravascular volume depletion can be harmful in patients with SAH.

Electrocardiographic Changes

Electrocardiographic (ECG) changes occur in at least one-half of patients with SAH, and nearly every type of abnormality has been described [128,129]. The most commonly reported ECG abnormalities include QT_c prolongation, symmetrically inverted T waves, nonspecific ST-T–wave changes, U waves, and left ventricular hypertrophy [130]. These abnormalities usually develop during the first 2–3 days after SAH and resolve over 1–2 weeks [128,131]. In the majority of patients with SAH, neurogenic ECG changes are clinically inconsequential. In a subset of patients with QT_c prolongation and inverted T waves, however, a reversible form of myocardial dysfunction can occur [130].

Patients with SAH who have neurogenic ECG changes may be at risk for cardiac arrhythmias. Minor rhythm disturbances, such as sinus tachycardia and bradycardia, occur in 35% of patients, with a peak occurrence on the second and third days after SAH [132]. Potentially life-threatening arrhythmias, including asystole, ventricular tachycardia, and hemodynamically significant atrial fibrillation, are seen in fewer than 5% of patients. Ventricular arrhythmias, which occur in 2% of patients, have been associated with severe QT-segment prolongation and hypokalemia [133].

Neurogenic Cardiac Injury

Echocardiographic studies have shown that a neurogenic form of left ventricular dysfunction occurs in nearly 10% of patients with acute SAH [130,134–136]. This form of cardiac injury, termed *neurogenic stunned myocardium*, occurs almost exclusively in poor-grade patients (Hunt and Hess grades III–V) and is typically found in association with borderline elevations (2–5%) of myocardial creatinine kinase. These patients have normal coronary arteries, and the abnormal wall motion invariably resolves over 2–6 weeks [137]. The pathologic substrate of neurogenic stunned myocardium appears to be contraction band necrosis, which results from intense sympathetic stimulation of the myocardium [129]. Neurogenic cardiac injury is important to diagnosis because patients may have hemodynamic dysfunction and be at increased risk for complications from triple-H therapy [138].

Neurogenic Pulmonary Edema

Neurogenic pulmonary edema is characterized by the sudden development of lung edema that occurs minutes to hours after SAH. It results from transiently elevated pulmonary vascular pressures, which can cause microvascular baro-trauma and loss of pulmonary capillary integrity, with resultant edema characterized by a high protein content. This normally noncardiogenic form of pulmonary edema can coexist with neurogenic left ventricular dysfunction, which can worsen the severity and duration of the pulmonary edema [139]. Acute sympathetically mediated injury to both the pulmonary vasculature and the heart may explain how myocardial dysfunction and noncardiogenic neurogenic pulmonary edema can coexist after SAH.

Outcomes after Subarachnoid Hemorrhage

Despite remarkable advances in surgical and intensive care management, SAH remains a devastating disease [140]. In 1989, a population-based study in Washington state found that 30 days after SAH, one-third of patients were dead, one-third had neurologic deficits, and one-third had a good recovery [141]. The prognosis for patients with SAH has improved since the 1980s, however, which most likely reflects advances in neurosurgery and neurocritical care. One tertiary care center reported a significant increase in the percentage of favorable outcomes in good-grade patients from 1983 to 1993 [142]. Similarly, a meta-analysis of population-based epidemiologic studies conducted worldwide from 1960 to 1992 reported a decreasing case-fatality rate [143]. Referral to a tertiary care center was associated with improved outcome after surgery for SAH in New York state from 1987 to 1993; hospital mortality was 43% lower in hospitals that treated more than 30 cases of SAH a year than in institutions that handled lower volumes [144].

Assessment of outcome after SAH is complicated by the fact that most patients with disabilities have subtle cognitive disturbances rather than the more severe physical handicaps that occur after stroke or traumatic brain injury [145,146]. For this reason, crude global assessment scales such as the Glasgow outcome score may not be appropriate for patients with SAH. A more relevant, standardized scale is needed that addresses the cognitive injury and social adjustment after SAH.

REFERENCES

1. Ingall TJ, Wiebers DO. Natural History of Subarachnoid Hemorrhage. In JP Whisnant (ed), Stroke: Populations, Cohorts, and Clinical Trials. Boston: Butterworth–Heinemann, 1993;174–186.
2. Broderick JP, Brott T, Tomsick T, et al. Intracerebral hemorrhage more than twice as common as subarachnoid hemorrhage. J Neurosurg 1993;78:188.
3. Davis PH, Hachinski V. Epidemiology of Cerebrovascular Disease. In DW Anderson (ed), Neuroepidemiology: A Tribute to Bruce Schoenberg. Boca Raton, FL: CRC, 1991;27–53.
4. Atkinson JL, Sundt TM Jr, Houser OW, et al. Angiographic frequency of anterior circulation intracranial aneurysms. J Neurosurg 1989;70:551.
5. Juvela S, Porras M, Heiskanen O. Natural history of unruptured intracranial aneurysms: a long-term follow-up study. J Neurosurg 1993;79:174.
6. Phillips LG, Whisnant JP, O'Fallon WM, et al. The unchanging pattern of subarachnoid hemorrhage in the community. Neurology 1980;30:1034.
7. Ingall TJ, Whisnant JP, Wiebers DO, et al. Has there been a decline in subarachnoid hemorrhage mortality? Stroke 1989;20:718.
8. Weir B. Epidemiology. In B Weir (ed), Aneurysms Affecting the Nervous System. Baltimore: Williams & Wilkins, 1987;19–53.

9. Wiebers D, Whisnant J, O'Fallon W. The natural history of unruptured aneurysms. N Engl J Med 1981;30:696.
10. Fox JL (ed). Intracranial Aneurysms (Vol 1). New York: Springer-Verlag, 1983.
11. Kassell NF, Torner JC, Haley EC Jr, et al. The International Cooperative Study on the Timing of Aneurysm Surgery. 1. Overall management results. J Neurosurg 1990;73:18.
12. Stehbens WE. The pathology of intracranial arterial aneurysms and their complications. In JL Fox (ed), Intracranial Aneurysms (Vol 1). New York: Springer-Verlag, 1983;272–357.
13. Ostergaard JR, Hog E. Incidence of multiple intracranial aneurysms: influence of arterial hypertension and gender. J Neurosurg 1985;63:49.
14. Rinne JK, Hernesniemi JA. De novo aneurysms: special multiple intracranial aneurysms. Neurosurgery 1993;33:981.
15. Kupersmith MJ, Hurst R, Berenstein A, et al. The benign course of cavernous carotid artery aneurysms. J Neurosurg 1992;77:690.
16. Crawford P, West C, Chadwick D. Arteriovenous malformation of the brain: natural history of unoperated patients. J Neurol Neurosurg Psychiatry 1986;49:1.
17. Austin G, Fisher S, Dickson D, et al. The significance of the extracellular matrix in intracranial aneurysms. Ann Clin Lab Sci 1993;23:97.
18. Kistler JP, Heros RC. Subarachnoid Hemorrhage Due to Ruptured Saccular Aneurysm. In AH Ropper, SF Kennedy (eds), Neurological and Neurosurgical Intensive Care. Rockville, MD: Aspen, 1988;219–232.
19. Schievink WI, Michels VV, Piepras DG. Neurovascular manifestations of heritable connective tissue disorders: a review. Stroke 1994;25:889.
20. Longstreth WT Jr, Nelson LM, Koepsell TD, et al. Subarachnoid hemorrhage and hormonal factors in women: a population-based case-control study. Ann Intern Med 1994;121:168.
21. Teunissen LL, Rinkel GJ, Algra A. Risk factors for subarachnoid hemorrhage: a systematic review. Stroke 1996;27:544.
22. Juvela S, Hillbom M, Numminen H, et al. Cigarette smoking and alcohol consumption as risk factors for aneurysmal subarachnoid hemorrhage. Stroke 1993;24:639.
23. Longstreth WT Jr, Nelson LM, Koepsell TD, van Belle G. Cigarette smoking, alcohol use, and SAH. Stroke 1992;23:1242.
24. Fogelholm R, Murros K. Cigarette smoking and subarachnoid hemorrhage: a population-based case-control study. J Neurol Neurosurg Psychiatry 1987;50:78.
25. Schievink WI, Katzmann JA, Piepgras DG, et al. Alpha-1–antitrypsin phenotypes among patients with intracranial aneurysms. J Neurosurg 1996;84:781.
26. Klatsky AL, Friedman GD, Siegelaub AB, Gerard MJ. Alcohol consumption and blood pressure: Kaiser Permanente multiphasic health examination data. N Engl J Med 1977;296:1194.
27. MacMahon SW. Alcohol and hypertension: implications for prevention and treatment [editorial]. Ann Intern Med 1986;105:124.
28. Fisher CM, Robertson GH, Ojemann RG. Cerebral vasospasm with ruptured saccular aneurysm: the clinical manifestations. Neurosurgery 1977;1:245.
29. Kassell NF, Kongable GL, Torner JC, et al. Delay in referral of patients with ruptured aneurysms to neurological attention. Stroke 1985;16:587.
30. Mayer PL, Awad IA, Todor R, et al. Misdiagnosis of symptomatic cerebral aneurysm: prevalence and correlation with outcome at four institutions. Stroke 1996;27:1558.
31. Garfinkle AM, Danys IR, Nicolle DA, et al. Terson's syndrome: a reversible cause of blindness following subarachnoid hemorrhage. J Neurosurg 1992;76:766.
32. Schievink WI, Karemaker JM, Hageman LM, van der Werf DJ. Circumstances surrounding aneurysmal subarachnoid hemorrhage. Surg Neurol 1989;32:266.
33. Adams H, Jergenson DD, Kassell NF, et al. Pitfalls in the recognition of subarachnoid hemorrhage. JAMA 1980;244:794.
34. Raps EC, Rogers JD, Galetta SL, et al. The clinical spectrum of unruptured intracranial aneurysms. Arch Neurol 1993;50:265.
35. Wiebers DO, Whisnant JP, Sundt TM Jr, et al. The significance of unruptured intracranial saccular aneurysms. J Neurosurg 1987;66:233.
36. Rinkel GJE, Wijdicks EFM, Vermeulen M, et al. The clinical course of perimesencephalic nonaneurysmal subarachnoid hemorrhage. Ann Neurol 1991;29:463.
37. van Gijn J, van Dongen KF, Vermeulen M, et al. Perimesencephalic hemorrhage. A nonaneurysmal and benign form of subarachnoid hemorrhage. Neurology 1985;35:493.
38. Hunt WE, Hess RM. Surgical risk as related to time of intervention in the repair of intracranial aneurysms. J Neurosurg 1968;28:14.

39. van Gijn J, van Dongen KJ. The time course of aneurysmal haemorrhage on computed tomograms. Neuroradiology 1982;23:153.
40. Vermeulen M, Hasan D, Blijenberg BG, et al. Xanthochromia after subarachnoid haemorrhage needs no revisitation. J Neurol Neurosurg Psychiatry 1989;52:826.
41. Satoh S, Kadoya S. Magnetic resonance imaging of subarachnoid hemorrhage. Neuroradiology 1988;30:361.
42. Alexander MSM, Dias PS, Uttley D. Spontaneous subarachnoid hemorrhage and negative cerebral panangiography. J Neurosurg 1986;64:537–542.
43. Beguelin C, Seiler R. Subarachnoid hemorrhage with normal cerebral panangiography. Neurosurgery 1983;13:409.
44. Forster DMC, Steiner L, Hakanson S, et al. The value of repeat pan-angiography in cases of unexplained subarachnoid hemorrhage. J Neurosurg 1978;48:712.
45. Duong H, Melancon D, Tampieri D, et al. The negative angiogram in subarachnoid haemorrhage. Neuroradiology 1996;38:15.
46. West HH, Mani RI, Eisenberg K, et al. Normal cerebral arteriography in patients with spontaneous subarachnoid hemorrhage. Neurology 1972;27:592.
47. Adams HP. Nonaneurysmal subarachnoid hemorrhage [editorial]. Ann Neurol 1991;29:461.
48. Huston J III, Nichols DA, Luetmer PH, et al. Blinded prospective evaluation of sensitivity of MR angiography to known intracranial aneurysms: importance of aneurysm size. AJNR Am J Neuroradiol 1994;15:1607.
49. Alberico RA, Patel M, Casey S, et al. Evaluation of the circle of Willis with three-dimensional CT angiography in patients with suspected intracranial aneurysms. AJNR Am J Neuroradiol 1995;16:1571.
50. Schievink WI, Schaid DJ, Rogers HM, et al. On the inheritance of intracranial aneurysms. Stroke 1994;25:2028.
51. Ronkainen A, Puranen MI, Hernesniemi JA, et al. Intracranial aneurysms: MR angiographic screening in 400 asymptomatic individuals with increased familial risk. Radiology 1995;195:35.
52. Ronkainen A, Hernesniemi J, Puranen M, et al. Familial intracranial aneurysms. Lancet 1997;349:380.
53. Chapman AB, Rubinstein D, Hughes R, et al. Intracranial aneurysms in autosomal dominant polycystic kidney disease. N Engl J Med 1992;327:916.
54. Ruggieri PM, Poulos N, Masaryk TJ, et al. Occult intracranial aneurysms in polycystic kidney disease: screening with MR angiography. Radiology 1994;191:33.
55. Orlowski JP, Shiesley D, Vidt DG, et al. Labetalol to control blood pressure after cerebrovascular surgery. Crit Care Med 1988;16:765.
56. Anile C, Zanghi F, Bracali A, et al. Sodium nitroprusside and intracranial pressure. Acta Neurochir 1981;58:203.
57. Allen G, Ahn H, Preziosi T, et al. Cerebral arterial spasm: a controlled trial of nimodipine in patients with subarachnoid hemorrhage. N Engl J Med 1983;308:619.
58. Pickard JD, Murray GD, Illingworth R, et al. Effect of oral nimodipine on cerebral infarction and outcome after subarachnoid haemorrhage; British Aneurysm Nimodipine Trial. BMJ 1989;298:636.
59. Baker CJ, Prestigiacomo CJ, Solomon RA. Short-term perioperative anticonvulsant prophylaxis for the surgical treatment of low-risk patients with intracranial aneurysms. Neurosurgery 1995;37:863.
60. Yasargil MG. Clinical Considerations, Surgery of the Intracranial Aneurysms and Results. In MG Yasargi (ed), Microneurosurgery. Stuttgart, Germany: Georg Thieme Verlag, 1984;1–32.
61. Sundt TM Jr. Results of Surgical Management. In TM Sundt Jr (ed), Surgical Techniques for Saccular and Giant Intracranial Aneurysms. Baltimore: Williams & Wilkins, 1990;19–25.
62. Spetzler RF, Hadley MN, Rigamonti D, et al. Aneurysms of the basilar artery treated with circulatory arrest, hypothermia, and barbiturate cerebral protection. Neurosurgery 1988;68:868.
63. Baumgartner WA, Silverberg GD, Ream AK, et al. Reappraisal of cardiopulmonary bypass with deep hypothermia and circulatory arrest for complex neurosurgical operations. Surgery 1983;94:242.
64. Solomon RA, Smith CR, Raps EC, et al. Deep hypothermic circulatory arrest for the management of complex anterior and posterior circulation aneurysms. Neurosurgery 1991;29:732.
65. Auer LM. Unfavorable outcome following early surgical repair of ruptured cerebral aneurysms—a critical review of 238 patients. Surg Neurol 1991;35:152.
66. Sundt TM, Whisnant JP. Subarachnoid hemorrhage from intracranial aneurysms: surgical management and natural history of disease. N Engl J Med 1978;299:116.
67. Kurtzke JF. Epidemiology of Cerebrovascular Disease. In FH McDowell, LR Kaplan (eds), Cerebrovascular Survey Report for the National Institute of Neurological and Communicative Disorders and Stroke. Bethesda, MD: National Institutes of Health, 1985;1–34.

68. Fogelholm R. SAH in middle Finland: incidence, early prognosis and indications for neurosurgical treatment. Stroke 1981;12:296.
69. Kassell NF, Torner JC, Jane JA, et al. The International Cooperative Study on the Timing of Aneurysm Surgery. Part 2: Surgical results. J Neurosurg 1990;73:37.
70. Bernardini GL, Mayer SA, Kossoff SB, et al. Anticoagulation and induced hypertension after endovascular treatment for ruptured intracranial aneurysms. Neurology 1999 (submitted).
71. Solomon RA, Fink ME, Pile–Spellman J. Surgical management of unruptured intracranial aneurysms. J Neurosurg 1994;80:440.
72. Romanov AP, Shcheglov VI. Intravascular Occlusion of Saccular Aneurysms of the Cerebral Arteries by Means of a Detachable Balloon Catheter. In H Krayenbuhl (ed), Advances and Technical Standards in Neurosurgery (Vol 9). Zurich: Springer-Verlag, 1982;25–48.
73. Fox AJ, Vinuela F, Pelz DM, et al. Use of detachable balloon for proximal artery occlusion in the treatment of unclippable cerebral aneurysms. J Neurosurg 1987;66:40.
74. Higashida RT, Halbach VV, Dowd CF, et al. Intracranial aneurysms: interventional neurovascular treatment with detachable balloons. Results in 215 cases. Radiology 1991;178:663.
75. Gobin YP, Vinuela F, Gurian JH, et al. Treatment of large and giant fusiform intracranial aneurysms with Guglielmi detachable coils. J Neurosurg 1996;84:55.
76. McDougall CG, Halback VV, Dowd CF, et al. Endovascular treatment of basilar tip aneurysms using electrolytically detachable coils. J Neurosurg 1996;84:393.
77. Byrne JV, Adams CB, Kerr RS, Molyneux AJ. Endosaccular treatment of inoperable intracranial aneurysms with platinum coils. Br J Neurosurg 1995;9:585.
78. Guglielmi G, Vinuela F, Sepetka I, et al. Electrothrombosis of saccular aneurysms via endovascular approach. Part 1: Electrochemical basis, technique, and experimental results. J Neurosurg 1991;75:1.
79. Fernandez Zubillaga A, Guglielmi G, Vinuela F, et al. Endovascular occlusion of intracranial aneurysms with electrically detachable coils: correlation of aneurysm neck size and treatment results. AJNR Am J Neuroradiol 1994;15:815.
80. Casasco AE, Aymard A, Gobin Y, et al. Selective endovascular treatment of 71 intracranial aneurysms with platinum coils. J Neurosurg 1993;73:3.
81. Vinuela G, Duckwiler G, Mawad M. Guglielmi detachable coil embolization of acute intracranial aneurysm: perioperative anatomical and clinical outcome in 403 patients. J Neurosurg 1997;86:475.
82. Sahs AL, Nibbelink DW, Torner JC (eds). Aneurysmal Subarachnoid Hemorrhage: Report of the Cooperative Study. Baltimore and Munich: Urban & Schwarzenberg, 1981.
83. Wijdicks EFM, Verneulen M, Murray GD, et al. The effects of treating hypertension following aneurysmal subarachnoid hemorrhage. Clin Neurol Neurosurg 1990;92:111.
84. Tovi D, Nilsson IM, Thulin CA. Fibrinolytic activity of the cerebrospinal fluid after subarachnoid hemorrhage. Acta Neurol Scand 1973;49:1.
85. Kassell NF, Torner JC, Adams HP. Antifibrinolytic therapy in the acute period following aneurysmal subarachnoid hemorrhage. Preliminary observations from the Cooperative Aneurysm Study. J Neurosurg 1984;61:225.
86. Vermeulen M, Lindsay KW, Cheah MF, et al. Antifibrinolytic treatment in subarachnoid hemorrhage. N Engl J Med 1984;311:432.
87. Kassell NF, Sasaki T, Colohan ART, et al. Cerebral vasospasm following aneurysmal subarachnoid hemorrhage. Stroke 1985;16:562.
88. Fisher CM, Kistler JP, Davis JM. Relationship of cerebral vasospasm to subarachnoid hemorrhage visualized by CT scanning. Neurosurgery 1980;6:19.
89. Ohman J, Servo A, Heiskanen O. Risk factors for cerebral infarction in good-grade patients after aneurysmal subarachnoid hemorrhage and surgery: a prospective study. J Neurosurg 1991;74:14.
90. Klebanoff LM, Fink ME, Solomon RA, et al. Management of cerebral vasospasm in the 1990's. Clin Neuropharmacol 1995;18:127.
91. Vermeulen M, Lindsay HW, van Gijn J. Cerebral Ischemia. In L Walton, CP Warlow, J van Gijn, (eds), Subarachnoid Hemorrhage. London: Saunders, 1992;69.
92. Mohr JP, Kase CS. Cerebral vasospasm. Part 1. In cerebral vascular malformations. Rev Neurol 1983;139:99.
93. Connay LW, McDonald LW. Structural changes of the intradural arteries following subarachnoid haemorrhage. J Neurosurg 1972;37:715.
94. Adams HP Jr, Kassell NF, Torner JC, et al. Predicting cerebral ischemia after aneurysmal subarachnoid hemorrhage: influences of clinical condition, CT results, and antifibrinolytic therapy: a report of the Cooperative Aneurysm Study. Neurology 1987;37:1586.
95. Baker CJ, Ortiz O, Solomon RA. Resolution of focal CT hypodense lesions in patients with SAH. Surg Neurol 1993;39:158.

96. Lennihan L, Petty GW, Fink ME, et al. Transcranial Doppler detection of anterior cerebral artery vasospasm. J Neurol Neurosurg Psychiatry 1993;56:906.

97. Sloan MA, Burch CM, Wozniak MA, et al. Transcranial Doppler detection of vertebrobasilar vasospasm following subarachnoid hemorrhage. Stroke 1994;25:2187.

98. Grosset DG, Staiton J, McDonald I, et al. Use of transcranial Doppler sonography to predict development of a delayed ischemic deficit after subarachnoid hemorrhage. J Neurosurg 1993;78:183.

99. Kimura T, Shinoda J, Funakoshi T. Prediction of cerebral infarction due to vasospasm following aneurysmal subarachnoid haemorrhage using acetazolamide-activated ^{123}I-IMP SPECT. Acta Neurochir 1993;123:125.

100. Mayer SA, Van Heertum RL, Tikofskky RS, et al. Presymptomatic detection of ischemia from vasospasm after subarachnoid hemorrhage with acetazolamide-activated SPECT. Stroke 1999 (in press).

101. Ohman J, Servoa A, Heiskanen O. Effect of intrathecal fibrinolytic therapy on clot lysis and vasospasm in patients with aneurysmal subarachnoid hemorrhage. J Neurosurg 1991;75:197.

102. Findlay JM, Kassell NF, Weir BK. A randomized trial of intraoperative, intracisternal tissue plasminogen activator for the prevention of vasospasm. Neurosurgery 1995;37:168.

103. Sasaki T, Ohta T, Kikuchi H, et al. A phase II clinical trial of recombinant human tissue-type plasminogen activator against cerebral vasospasm after aneurysmal subarachnoid hemorrhage. Neurosurgery 1994;35:597.

104. Usui M, Saito N, Hoya K, et al. Vasospasm prevention with postoperative intrathecal thrombolytic therapy: a retrospective comparison of urokinase, tissue plasminogen activator, and cisternal drainage alone. Neurosurgery 1994;34:235.

105. Steinberg GK, Vanefsky MA, Marks MP, et al. Failure of intracisternal tissue plasminogen activator to prevent vasospasm in certain patients with aneurysmal subarachnoid hemorrhage. Neurosurgery 1994;34:809.

106. Philippon J, Grab R, Dagreou F, et al. Prevention of vasospasm in subarachnoid haemorrhage. A controlled study with nimodipine. Acta Neurochir 1986;82:110.

107. Petruk KC, West M, Mohr G, et al. Nimodipine treatment in poor-grade aneurysm patients. Results of a multicenter double-blind placebo controlled trial. J Neurosurg 1988;86:505.

108. Steinke DE, Weir BKA, Findlay JM, et al. A trial of the 21-aminosteroid U74006F in a primate model of chronic cerebral vasospasm. Neurosurgery 1989;24:179.

109. Vollmer DG, Kassell NF, Hongo K, et al. Effect of the nonglucocorticoid 21-aminosteroid U74006F on experimental cerebral vasospasm. Surg Neurol 1989;31:190.

110. Haley EC, Kassell NF, Apperson-Hansen C, et al. A randomized, double-blind, vehicle-controlled trial of tirilazad mesylate in patients with aneurysmal subarachnoid hemorrhage: a cooperative study in North America. J Neurosurg 1997;86:467.

111. Kassell NF, Peerless SJ, Durward QJ, et al. Treatment of ischemic deficits from vasospasm with intravascular volume expansion and induced arterial hypertension. Neurosurgery 1982;11:337.

112. Levy M, Giannotta S. Cardiac performance indices during hypervolemic therapy for cerebral vasospasm. J Neurosurg 1991;75:27.

113. Higashida RT, Halback VV, Dowd CF, et al. Intravascular balloon dilation therapy for intracranial arterial vasospasm: patient selection, technique, and clinical results. Neurosurg Rev 1992;15:89.

114. Newell DW, Eskridge LJM, Mayberg MR, et al. Angioplasty for the treatment of symptomatic vasospasm following subarachnoid hemorrhage. J Neurosurg 1989;71:654.

115. Barnwell SL, Higashida RT, Halbach VV, et al. Transluminal angioplasty of intracerebral vessels for cerebral arterial spasm: reversal of neurological deficits after delayed treatment. Neurosurgery 1989;25:424.

116. Rinkel GJE, Wijdicks EFM, Ramos LMP, et al. Progression of acute hydrocephalus in subarachnoid haemorrhage: a case report documented by serial CT scanning. J Neurol Neurosurg Psychiatry 1990;53:354.

117. Hasan D, Verneulen M, Wijdicks EFM, et al. Management problems in acute hydrocephalus after subarachnoid hemorrhage. Stroke 1989;20:747.

118. Mayhall CG, Archer NH, Lamb VA, et al. Ventriculostomy-related infections. A prospective epidemiologic study. N Engl J Med 1984;310:553.

119. Holloway KL, Barnes T, Choi S, et al. Ventriculostomy infections: the effect of monitoring duration and catheter exchange in 584 patients. J Neurosurg 1996;85:419.

120. Hasan D, Lindsay KW, Vermeulen M. Treatment of acute hydrocephalus after SAH with serial lumbar puncture. Stroke 1991;22:190.

121. Yasargil MG, Yonekawa Y, Zumstein B, Stahl H-J. Hydrocephalus following spontaneous subarachnoid hemorrhage: clinical features and treatment. J Neurosurg 1973;39:474.

122. Vale RL, Bradley EL, Fisher WS. The relationship of subarachnoid hemorrhage and the need for postoperative shunting. J Neurosurg 1997;86:462.
123. Hasan D, Schonck RS, Avezaat CJ, et al. Epileptic seizures after subarachnoid hemorrhage. Ann Neurol 1993;33:286.
124. Wijdicks EFM, Vermeulen M, ten Haaf JA, et al. Volume depletion and natriuresis in patients with a ruptured intracranial aneurysm. Ann Neurol 1985;18:211.
125. Dóczi T, Bende J, Huska E, et al. Syndrome of inappropriate secretion of antidiuretic hormone after subarachnoid hemorrhage. Neurosurgery 1981;4:394.
126. Mayer SA, Solomon RA, Fink ME, et al. Physiologic determinants of renal salt wasting in subarachnoid hemorrhage. Ann Neurol 1994;36:263.
127. Diringer MN, Wu KC, Verbalis JG, et al. Hypervolemic therapy prevents volume contraction but not hyponatremia following subarachnoid hemorrhage. Ann Neurol 1992;31:543.
128. Brouwers PJAM, Wijdicks EFM, Hasan D, et al. Serial electrocardiographic recording in aneurysmal subarachnoid hemorrhage. Stroke 1989;20:1162.
129. Mayer SA, Swarup R. Neurogenic cardiac injury after SAH. Curr Op Anesth 1996;9:356.
130. Mayer SA, LiMandri G, Sherman D, et al. Electrocardiographic markers of abnormal left ventricular wall motion in acute SAH. J Neurosurg 1995;83:889.
131. Hunt D, McRae C, Zapf P. Electrocardiographic and serum enzyme changes in subarachnoid hemorrhage. Am Heart J 1969;77:479.
132. Solensky NJ, Haley EC, Kassell NF, et al, and the participants of the Multicenter, Cooperative Aneurysm Study. Medical complications of aneurysmal subarachnoid hemorrhage: a report of the Multicenter, Cooperative Aneurysm Study. Crit Care Med 1995;23:1007.
133. Andreoli A, Di Pasquale G, Pinelli G, et al. Subarachnoid hemorrhage: frequency and severity of cardiac arrhythmias. Stroke 1987;18:558.
134. Davies KR, Gelb AW, Manninen PH, et al. Cardiac function in aneurysmal subarachnoid haemorrhage: a study of electrocardiographic and echocardiographic abnormalities. Br J Anaesth 1991;67:58.
135. Pollick C, Cujec B, Parker S, et al. Left ventricular wall motion abnormalities in subarachnoid hemorrhage: an echocardiographic study. J Am Coll Cardiol 1988;12:600.
136. Sato K, Masuda T, Kikuno T, et al. Left ventricular asynergy and myocardial necrosis accompanied by subarachnoid hemorrhage: contribution of neurogenic pulmonary edema [Japanese]. J Cardiol 1990;20:359.
137. Kono T, Morita H, Kuroiwa T, et al. Left ventricular wall motion abnormalities in patients with subarachnoid hemorrhage: neurogenic stunned myocardium. J Am Coll Cardiol 1994;24:636.
138. Mayer SA, Sherman D, Fink ME, et al. Myocardial injury and left ventricular dysfunction in acute subarachnoid hemorrhage. Ann Neurol 1993;34:288.
139. Mayer SA, Fink ME, Homma S, et al. Cardiac injury associated with neurogenic pulmonary edema following subarachnoid hemorrhage. Neurology 1994;44:815.
140. Ropper AH, Zervas NT. Outcome 1 year after subarachnoid hemorrhage from cerebral aneurysm. Management morbidity, mortality, and functional status in 112 consecutive good-risk patients. J Neurosurg 1984;60:909.
141. Longstreth WT Jr, Nelson LM, Koepsell TD, et al. Clinical course of spontaneous subarachnoid hemorrhage: a population–based study in King County, Washington. Neurology 1993;43:712.
142. Le Roux PD, Elliot JP, Downey L, et al. Improved outcome after rupture of anterior circulation aneurysms: 10-year review of 224 good-grade patients. J Neurosurg 1995;83:394.
143. Hop JW, Rinkel GLE, Algra A, et al. Case-fatality rates and functional outcome after subarachnoid hemorrhage: a systematic review. Stroke 1997;28:660.
144. Solomon RA, Mayer SA, Tarmey J. The relationship between the volume of craniotomies for cerebral aneurysm performed at New York state hospitals and in-hospital mortality. Stroke 1996;27:13.
145. Sonesson B, Ljunggren B, Saveland H, et al. Cognition and adjustment after late and early operation for ruptured aneurysm. J Neurosurg 1987;21:279.
146. Vilkki J, Holst P, Ohman J, et al. Cognitive deficits related to computed tomographic findings after surgery for a ruptured intracranial aneurysm. Neurosurgery 1989;25:166.

11
Chronic Respiratory Failure of Neurogenic Origin

Robin S. Howard and Adrian J. Williams

Respiratory insufficiency is the inability to maintain adequate ventilation to match acid-base status and oxygenation to metabolic requirements. The initial abnormality may be intermittent nocturnal hypoventilation that leads to hypercapnia and hypoxia. This eventually persists while the patient is awake, and symptoms can develop concurrently. Respiratory failure is defined as a Pao_2 of less than 8.0 kPa (60 mm Hg) or a $Paco_2$ greater than 6.7 kPa (50 mm Hg), or both [1]. Respiratory insufficiency can develop during the course of many neurologic disorders. It occurs most commonly as a consequence of neuromuscular weakness but can also accompany disturbances of brain stem function or interruption of descending respiratory pathways. Respiratory failure can occur during the course of acute and potentially treatable or self-limiting disorders (e.g., Guillain-Barré syndrome, myasthenia gravis, polymyositis), after an acute insult that results in permanent disability (e.g., spinal cord injury), or as a result of progressive disease (e.g., muscular dystrophy, motor neuron disease). In a number of apparently stable disorders (e.g., poliomyelitis), late deterioration can lead to the development of respiratory failure many years after the acute illness [2]. Previously unsuspected respiratory insufficiency may present as failure to wean from elective, perioperative mechanical ventilation [3].

It is important to recognize patients at risk of respiratory failure, because providing appropriate support reduces morbidity and mortality, allowing survival for prolonged periods with or without respiratory support [4,5]. The decision to assist ventilation in acute neurologic disorders is usually straightforward. More difficult issues are raised in progressive neuromuscular disease, however, particularly if associated with bulbar weakness. In this situation, an accurate diagnosis and prognosis are essential to determine the aims and type of ventilatory support. For example, noninvasive support in motor neuron disease can alleviate distressing symptoms of breathlessness and orthopnea without preventing the development of aspiration and bronchopneumonia, while ventilation via a cuffed tracheostomy can protect the airway and prolong survival inappropriately in the face of severe or total paralysis. Ethical considerations in providing ventilatory

249

support in progressive neuromuscular disease are complex and depend on detailed individual assessment and discussion with the patient and family.

CLINICAL FEATURES OF RESPIRATORY INSUFFICIENCY AND FAILURE

Symptoms

Respiratory insufficiency can develop insidiously, presenting few symptoms other than the universal increase in exertional dyspnea associated with advancing age. In neurologic disease, the decrease in functional respiratory reserve becomes significant when regular daily activities, such as walking or sleeping, cause hypercapnia. Hypoxia on exercise can occur in neurologic conditions, such as postpolio, when motor neurons innervating limb musculature are relatively less affected than those that innervate respiratory muscles. More commonly, hypercapnia first occurs during sleep. Nocturnal hypoventilation or sleep apnea may initially be asymptomatic but, if persistent, is characterized by insomnia, daytime hypersomnolence and lethargy, morning headaches, reduced mental concentration, depression, anxiety, or irritability. Symptoms of obstructive sleep apnea (OSA) are similar, but the patient or his or her partner often complains of snoring, abnormal sleep movements, and disturbed sleep with distressing dreams. Patients with progressive diaphragm weakness are often first aware of respiratory difficulty during jerky motion, as occurs in horseback riding, driving over rough surfaces, or swimming in rough seas. Orthopnea can be severe, with patients often refusing to lie supine for the clinical examination, claiming that the supine position causes backache, claustrophobia, or panic attacks. This can make recognition of the clinical signs uncertain. Nocturnal orthopnea is usually severe and can mimic paroxysmal nocturnal dyspnea. Excessive nocturnal salivation with crusting of the lips is sometimes present.

Clinical Signs

Clinical signs are often absent in the early stages, which can lead to the condition of respiratory failure being missed. As the condition progresses, the patient may have an unexplained tachycardia, an accentuated second heart sound over the pulmonary valve area, and signs of polycythemia. Obesity is often present in individuals with OSA, increased accessory muscle activity and diaphragmatic weakness occurs, or paralysis causes paradoxical movement of the abdominal wall with inspiratory indrawing of the lower lateral rib margin when the patient is supine or near supine.

As the condition progresses, the full picture of respiratory failure is present. This is closely similar to cor pulmonale, which can lead to inappropriate treatment if the neurologic etiology is not appreciated. Sudden unexpected death may then occur [6].

Bulbar dysfunction is revealed by clinical signs of lesions of the ninth and tenth cranial nerves, including loss of posterior pharyngeal wall sensation, reduced palatal movement and pharyngeal reflex, poor cough, impaired speech, and ineffective swallowing [7]. However, clinical signs of bulbar dysfunction are not always a good guide to the development of aspiration [8,9].

INVESTIGATIONS

In progressive neuromuscular disease, vital capacity (VC) falls because of respiratory muscle weakness or fatigue, or both, and reduced chest wall and lung compliance [10–12], resulting from microatelectasis [13] and restriction of chest wall movement [14]. This is associated with reduced total lung compliance and preserved residual volume. Diaphragm weakness is associated with a marked fall (greater than one-third) in VC when the patient is sitting or lying down [14,15]. Regular measurements of VC (erect and supine) allow assessment of the extent and progression of respiratory muscle weakness. Carbon monoxide transfer is normal when corrected for volume.

Chest radiographs may show clinically unsuspected unilateral or bilateral diaphragmatic paresis, aspiration pneumonitis, or bronchopneumonia. Fluoroscopic screening performed with the patient in the supine position may show paradoxical upward movement of the paralyzed diaphragm during inspiration or, preferably, during short, sharp submaximal sniff. Hemidiaphragm excursion can also be assessed using ultrasound [16–18].

Waking arterial blood gas tensions are often virtually normal during the early stages of neurologic respiratory insufficiency, even when significant nocturnal hypoventilation is occurring. Pao_2 may be slightly reduced, leading to the erroneous suspicion of intrinsic lung disease. As the condition progresses, daytime $Paco_2$ becomes elevated. Arterial gas tension monitoring by indwelling arterial catheter is necessary to show progressive nocturnal hypoventilation. Surface $Paco_2$ electrodes can produce misleading results when used overnight because of changes in skin temperature and blood flow that occur during sleep. Nocturnal oximetry can be helpful, but its role is limited because desaturation is a late feature of progressive nocturnal hypoventilation. Nevertheless, oximetry is the measurement of choice to detect periodic sleep apnea. However, detailed analysis of the mechanisms of sleep-induced respiratory failure require full polysomnography [19].

When the lung is normal, transpulmonary pressure is low and static inspiratory and expiratory pressures measured at the mouth reflect pleural pressure, thus providing a valuable method of measuring global inspiratory and expiratory muscle strength [20,21]. Transdiaphragmatic pressure can be determined from esophageal and gastric pressures during maximum sniff using balloon transducers passed nasogastrically [22]. The maximum nasopharyngeal pressure measured nasally during maximum sniff can also provide a close reflection of transdiaphragmatic pressure [23].

Phrenic nerve function can be assessed by direct electrical phrenic nerve stimulation in the patient's neck by measuring conduction time and compound muscle action potential (CMAP) using surface or percutaneous recording or by measuring twitch transdiaphragmatic pressure [24–28]. The amplitude and area of diaphragmatic response may be more sensitive than latency in detecting phrenic nerve paresis. Intercostal nerve conduction studies and electromyography (EMG) may also allow assessment of latency, CMAP, f-wave latencies, and patterns of intercostal muscle activities [29]. Supramaximal bilateral phrenic nerve stimulation can also be achieved by transcortical or cervical magnetic stimulation [30]. These techniques are well tolerated and allow assessment of central motor conduction in addition to measuring the latency and amplitude of motor evoked potentials and transdiaphragmatic pressure. Needle EMG from the diaphragm is safe, causes little discomfort, and provides good recording of diaphragmatic activity. In particular, the spontaneous breathing pattern, the appearance, and the firing patterns of the motor units can be observed. Spontaneous activity, myotonia, polyphasic motor units, and decreased recruitment can be shown [31–38].

PATHOPHYSIOLOGY

Respiratory muscle weakness, bulbar failure, or disturbance of the central control of respiration contributes to nocturnal hypoventilation and can precipitate respiratory insufficiency [7,39,40]. Although the effects of respiratory failure caused by neuromuscular disease can become obvious, the initial abnormality is disordered breathing during sleep, and this remains the critical period for respiratory compromise and sudden death [41].

Respiratory Muscles

Inspiratory and expiratory muscle weakness do not necessarily develop in parallel. In many conditions, the diaphragm is preferentially affected (e.g., motor neuron disease). Adequate ventilation during rapid eye movement sleep is largely dependent on diaphragm function, and episodic hypoventilation or central sleep apnea is inevitable if the diaphragm is paralyzed [41]. In Duchenne's muscular dystrophy, however, expiratory muscles tend to become weak earlier than inspiratory muscles [42], leading to an impaired ability to cough, which in turn precipitates aspiration and bronchopneumonia, particularly if associated bulbar weakness is present.

The consequences of respiratory muscle weakness, which can be exacerbated by scoliosis, include widespread atelectasis, reduced compliance, ventilatory perfusion inequality, and impaired airway patency. The muscles are inevitably working closer to their fatigue threshold [43] at a critical level of pulmonary function, and the addition of any respiratory load, such as respiratory tract infection, aspiration pneumonitis, diaphragmatic splinting in pregnancy, or abdominal distention, can precipitate fatigue and respiratory failure [44,45]. Weakness of abdominal muscles also reduces the capacity to cough, as does abdominal distention caused by ileus, constipation, or bladder distention. Other factors that can precipitate respiratory deterioration in patients who are functioning with reduced reserve include obesity, anesthesia, sedative drugs, surgery, tracheostomy complications, and general medical disorders [2].

Sleep Apnea and Alveolar Hypoventilation

Periodic apnea is conventionally divided into OSA, central sleep apnea, and nocturnal hypoventilation. In *obstructive apnea*, upper airway obstruction is present despite normal movement of the intercostals and diaphragm. In *central apnea*, all respiratory phased movements are absent [46]. Considerable evidence exists that similar mechanisms underlie different forms of apnea [47]. It is important to emphasize that the upper airway respiratory muscles (genioglossus, tensor palatini, and stylopharyngeus) behave like more conventional respiratory muscles, with activities phasically modulated during inspiration and expiration and by classic respiratory stimuli. Thus, OSA is thought to occur when the motor drive to the upper airway muscles is inadequate despite the presence of effective diaphragmatic contractions, and central apnea is a closely related but more severe phenomenon, with inadequate drive to both the upper airway muscles and the diaphragm. OSA is exacerbated by coexisting factors, including obesity; structural abnormalities of the upper airway; depressant drugs and alcohol; supine position; and endocrine, metabolic, musculoskeletal, and autonomic disturbances. In addition to the disturbance of sleep architecture caused by microarousals, OSA leads to progressive hypoxia and hypercapnia; eventually, untreated hypercapneic respiratory failure develops, associated with pulmonary and systemic hypertension, congestive cardiac failure, and polycythemia [6].

Alveolar hypoventilation is characterized by a reduced ventilatory response to carbon dioxide and consequent carbon dioxide retention in the absence of primary pulmonary disease. Progressive reduction in the tidal volume and reduced hypoxic and hypercapneic drive that can culminate in central apnea occur. These effects occur primarily during sleep, but hypercapnia can persist while the patient is awake, with the development of respiratory failure [42]. Nocturnal alveolar hypoventilation may be caused by a central lesion of the automatic pathway or respiratory muscle weakness. Most causes of severe diaphragm weakness lead to alveolar hypoventilation during rapid eye movement sleep, culminating in hypercapnia [15].

Central Control of Respiration in Humans

Precise anatomic localization of specific respiratory function in humans has proved elusive because lesions are rarely isolated, and, even with newer imaging techniques, antemortem localization is imprecise. Furthermore, techniques of studying the patterns of acute respiratory disturbance are relatively insensitive, and accurate diagnosis of respiratory insufficiency has led to earlier therapeutic intervention with controlled ventilation. The neural substrate of respiratory control probably has considerable redundancy and plasticity; for example, congenital, long-standing, or slowly progressive and destructive mass lesions can have little or no functional consequence (Figure 11.1), whereas acute, discrete lesions in a similar distribution can lead to profound respiratory impairment. Finally, much of the literature is flawed because extensive experimental animal work has been applied to humans without any evidence for analogous, anatomicophysiologic correlates.

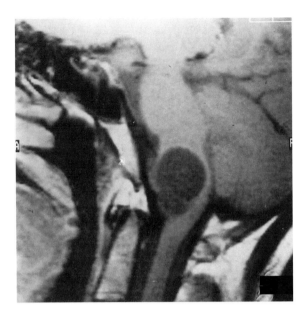

Figure 11.1 Large congenital developmental cyst causing massive distortion of the medulla. Despite the size of the space-occupying lesion and the extent of tissue destruction, no respiratory compromise occurred. This was presumably because the lesion had been present throughout growth, allowing for the development of alternative respiratory pathways.

Neural control of respiration in humans has been considered to depend on three largely anatomically and functionally independent pathways [39], although it is clear that these systems must interact with one another [48,49].

Behavioral (Voluntary) Control

Behavioral (voluntary) control operates during wakefulness and allows voluntary modulation of respiration in response, for example, to speaking, singing, breath-holding, and straining. Techniques of central motor stimulation and functional imaging have confirmed that the respiratory muscles are activated behaviorally, with phrenic motor neurons being controlled by rapidly conducting, oligosynaptic pathways from the contralateral motor cortex. Inspiratory muscles have a direct representation in the primary motor cortex, premotor cortex, supplementary motor area, and thalamus, whereas for active expiration the areas are more extensive and involve limbic cortex [50–54]. Stimulation of large areas of the limbic cortex inhibits respiration by slowing the respiratory rate [55], while both rate and tidal volume are increased by simultaneous bilateral stimulation of the anterior amygdala [56].

Voluntary control can be impaired by bilateral lesions affecting the descending corticospinal or corticobulbar tract [7]. This is particularly seen in association with destructive lesions of the basal pons or of the medullary pyramids and adjacent ventromedial portion, which can result in the "locked-in" syndrome (Figure 11.2). Selective interruption of the voluntary pathways in humans leads to a strikingly regular and unvarying respiratory pattern during wakefulness as well as sleep, with loss of the ability to take a deep breath, hold the breath, cough voluntarily, or initiate any kind of volitional respiratory

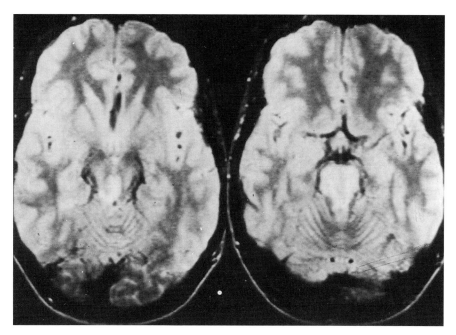

Figure 11.2 T2-weighted magnetic resonance imaging scans in a patient with locked-in syndrome shows extensive pontine infarction owing to basilar occlusion.

movement. The tidal volume remains responsive to carbon dioxide, and a reflex cough is preserved.

Metabolic (Automatic) Respiration

Metabolic (automatic) respiration is the homeostatic pathway by which ventilation can be mediated to maintain acid-base status and oxygenation to the metabolic requirements. Automatic control is mediated by localized areas in the dorsolateral tegmentum of the pons and medulla in the region of the nucleus tractus solitarius and nucleus retroambigualis (for review, see reference 7). As a consequence of lesions in this area, automatic respiratory control is disrupted; the patient is voluntarily able to maintain his or her respiratory pattern and breaths normally while awake and alert, but during sleep there is a sudden or progressive decline in tidal volume and respiratory rate culminating in sleep apnea [57].

Abnormal patterns of rate and rhythm are also often a reflection of impaired automatic ventilatory control. Many of these patterns were first described as manifestations of progressive central brain stem herniation and were considered to have fairly precise localizing values patterns [58]. However, these phenomena are now seen less commonly because controlled ventilation is instituted earlier in patients with neurogenic respiratory insufficiency. Primary central neurogenic hyperventilation, characterized by rapid, regular hyperventilation, persists in the face of alkalosis, elevated Po_2, and low Pco_2 and in the absence of any pulmonary

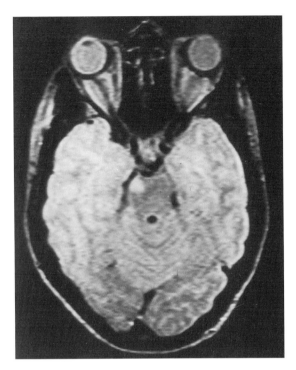

Figure 11.3 T2-weighted magnetic resonance imaging scan in a patient with an acute exacerbation of multiple sclerosis shows a focal high signal pontine lesion. An apneustic pattern of respiration developed that persisted for 6 days.

or airway disorder. It is extremely rare, and the few cases in the literature have been associated with either lymphoma or infiltrating glioma [59,60]. Hyperventilation in the seriously ill patient is common but is owing to intrinsic pulmonary involvement, leading to ventilation-perfusion ratio mismatch, pulmonary shunting, and increased vagally mediated reflexes [61–63]. In apneustic breathing, there are sustained inspiratory cramps with a prolonged pause at full inspiration or alternating brief end-inspiratory and expiratory pauses. The pattern has been associated with bilateral tegmental infarcts or demyelinating lesions in the pons (Figure 11.3). In cluster breathing, respiration occurs in irregular bursts separated by variable periods of apnea; the regularity and decrescendo-crescendo pattern of Cheyne-Stokes respiration is absent, and the cycle time is much shorter. Ataxic respiration is characterized by a completely irregular respiratory cycle of variable frequency and tidal volume alternating with periods of apnea; it is particularly associated with medullary compression owing to rapidly expanding lesions and may be an important sign of impending respiratory arrest.

Hiccups consist of brief bursts of intense inspiratory activity involving the diaphragm and inspiratory intercostal muscles with reciprocal inhibition of the expiratory intercostals [64,65]. Glottic closure occurs almost immediately after the onset of diaphragmatic contraction, thus minimizing the ventilatory effect. Intractable hiccups may be the result of structural or functional disturbances of the medulla or afferent or efferent connections with the respiratory muscles. They may be associated with structural lesions of the medulla, including infarction in the territory of the posterior inferior cerebellar artery, tumor, tuberculoma, abscess, syrinx, hematoma, and demyelination. Development of hiccups in this context may anticipate the development of irregularities of the respiratory rhythm, culminating in respiratory arrest.

Limbic (Emotional) Control

Limbic (emotional) control accounts for the preservation of respiratory modulation to emotional stimuli, including laughing, coughing, and anxiety, despite loss of voluntary control. This implies that descending limbic influences on automatic respiration are anatomically and functionally independent of the voluntary respiratory system. Munschauer and associates [66] described a patient with locked-in syndrome owing to infarction of the basal pons. This led to loss of voluntary control with normal carbon dioxide responses but preservation of respiratory modulation to emotional stimuli, including laughing, coughing, and anxiety. Such a descending pathway, mediating limbic control of respiration, lay either in the pontine tegmentum or lateral basis pontis.

PATTERNS OF RESPIRATORY IMPAIRMENT CAUSED BY NEUROLOGIC DISORDERS

Cortex

Apnea and prolonged expiratory apneusis are common occurrences during complex partial and generalized seizures. They may be associated with upper airway obstruction, laryngospasm, and masseter spasm, leading to hypoxemia and cyanosis. Isolated apnea may be an ictal phenomenon, requiring prolonged ventilation, and can contribute to sudden unexpected death in epileptic patients [67–70].

Patients with bilateral hemispheric cerebrovascular disease show an increased respiratory responsiveness to carbon dioxide and are liable to develop Cheyne-Stokes respiration, suggesting disinhibition of lower respiratory centers [71]. Diffuse cortical vascular disease can also lead to a selective inability of voluntary breathing (respiratory apraxia). Reduced chest wall movement and reduced contralateral diaphragmatic excursion, particularly during voluntary breathing, have been described after cortical vascular events.

Brain Stem

The effects of brain stem dysfunction on respiration depend on the pathology, localization, and speed of onset of the lesion (see Figure 11.1). In patients with bulbar lesions, particularly vascular or demyelinating, the combination of impaired swallow, abnormalities of the respiratory rhythm, reduced VC, and reduced or absent triggering of a cough reflex all increase the risk of aspiration pneumonia [72]. Nocturnal upper airway occlusion can also contribute to respiratory impairment.

The most common cause of brain stem lesions that disrupt respiration is cere-brovascular disease. Unilateral or bilateral lateral tegmental infarcts in the pons (at or below the level of the trigeminal nucleus) lead to apneustic breathing and impairment of carbon dioxide responsiveness, while similar lesions in the medulla (e.g., lateral medullary syndrome) can result in acute failure of automatic respiration [73,74]. Infarction of the basal pons (locked-in syndrome) or of the pyramids and the adjacent ventromedial portion of the medulla can lead to com-plete loss of the voluntary system with a highly regular breathing pattern but a complete inability to initiate any spontaneous respiratory movements [75] (see Figure 11.2).

Respiratory abnormalities may be associated with encephalitis involving the brain stem, in particular encephalitis lethargica. A variety of patterns occur dur-ing the acute phase and after recovery, including alveolar hypoventilation, cen-tral sleep apnea, and respiratory dysrhythmias such as tachypnea, myoclonic jerking of the diaphragm, apneusis, and ratchet and cluster breathing [76]. Res-piratory failure has also been described as a result of postrubeolar and varicella encephalomyelitis and acute disseminated encephalomyelitis.

Brain stem tumors can lead to automatic respiratory failure or central neuro-genic hyperventilation. Although aspiration and bronchopneumonia are com-mon complications of acute bulbar demyelination, multiple sclerosis has only rarely been associated with central disorders of respiratory rate and rhythm (see Figure 11.3). Acute loss of the automatic system has been associated with large, demyelinating lesions in the region of the medial lemniscus and loss of the vol-untary control system with evidence of an acute demyelinating lesion at the cer-vicomedullary junction [72]. A further respiratory abnormality seen in patients with acute demyelinating brain stem lesions is the tonic seizure described by Matthews [77]. This attack may take the form of paroxysmal hyperventilation precipitated by changes in posture [72].

Additional clinical causes of automatic respiratory failure owing to brain stem disorders include other central nervous system infections such as *Borrelia* and *Lis-teria*; postinfectious encephalomyelitis; and malignant disease, either primary or secondary or as a paraneoplastic brain stem encephalitis with anti-human anti-bodies that can cause central alveolar hypoventilation and central sleep apnea cul-minating in respiratory failure [78]. In Leigh's disease, automatic respiratory failure has been associated with ataxic or cluster breathing and sleep apnea [79]. Reye's syndrome with medullary involvement has also been associated with pro-longed periods of nocturnal apnea and decreased ventilatory response to carbon dioxide, necessitating ventilatory support. Chronic alveolar hypoventilation that cannot be explained in terms of obesity or respiratory or musculoskeletal disor-ders has been termed *Ondine's curse* [80]. In infants, it may be associated with evi-dence of other malformations of the neural crest (ganglioneuroma, multiple ganglioblastoma, Hirschsprung's disease) (for review, see reference 81).

Involuntary Movements of the Respiratory Muscles

A number of patterns of involuntary movements of the respiratory musculature can interfere with ventilation. These include laryngeal dyskinesia or dystonia, which are characterized by paradoxical adduction of the vocal cords that is often precipitated by neuroleptics; patients may present with wheezing, stridor, and exertional dyspnea. In diaphragm flutter, frequent, spontaneous contractions of the diaphragm that are unrelated to inspiration occur; otherwise the diaphragm moves normally. It is associated with dyspnea, severe inspiratory stridor, pain in the thoracic and abdominal wall, and epigastric pulsation. In diaphragmatic or respiratory myoclonus, which is often associated with palatal myoclonus, there are frequent but irregular bilateral diaphragmatic contractions that also involve external intercostal muscles and suppress normal respiratory movements [82]. Paroxysmal nocturnal dystonia presents with stereotypic body movements during sleep with tachycardia, respiratory irregularities, and frequent, repetitive transient arousals, and patients complain of excessive daytime somnolence [83]. Dystonia of the abdominal wall ("belly dancer's dystonia") occasionally presents with breathlessness; it is abolished by breath-holding and deep inspiration [84].

Autonomic Failure

Multisystem atrophy is a global term that includes many neurodegenerative disorders [85]. A characteristic feature is paresis of the vocal cord abductors (posterior cricoarytenoids); the cords lie closely opposed, leading to severe upper airway limitation during sleep and giving rise to the characteristic presenting feature of severe nocturnal stridor [86]. Other factors also contribute to the development of respiratory insufficiency. These include abnormalities of rate, rhythm, and amplitude during sleep and a reduction in central respiratory drive, leading to OSA owing to upper airway occlusion and central sleep apnea caused by loss of automatic control. The abnormal respiratory patterns include Cheyne-Stokes respiration, periodic breathing, inspiratory gasps, apneustic breathing, and respiratory arrest. A further important factor is the accompanying autonomic failure, which contributes to impaired cardiorespiratory control mechanisms [87,88].

Extrapyramidal and Cerebellar Disorders

Respiratory abnormalities similar to multisystem atrophy may be associated with olivopontocerebellar degeneration with marked autonomic involvement. Considerable evidence also exists that cerebellar lesions or cerebellar degenerative disorders lead to sleep fragmentation and apnea.

A variety of respiratory disturbances have been described in idiopathic Parkinson's disease, although they are rarely symptomatic. A defect of voluntary control is suggested by impaired breath-holding, but there may also be impairment of respiratory muscle function owing to bradykinesia or rigidity and airflow obstruction caused by laryngeal stridor [89]. Laryngeal and respiratory muscles can also be affected by focal or segmental dystonia. Steele-Richardson-Olszewski syndrome (progressive supranuclear palsy) is characterized by a profound disturbance of supranuclear, ocular, bulbar, and respiratory control. Impairment and, eventually, complete loss of voluntary respiratory control occurs, although nocturnal ventilation is preserved [90].

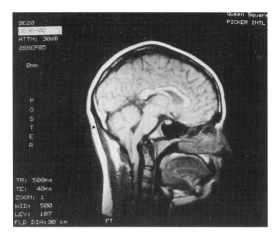

Figure 11.4 T1-weighted magnetic resonance imaging scan shows Arnold-Chiari type I malformation in a patient with nocturnal hypoventilation.

Foramen Magnum Lesions

Foramen magnum lesions are an important cause of acute or subacute respiratory insufficiency. Cerebellar ectopia and syringomyelia can present with either progressive nocturnal hypoventilation, OSA, or sudden respiratory arrest, usually precipitated by some intercurrent event [91] (Figure 11.4). In patients with rheumatoid atlantoaxial dislocation, clinically unsuspected hypoventilation and sleep apnea are common if severe medullary compression occurs, and this may contribute to the high mortality of the condition (Figure 11.5). Respiratory com-

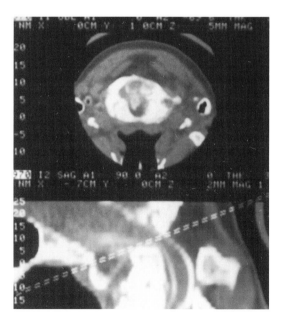

Figure 11.5 Computed tomographic myelogram shows atlantoaxial dislocation with erosion of the dens owing to rheumatoid disease. Severe medullary compression exists, and this was associated with nocturnal apnea.

Figure 11.6 T2-weighted magnetic resonance imaging scan shows a high signal lesion owing to infarction, affecting the anterior spinal cord and extending from C1 to C6.

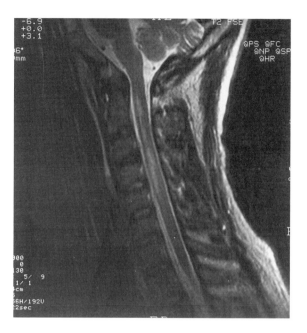

plications may be caused by abnormalities in automatic ventilatory control, involvement of descending ventrolateral automatic or corticospinal voluntary pathways, upper airway obstruction, or aspiration associated with bulbar weakness. Similar respiratory abnormalities may be associated with achondroplasia, osteogenesis imperfecta, and foramen magnum meningioma.

Spinal Cord

Traumatic, demyelinating, or vascular lesions of the spinal cord, particularly at high cervical levels, can selectively affect respiratory control [72]. Lesions of the anterior pathways, particularly descending reticulospinal, as occurred after cordotomy, lead to loss of automatic control and sudden nocturnal death from apnea. Involvement of the dorsolateral corticospinal tracts can lead to automatic respiration (Figures 11.6 and 11.7).

Respiratory effects of traumatic or vascular lesions of the spinal cord depend on the timing of onset and the extent of involvement of the phrenic nerve supply (C3–C5). Complete lesions usually lead to sudden respiratory arrest and death unless immediate resuscitation is available. Patients with lesions at or above C3 and some patients with lesions at a lower level may require prolonged or even permanent ventilator support [92] (Figure 11.8). Quadriparetic patients with levels below C4 lose intercostal and abdominal muscle function while maintaining diaphragm and spinal accessory muscles. Progressive diaphragm fatigue is an important factor in predisposing to intercurrent respiratory infection. Other complications that lead to respiratory problems include impaired cough effectiveness, increased physiologic arteriovenous shunting, and ventilation-perfusion ratio mismatching.

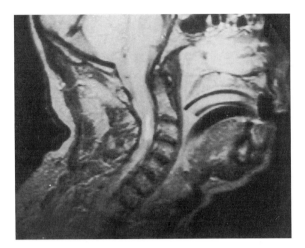

Figure 11.7   Magnetic resonance imaging scan shows a high signal lesion at the C3 level owing to infarction confined to the anterior two-thirds of the cord.

Anterior Horn Cell

During acute poliomyelitis, respiratory insufficiency occurs as a result of respiratory muscle weakness or involvement of the central respiratory control mechanisms. Respiratory insufficiency can develop many years after poliomyelitis, even in the absence of any obvious respiratory involvement during the acute illness or convalescent phase. This usually manifests as progressive nocturnal hypoventilation owing to respiratory muscle weakness and fatigue, particularly with decreased compliance caused by kyphoscoliosis. Other contributory factors include pregnancy, alcohol, and sedative drugs. Development of progressive nocturnal hypoventilation is often insidious; the patient may have no symptoms until a respiratory tract infection supervenes to precipitate respiratory failure or even arrest [2,93].

Respiratory insufficiency is the common terminal event in motor neuron disease either owing to respiratory muscle or bulbar weakness, leading to hypoventilation, aspiration, bronchopneumonia, or pulmonary emboli. An important proportion of patients with motor neuron disease develop respiratory insufficiency early in the course of the disease and present with respiratory failure or even respiratory arrest. The most common cause of respiratory symptoms is generalized respiratory muscle weakness, often with predominant diaphragm paresis. Nocturnal hypoventilation and both central and OSA have been demonstrated in the pseudobulbar form of motor neuron disease [94]. Similarly, ventilatory failure has been described in all three forms of proximal spinal muscular atrophy as a consequence of weakness of respiratory and bulbar muscles and, in the younger onset, progressive scoliosis. Respiratory embarrassment owing to persistent muscle contraction can also occur during acute tetanus, and apnea is a well-recognized complication.

Peripheral Nerves

The incidence of respiratory failure that requires mechanical ventilation in Guillain-Barré syndrome is approximately 20%. Ventilatory failure is primar-

Figure 11.8 **A.** Magnetic resonance imaging shows an extensive, long, intrinsic anterior cervical cord lesion owing to infarction with no brain stem involvement.

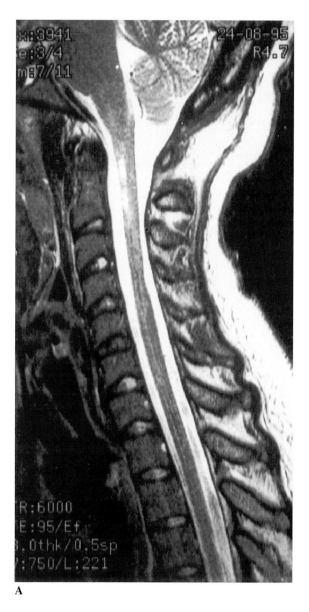

A

ily caused by inspiratory muscle weakness, although weakness of the abdominal and accessory muscles of respiration, retained airway secretion leading to aspiration, and atelectasis are all contributory factors. Associated bulbar weakness and autonomic instability contribute to the necessity for control of the airway and ventilation [95,96]. Prolonged phrenic nerve conduction time or conduction block can predict impending ventilatory failure, and those patients with axonal degeneration have prolonged recovery and increased morbidity and mortality [97,98].

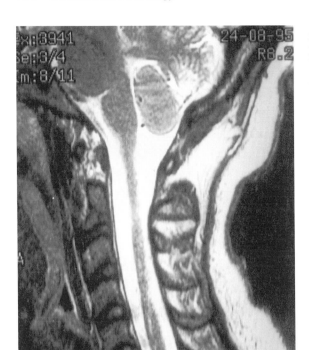

Figure 11.8 (continued)
B. Repeat magnetic resonance imaging scan shows an atrophic spinal cord in the cervical region.

B

Neuralgic amyotrophy can present with dyspnea and orthopnea owing to selective or isolated involvement of the phrenic nerve causing unilateral or bilateral diaphragm paresis [99]. Predominant phrenic nerve involvement can occur in neuropathies associated with underlying carcinoma, diphtheria, and herpes zoster–varicella, and after immunization. Acute respiratory failure is also a feature of vasculitic, acute porphyric, and toxic neuropathies [98]. Similarly, diaphragmatic weakness has been described in hereditary sensorimotor neuropathy [100], and this is associated with reduced transdiaphragmatic pressures and undetectable phrenic nerve conduction. However, phrenic nerve involvement occurs most commonly as a result of trauma during thoracic surgery, hypothermia, or direct involvement by neoplasm [101,102].

Critical illness polyneuropathy is characterized by symmetric weakness of respiratory muscles and of muscles of the upper and lower extremities. Muscle wasting, hyporeflexia, and sensory loss can occur. Phrenic nerve studies show axonal loss, and needle EMG demonstrates evidence of diaphragm denervation correlating with the duration of mechanical ventilation [3].

Neuromuscular Junction

Respiratory failure in myasthenia gravis often results from a myasthenic crisis (usually precipitated by infection) but is also associated with cholinergic crisis, thymectomy, or steroid myopathy. Associated bulbar weakness predisposes to aspiration and acute respiratory failure, necessitating urgent intubation and ventilation. Expiratory and inspiratory intercostal and diaphragm weakness is common, even when only mild peripheral muscle weakness is present [103]. Respiratory impairment is also an important feature in Lambert-Eaton myasthenic syndrome, in which it can be precipitated by anesthesia [104]. Diaphragm and expiratory intercostal weakness is relatively common and can be relieved by 3,4-diaminopyrimidine or treatment of the underlying tumor. In botulism, respiratory muscle weakness and aspiration leading to arrest are common, and urgent and prolonged ventilatory support may be necessary, as the prognosis is generally good.

Muscle

Respiratory muscle weakness is a common cause of morbidity and mortality in muscular dystrophies [105]. In Duchenne's muscular dystrophy, diaphragmatic weakness is not prominent, but chronic respiratory insufficiency is caused by intercostal weakness, scoliosis, reduced lung compliance, aspiration, and repeated infections [45]. Respiratory dysfunction in Becker's muscular dystrophy is rare and is associated with global respiratory muscle weakness. In limb girdle dystrophies, the major pattern of respiratory involvement is gradual, and progressive global weakness of the respiratory muscles is compounded by scoliosis; however, in both limb girdle dystrophies and facioscapulohumeral dystrophy there may be selective diaphragm involvement, and respiratory tract infections are common despite the absence of clinically overt bulbar weakness [106]. In contrast, acid maltase deficiency is characterized by early and selective diaphragm weakness, often with minimal involvement of other respiratory and bulbar musculature [107]. Congenital myopathies, including mitochondrial and nemaline myopathy, may present with respiratory insufficiency or develop alveolar hypoventilation early in the course of the disease [106]. Progressive scoliosis and restrictive ventilatory insufficiency are important complications of Emery-Dreifuss muscular dystrophy and rigid spine syndrome. Complex abnormalities of automatic control also occur in mitochondrial cytopathy; in particular, the phenotype of Leigh's disease. In our experience, these patients show patterns of respiratory insufficiency associated with failure of automatic control, bulbar weakness, and cardiac and respiratory muscle weakness in addition to multiple metabolic abnormalities, including recurrent lactic acidosis [108]. In dystrophia myotonica, respiratory involvement is multifactorial [36]. Respiratory muscle weakness can affect both the diaphragm and expiratory muscles, leading to a poor cough, restrictive lung defect, and alveolar hypoventilation; little evidence exists that myotonia of the respiratory muscles is a significant factor. A central abnormality contributes to alveolar hypoventilation, as can a reduced ventilatory response to carbon dioxide in the absence of carbon dioxide retention, hypersomnolence, and an undue sensitivity to anesthetics and sedatives. This is confirmed by central motor stimulation showing reduced diaphragm CMAP and increased excitatory threshold. Respiratory symptoms develop late in the course of the disease in association with severe respiratory muscle and bulbar weakness, myotonia, and systemic features. Hypersomnolence is the most common presenting symptom, frequently occurring in the absence of hypoventilation. Cardiomyopathy may also be important in sudden, unexpected death in these patients [106].

Respiratory muscle weakness also occurs in the inflammatory myopathies, such as polymyositis, dermatomyositis, inclusion body myositis, and sarcoidosis [109], as well as endocrine myopathies, including Addison's disease, acromegaly, thyrotoxicosis, and myxedema [40], and electrolyte disorders (hypokalemia, hypophosphatemia, hypomagnesemia) and amyloidosis. Acute rhabdomyolysis owing to alcohol abuse, viral infections, *Mycoplasma*, and drugs, such as cholesterol-lowering agents, can cause respiratory failure.

MANAGEMENT OF CHRONIC RESPIRATORY FAILURE OF NEUROMUSCULAR ORIGIN

For the efficient management of respiratory failure in diseases of neuromuscular origin, it is essential to anticipate or recognize at an early stage the critical warning signs. Integral to this management strategy has been the development of augmented alveolar ventilation by noninvasive techniques, which now form the mainstay of treatment. Notwithstanding the ease and acceptability of these current methods, the criteria for intervention remain those of symptoms of excessive daytime sleepiness, morning headaches, and cognitive impairment in the presence of demonstrated sleep-disordered breathing. The degree of physiologic disturbance, such as the severity of desaturations and cardiovascular consequences, may modify the decision to intervene, and as information has accumulated about the natural history of respiratory failure in neuromuscular disease, prophylactic assisted ventilation can be considered.

The following should be considered risk factors for development of acute respiratory failure in patients with neuromuscular diseases:

1. Development of diaphragmatic weakness. This may be evident by clinical signs of respiratory paradox, a standing-to-supine fall in VC of greater than 15%, or the development of low inspiratory pressures.
2. A VC that is less than 30% of predicted.
3. An accelerated decline in VC.

The preceding may or may not themselves be related to alterations in respiratory pressures as measured at the mouth—that is, maximum inspiratory and maximum expiratory. Although the latter are inherently quite variable and poorly predictive, they may be useful as a way of following patients. It has been said that a maximum inspiratory pressure of less than 30% of predicted or a maximum expiratory pressure of less than 70 cm H_2O is indicative of the development of respiratory failure. In addition, weakness of the expiratory muscles with the development of a poor cough can predispose to respiratory tract infections, and another factor is an associated scoliosis, which also impairs respiratory defense against infection.

HISTORICAL PERSPECTIVES

From the mid-nineteenth century to the beginning of the twentieth century, a large number of negative pressure ventilators were developed [110–112]. A century later, these ventilators, particularly the iron lung, served as the mainstay of ventilatory support during the polio epidemics [110]. The epidemics in particular led to the development of additional ventilatory modes, which are discussed in the following section. Notwithstanding the efficacy of such negative pressure ventilation in the polio epidemics, it became appreciated that many acutely ill patients could be ventilated more effectively and with lower mortality using positive-pressure ventilation administered by an endotracheal tube [111]. As a result, the use of noninvasive negative pressure systems declined in the 1950s and 1960s. Since the early 1980s, however, interest in the application of mechanical ventilation without an endotracheal tube or tracheostomy has increased based on two occurrences: first, the recognition that diurnal symptoms of nocturnal respiratory insufficiency can be alleviated with limited (<24 hours/day) assisted ventilation, which is usually nocturnal; and second, the development of delivery systems that are convenient. The latter arose out of the invention of nasal masks that were capable of applying continuous positive airway pressure to the patient's nose [112]. Before the use of positive-pressure ventilation through such masks, noninvasive positive-pressure ventilation had been limited to delivery by mouthpieces or full face masks, both of which have their inherent disadvantages [113].

In tandem with the introduction of nocturnal positive-pressure ventilation through the patient's nose, advances in equipment for delivering these positive pressures occurred. Not least was the introduction of bilevel positive airway pressure as a more comfortable form of continuous positive airway pressure for the treatment of OSA, thus creating a pressure ventilator (Bi-Pap, Respironics, Murrysville, PA).

These developments led to a proliferation of studies evaluating noninvasive ventilation in both acute and chronic respiratory failure. Benefits to the management of respiratory failure of neuromuscular origin have been substantial.

METHODS OF ASSISTED VENTILATION

Noninvasive assisted ventilation (without an endotracheal or tracheostomy tube) encompasses the following three distinct modalities:

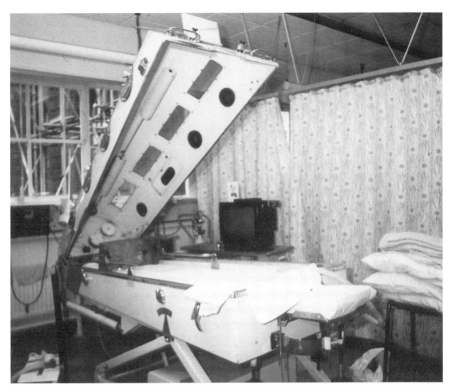

Figure 11.9   The Kelleher iron lung.

Negative-Pressure Ventilation

Pressure change applied to the patient's trunk, but not his or her head, is usually referred to as *negative-pressure ventilation* (although this term is not satisfactory because it can involve positive pressure as well). The basic device is the tank ventilator or iron lung. Despite its size and antiquity—it was first described in 1929 by Philip Drinker and therefore is occasionally called a "Drinker"—the iron lung retains a limited role today [114]. In principle, it consists of an opening chamber in which the patient's whole body is placed with only his or her head protruding. An airtight collar fits around the patient's neck, and the chamber is intermittently evacuated by a large bellows, causing air to pass in and out of the patient's lungs (Figure 11.9). Its current use is confined, however, to three circumstances:

1. In acute exacerbations of chronic obstructive lung disease, particularly when an interface between the ventilator and patient through traditional masks has failed
2. As a means of providing noninvasive, assisted ventilation for periods to allow the nasal airway to be "rested"
3. In those patients in whom the iron lung has been the mainstay of their assisted ventilation, having been introduced before the availability of other convenient systems—that is, positive pressure ventilation

An additional negative-pressure device is the cuirass shell. This is a limited system of delivering negative pressure to the respiratory bellows. The shell is applied tightly to the patient's thorax and upper abdomen, and negative pressure applied to this produces the same inflow of air into the patient's lungs. The advantages of this form of negative-pressure ventilation lie in the access to the rest of the individual, which the iron lung does not allow with ease, but with the disadvantage that the application of efficient ventilation is slightly less easy to obtain.

Although negative-pressure ventilation is an old technique and is used as such, new developments in available equipment, specifically the Hayek oscillator (Flexo Medical Instruments, Zurich, Switzerland), have led to a revival of this method. The Hayek uses negative pressure in the way of the old systems but also has the ability to ventilate at relatively high rates and to apply end-expiratory positive pressure to the patient's thorax and abdomen. We have used such a system to ventilate patients with neuromuscular disease during bronchoscopies or as a means of resting the nasal airway.

Drawbacks to negative-pressure ventilation include a lack of portability of the systems used along with a physiologic effect of increasing the prevalence of obstructive apneas during sleep, as negative pressure applied to the thorax leads to an increased tendency to collapse the upper airway in the region of the velopharynx. In addition, negative-pressure ventilators may not lend themselves to use with patients who have major thoracic deformities.

Positive-Pressure Ventilation

Positive-pressure ventilation is without doubt the most efficient form of assisted ventilation and was also first applied in the polio epidemics [111]. For continuous use, or, in practical terms, more than 16 hours a day, a connection to the patient's trachea via cuffed endotracheal tube or directly by tracheostomy is required. For such long-term use, positive pressure is generated by machines of two principal types. Those that deliver a preset volume per breath (volumes/cycle) can be set to deliver a constant respiratory minute volume or, more commonly, set to respond to respiratory efforts as well (assist control ventilation). Volume ventilation is particularly indicated when the compliance of the respiratory system is reduced, as might occur in severe restrictive lung disease, or, more important, when the compliance is variable, as occurs in children, and mandated alveolar ventilation is required.

Machines that deliver a predetermined pressure are now more common. Assisted ventilation in the intensive care unit is currently much more frequently provided in this form as so-called pressure-support ventilation. The advantages lie in the ability of the patient to vary tidal volume on a breath-to-breath basis. These ventilators are leak compensating, which provides another advantage, because intermittent speech during the inspiratory stroke of the ventilator can be accomplished. They are particularly suitable for long-term use in neurologic disease and are usually simple and reliably constructed, making them suitable for home use. These ventilators have commonly been used to deliver positive pressure through nasal masks, so-called nasal intermittent positive-pressure ventilation [112].

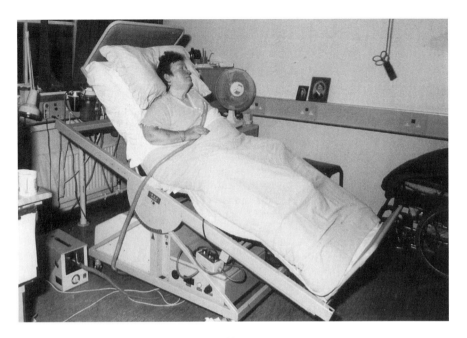

Figure 11.10   Rocking bed, inspiratory position.

Body Ventilators

If the interface surrounding the patient (for negative-pressure ventilation) or at the face (for positive-pressure ventilation) fails or is resisted, it is possible to adequately ventilate by means of less direct methods. The idea that breathing could be assisted by rocking a patient's head up and down first occurred to Eve (1932), who used the family rocking chair when trying to help a diphtheritic child [115,116]. He adapted it for resuscitation, and for many years it was known as Eve's rocking method. A mechanical rocking bed was described by Schuster and Fischer-Williams [116], and the technique has remained popular and effective in patients whose respiratory weakness is predominantly diaphragmatic [117] (Figure 11.10). It is the only method of respiratory assistance that leaves the patient unconnected to an apparatus. Although diaphragmatic weakness commonly involves the crura, it is unusual for rocking-bed users to experience reflux. One disadvantage is engineering problems in receiving a smooth motion.

Body ventilators are variably tolerated and, as with the negative-pressure devices, are not portable and are less efficient. Steljes et al. [118] have reported that, while using a rocking bed, sleep efficiency was poor with an increase in stage 1 and wake during sleep, a consequence of the repeated motions. However, some of our patients have described their sleep as refreshing and have no desire to switch to another form of ventilation.

An additional method of moving the diaphragm without the application of pressure changes to the patient's thorax is by way of an abdominal binder. This is an inflatable corset applied to the patient's abdomen and lower chest. When rhythmically inflated, it augments expiration. Its unique value is for severe respiratory dependence in patients with paralysis of both diaphragm and abdominal wall and the assistance it gives by day when patients are sitting. The weight of the abdominal contents descending provides adequate inspiration.

An important nonmechanical respiratory support method is glossopharyngeal (frog)-breathing. This uses the patient's mouth and pharynx to inflate his or her passive chest [119–121]. Serial incremental inflation of the lungs is produced by gulping air into the oropharynx, closing the mouth and soft palate, opening the larynx, and forcing the air from the pharynx to the trachea. The vocal cord is then closed and the process repeated. By learning this method, a patient can often take a deep breath that is three or four times the amount of his or her VC. This technique greatly assists coughing and maintains mobility of the costovertebral and sternocostal joints. It is a useful adjunct to breathing in poliomyelitis, and many patients are able to manage prolonged periods of the day by glossopharyngeal breathing alone; 50–60 adult boluses can be delivered to the lungs that breathe 1 second or less, leading to a possible minute ventilation of 5–6 liters.

DEFINITIONS

Ventilation is normally achieved by variations in transpulmonary pressure brought about by the action of the respiratory muscles. In normal inspiration, a minor negative pressure within the pleural space (of 4–5 cm H_2O) achieves the inspiration of a tidal volume. Expiration is accomplished by spontaneous recoil, occasionally assisted by expiratory muscles, including the abdominal wall. Continuous positive airway pressure is the application of a continuous positive pressure to the system with the previously described fluctuations on the background of this positive pressure. Reduction in this positive pressure during expiration leads to bilevel positive airway pressure. This system was first developed to provide more comfortable levels of continuous positive airway pressure for those patients with difficult-to-control OSA and the requirement for high pressures, in doing so creating a "ventilator," the difference between inspiratory and expiratory positive airway pressures lending energy to the system—that is, assisted ventilation. The absence of any expiratory positive airway pressure produces intermittent positive-pressure ventilation, the standard method of assisted ventilation in the intensive care unit and elsewhere.

SUCCESS OF NONINVASIVE VENTILATION

Use of noninvasive ventilation in patients with chronic respiratory insufficiency of neuromuscular origin has a long track record. Numerous patients with paralytic poliomyelitis were sustained for years or even decades by noninvasive ventilators despite severe respiratory muscle dysfunction. In the early 1980s, nocturnal use of negative pressure ventilators was associated with sustained improvement in daytime gas exchange and symptoms of hypoventilation in patients with respiratory failure owing to neuromuscular disease as well as chest wall deformities and central hypoventilation. More recently, similar studies using the nasal mask have appeared confirming the earlier findings [19]. These studies have consistently demonstrated that the use of noninvasive ventilation for as little as 6–8 hours a night lowers the daytime $PaCO_2$, and as a consequence raises daytime PaO_2 and eliminates symptoms of morning headache and hyposomnolence. These uncontrolled studies are uniform in demonstrating the benefits such that randomized studies now seem unnecessary [45,122–125].

The success of intermittent noninvasive ventilation (usually nocturnal) in large part lies with the acceptability of the device to the patient. The choice of ventilator is less important than that of the interface. The time needed to accommodate the patient to the relevant mask is well spent. These masks can be applied around the patient's nose with a pneumatic seal produced by positive pressure. They can also be introduced into the nares in the form of nasal pillows or can be applied at the nares in the form of a nasal sling. Having more than one form of mask available is an advantage, although it adds to the cost. It is convenient to initiate assisted ventilation during a diurnal waking trial. This establishes not only the comfort but also the level of pressure required to maintain adequate ventilation. During the initial nocturnal trials, ventilation can be reasonably monitored by nocturnal oxygen saturation to identify periods of underventilation. Monitoring of this and the patient's symptoms is a sufficient guide to the adequacy of ventilatory assistance.

After stabilization on nocturnal ventilation, problems frequently arise relating to nasal stuffiness that can be managed by humidification or a trial of nasal steroids or nasal ipratropium. It is usually possible to overcome these reactions, although very occasionally a period of rest off the ventilator is indicated. We have found it particularly useful at these times to consider other modes of ventilation, including the cuirass, the iron lung, and even the rocking bed.

HOW DOES INTERMITTENT NONINVASIVE VENTILATION WORK?

Hill [126] has proposed three theories to explain how as little as 4–6 hours of nightly noninvasive ventilation improves daytime symptoms and gas exchange:

1. The intermittent rest of the fatigued muscles restores function, leading to improved daytime gas exchange and symptoms [40,43].
2. Intermittent ventilatory assistance improves daytime gas exchange by increasing lung compliance [11,13].
3. Respiratory control is blunted during the development of chronic respiratory failure and can be restored by nocturnal noninvasive ventilation.

In more recent studies, Hill [126] withdrew nocturnal ventilation for a week in patients with neuromuscular disease whose respiratory failure had been stabilized by nocturnal ventilation for at least 6 months. During the nonventilated phase, nocturnal hypoventilation worsened and symptoms recurred, but VC and the respiratory muscle strength did not change. This suggests that variation of nocturnal hypoventilation with resetting of the respiratory center's sensitivity to carbon dioxide may be the most important of the three mechanisms.

HOME MECHANICAL VENTILATION

When respiratory failure in neuromuscular disease is irreversible, long-term assisted ventilation may need to be continued on an almost daily basis. Those patients who require near continuous assisted ventilation usually have a tracheostomy (instances occur in our unit when continuous noninvasive ventilation is applied by cuirass or tank ventilator, or both, but these are rare). Lesser ventilatory needs can be met by noninvasive systems, with resulting simplification of home care [127–130]. Indeed, for patients who are able to apply the nosepiece setup themselves, assisted ventilation may not require additional support services in the home environment, but rather the backup of a respiratory team to deal with the patients' physical and psychological requirements as well as equipment maintenance. This can be done by regular visits to the center or through home visits by technicians.

When the application of nocturnal ventilation or, in addition, some diurnal ventilation requires the help of other individuals because of the patient's disability, additional training and expertise on the part of caregivers are necessary.

REFERENCES

1. Sykes MK, McNicol MW, Campbell EJM. Introduction. In MK Sykes, MW McNicol, EJM Campbell (eds), Respiratory Failure. Oxford, UK: Blackwell Scientific, 1976;i–xv.
2. Howard RS, Wiles CM, Spencer GT. The late sequelae of poliomyelitis. QJM 1988;66:219.
3. Bolton CF. Muscle weakness and difficulty in weaning from the ventilator in the critical care unit. Chest 1994;106:1.
4. O'Donohue WJ, Baker JP, Bell GM, et al. Respiratory failure in neuromuscular disease. Management in a respiratory intensive care unit. JAMA 1976;235:733.
5. Douglas JG, Fergusson RJ, Crompton GK, Grant IWB. Artificial ventilation for neurological disease; retrospective analysis 1972–1981. BMJ 1983;286:1943.
6. Stradling JR, Philipson EA. Breathing disorders during sleep. QJM 1986;225:3.
7. Howard RS, Newsom Davis J. The Neural Control of Respiratory Function. In R Crockard, R Hayward, JT Hoff (eds), Neurosurgery—the Scientific Basis of Clinical Practice (2nd ed). Oxford, UK: Blackwell Scientific, 1992;318–336.
8. Linden P, Siebens AA. Dysphagia: predicting laryngeal penetration. Arch Phys Med Rehabil 1983;64;281.
9. Splaingard ML, Hutchins B, Sulton LD, Chaudhuri G. Aspiration in rehabilitation patients: videofluoroscopy vs bedside clinical assessment. Arch Phys Med Rehabil 1988;69:637.
10. De Troyer A, Borenstein S, Cordier R. Analysis of lung volume restriction in patients with respiratory muscle weakness. Thorax 1980;35:603.
11. Estenne M, Heilporn A, Delhez L, et al. Chest wall stiffness in patients with respiratory muscle weakness. Am Rev Respir Dis 1983;128:1002.
12. Seresier DE, Mastaglia FL, Gibson GJ. Respiratory muscle function and ventilatory control. I. In patients with motor neurone disease. II. In patients with myotonic dystrophy. QJM 1982;202:205.
13. Gibson GJ, Pride NB, Newsom Davis J, Loh L. Pulmonary mechanics in patients with respiratory muscle weakness. Am Rev Respir Dis 1977;115:389.
14. Loh L, Goldman M, Newsom Davis J. The assessment of diaphragm function. Medicine (Baltimore) 1977;56:165.
15. Newsom Davis J, Goldman M, Loh, L, Casson M. Diaphragm function and alveolar hypoventilation. QJM 1976;457:87.
16. Ueki J, De Bruin PF, Pride NB. In vivo assessment of diaphragm contraction by ultrasound in normal subjects. Thorax 1995;50:1157.
17. Houston JG, Morris AD, Grosset DG, et al. Ultrasonic evaluation of movement of the diaphragm after acute cerebral infarction. J Neurol Neurosurg Psychiatry 1995;58:738.

18. Cohen E, Mier A, Heywood P, et al. Diaphragmatic movement in hemiplegic patients measured by ultrasonography. Thorax 1994;49:890.
19. Bye PTP, Ellis ER, Issa FG, et al. Respiratory failure and sleep in neuromuscular disease. Thorax 1990;45:241.
20. Black LF, Hyatt RE Maximal respiratory pressures: normal values and relationship to age and sex. Am Rev Respir Dis 1969;99:696.
21. Black LF, Hyatt RE. Maximal static respiratory pressures in generalized neuromuscular disease. Am Rev Respir Dis 1971;103:641.
22. Miller JM, Moxham J, Green M. The maximal sniff in the assessment of diaphragm function in man. Clin Sci 1985;69:91.
23. Polkey MI, Green M, Moxham J. Measurement of respiratory muscle strength. Thorax 1995;50:1131.
24. Chen R, Collins S, Remtulla H, et al. Phrenic nerve conduction study in normal subjects. Muscle Nerve 1995;18:330.
25. Mills GH, Kyroussis D, Hamnegard CH, et al. Unilateral magnetic stimulation of the phrenic nerve. Thorax 1995;50:1162.
26. Hamnegard CH, Wragg S, Kyroussis D, et al. Mouth pressure in response to magnetic stimulation of the phrenic nerves. Thorax 1995;50:620.
27. Ferguson GT. Use of twitch pressures to assess diaphragmatic function and central drive. J Appl Physiol 1994;77:1705.
28. Wragg S, Aquilina R, Moran J, et al. Comparison of cervical magnetic stimulation and bilateral percutaneous electrical stimulation of the phrenic nerves in normal subjects. Eur Respir J 1994;7:1788.
29. Misra VP, Howard RS, Youl BD. Techniques for the neurophysiological evaluation of respiratory function. J Neurol Neurosurg Psychiatry 1997;62:215.
30. Zifko U, Remtulla H, Power K, et al. Transcortical and cervical magnetic stimulation with recording of the diaphragm. Muscle Nerve 1996;19:614.
31. Chen R, Collins SJ, Remtulla H, et al. Needle EMG of the human diaphragm: power spectral analysis in normal subjects. Muscle Nerve 1996;19:324.
32. Bolton CF. AAEM minimonograph: 40: clinical neurophysiology of the respiratory system. Muscle Nerve 1993;16:809.
33. Bolton CF, Grand'Maison F, Parkes A, Shkrum M. Needle electromyography of the diaphragm. Muscle Nerve 1992;15:678.
34. Silverman JL, Rodriquez AA. Needle electromyographic evaluation of the diaphragm. Electromyogr Clin Neurophysiol 1994;34:509.
35. Saadeh PB, Crisafulli CF, Sosner J, Wolf E. Needle electromyography of the diaphragm: a new technique. Muscle Nerve 1993;16:15.
36. Zifko UA, Hahn AF, Remtulla H, et al. Central and peripheral studies in myotonic dystrophy. Brain 1996;119:1911.
37. Misra VP, Howard RS, Youl BD. Neurophysiological examination of respiratory muscle function in myotonic disorders. J Neurol Neurosurg Psychiatry 1995;59:216A.
38. Misra VP, Youl BD, Howard RS. A technique for the assessment of intercostal nerve function. J Neurol Neurosurg Psychiatry 1996;60:122A.
39. Plum E. Neurological Integration of Behavioural and Metabolic Control of Breathing. In R Parker (ed), Breathing: Hering Breuer Centenary Symposium. London: Churchill, 1970;314–332.
40. Laroche CM, Moxham J, Green M. Respiratory muscle weakness and fatigue. QJM 1989;71:373.
41. Phillipson EA, Bowes G. Control of Breathing during Sleep. In AP Fishman (ed), Handbook of Physiology, The Respiratory System (Vol II). Bethesda, MD: American Physiological Society, 1986;649–674.
42. Inkley SR, Oldenburg FC, Vignos PJ. Pulmonary function in Duchenne muscular dystrophy related to stage of disease. Am J Med 1974;56:297.
43. Moxham J. Respiratory muscle fatigue: mechanisms, evaluation and therapy. Br J Anaesth 1990;65:45.
44. Kreitzer SM, Saunders NA, Tyler HR, Ingram RH. Respiratory function in amyotrophic lateral sclerosis. Am Rev Respir Dis 1978;117:443.
45. Smith PEM, Edwards RHT, Calverley PMA. Mechanisms of sleep disordered breathing in chronic neuromuscular disease: implications for management. QJM 1991;81:961.
46. Douglas NJ. Control of breathing during sleep. Clin Sci 1984;67:465.
47. Douglas NJ. Breathing during Sleep in Adults. In DC Flenley, TL Petty (eds), Recent Advances in Respiratory Medicine, 4. Edinburgh, UK: Churchill Livingstone, 1986;231–248.
48. Murphy K, Mier A, Adams L, Guz A. Putative cerebral cortical involvement in the ventilatory response to inhaled CO_2 in conscious man. J Physiol 1990;420:1.

49. Orem J, Netick A. Behavioral control of breathing in the cat. Brain Res 1986;366:238.
50. Gandevia SC, Rothwell JC. Activation of the human diaphragm from the motor cortex. J Physiol 1987;384:109.
51. Macefield G, Gandevia SC. The cortical drive to human respiratory muscles in the awake state assessed by premotor cerebral potentials. J Physiol 1991;439:545.
52. Colebach JG, Adams L, Murphy K, et al. Regional cerebral blood flow during volitional breathing in man. J Physiol 1991;443:91.
53. Maskill D, Murphy K, Mier A, et al. Motor cortical representation of the diaphragm in man. J Physiol 1991;443:105.
54. Ramsay SC, Adams L, Murphy K, et al. Regional cerebral blood flow during volitional expiration in man: a comparison with volitional inspiration. J Physiol 1993;461:85.
55. Kaarda BR. Cingulate, Posterior Orbital, Anterior Insular and Temporal Pole Cortex. In HW Magoun (ed), Handbook of Physiology (Sec 1), Neurophysiology (Vol 2). Washington, DC: American Physiological Society, 1960;1345–1372.
56. Pool JL, Ranshoff J. Autonomic effects on stimulating rostral portion of cingulate gyri in man. J Neurophysiol 1949;12:385.
57. Baker AB, Matzke H, Brown JR. Poliomyelitis; III. Bulbar poliomyelitis. A study of medullary function. Arch Neurol Psychiatry 1950;63:257.
58. Plum F, Posner JR. Diagnosis of Stupor and Coma. Philadelphia: Davis, 1983.
59. Rodriguez M, Beale PL, Marsh HM, Okazaki H. Central neurogenic hyperventilation in an awake patient with brainstem astrocytoma. Ann Neurol 1982;11:625.
60. Pauzner R, Mouallem M, Sadeh M, et al. High incidence of primary cerebral lymphoma in tumor induced central neurogenic hyperventilation. Arch Neurol 1989;46:510.
61. Mazzara JT, Ayres SM, Grace WJ. Extreme hypocapnia in the critically ill patient. Am J Med 1974;56:450.
62. North JB, Jennett S. Abnormal breathing patterns associated with acute brain damage. Arch Neurol 1974;31:338.
63. Leigh RJ, Shaw DA. Rapid, regular respiration in unconscious patients. Arch Neurol 1976;33:356.
64. Newsom Davis J. An experimental study of hiccup. Brain 1970;93:851.
65. Howard RS. The causes and treatment of intractable hiccups. BMJ 1992;305:1237.
66. Munschauer FE, Mador MJ, Ahuja A, Jacobs L. Selective paralysis of voluntary but not limbically influenced automatic respiration. Arch Neurol 1991;48:1190.
67. Nelson DA, Ray CD. Respiratory arrest from seizure discharges in limbic system. Arch Neurol 1968;19:199.
68. Coulter DL. Partial seizures with apnea and bradycardia. Arch Neurol 1984;41:173.
69. Shorvon SJ. Tonic clonic status epilepticus. J Neurol Neurosurg Psychiatry 1993;56:125.
70. Nashef L, Walker F, Allen P, et al. Apnoea and bradycardia during epileptic seizures: relation to sudden death in epilepsy. J Neurol Neurosurg Psychiatry 1996;60:297.
71. Tobin MJ, Snyder JV. Cheyne-Stokes respiration revisited. Controversies and implications. Crit Care Med 1984;12:882.
72. Howard RS, Wiles CM, Hirsch NP, et al. Respiratory involvement in multiple sclerosis. Brain 1992;115:479.
73. Bogousslavsky J, Khurana R, Deruaz JP, et al. Respiratory failure and unilateral caudal brainstem infarction. Ann Neurol 1990;28:668.
74. Levin BE, Margolis G. Acute failure of automatic respiration secondary to a unilateral brainstem infarct. Ann Neurol 1977;1:583.
75. Devereaux MW, Keane JR, Davis RL. Automatic respiratory failure associated with infarction of the medulla. Arch Neurol 1973;29:4652.
76. Howard RS, Lees AJ. Encephalitis lethargica—four recent cases. Brain 1987;110:19.
77. Matthews WB. Tonic seizures in disseminated sclerosis. Brain 1958;81:193.
78. Ball JA, Warner T, Howard RS, et al. Central alveolar hypoventilation associated with paraneoplastic brainstem encephalitis and anti-Hu antibodies. J Neurol 1994;241:561.
79. Cumminskey J, Guilleminault C, Davis R, et al. Automatic respiratory failure: sleep studies and Leigh's disease. Neurology 1987;37:1876.
80. Mellins RB, Balfour HH, Turino GM, Winters RW. Failure of automatic control of ventilation (Ondine's curse). Medicine 1970;49:487.
81. Howard RS. Patterns of Respiratory Impairment in Neurological Disease. In H Bostock, PA Kirkwood, AH Pullen (eds), Neurobiology and Disease: Contributions from Clinical Neuroscience to Clinical Neurology. Cambridge: Cambridge University Press, 1996;348–356.
82. Chen R, Remtulla H, Bolton CF. Electrophysiological study of diaphragmatic myoclonus. J Neurol Neurosurg Psychiatry 1995;58:480.

83. Maccario M, Lustman LI. Paroxysmal nocturnal dystonia presenting as excessive daytime somnolence. Arch Neurol 1990;47:291.
84. Iliceto G, Thompson PD, Day L, et al. Diaphragmatic flutter, the moving umbilicus syndrome, and "belly dancer's" dyskinesia. Movement Disorders 1990;5:15.
85. Quinn NP. Multiple system atrophy—the nature of the beast. J Neurol Neurosurg Psychiatry 1990;53(suppl):78.
86. Bannister R, Gibson W, Michaels L, Oppenheimer DR. Laryngeal abductor paralysis in multiple system atrophy. Brain 1981;104:51.
87. Chokroverty S. The Assessment of Sleep Disturbance in Autonomic Failure. In R Bannister, CJ Mathias (eds), Autonomic Failure (3rd ed). Oxford, UK: Oxford Medical, 1992;442–461.
88. Munschauer FE, Loh L, Bannister R, Newsom-Davis J. Abnormal respiration and sudden death during sleep in multiple system atrophy with autonomic failure. Neurology 1990;40:677.
89. Apps MCP, Sheaff PC, Ingram DA, et al. Respiration and sleep in Parkinson's disease. J Neurol Neurosurg Psychiatry 1985;48:1240.
90. De Bruin VS, Machedo C, Howard RS, et al. Nocturnal and respiratory disturbance in Steele-Richardson-Olszewski syndrome (SROS). Postgrad Med J 1996;72:293.
91. Fish DR, Howard RS, Wiles CM, Symon L. Respiratory arrest: a complication of cerebellar ectopia in adults. J Neurol Neurosurg Psychiatry 1988;4:717.
92. Howard RS, Thorpe J, Barker R, et al. Respiratory insufficiency due to high anterior cervical cord infarction. J Neurol Neurosurg Psychiatry 1998;64:358.
93. Kidd D, Howard RS, Williams AJ, et al. Late functional deterioration following paralytic poliomyelitis. QJM 1997;90:189.
94. Howard RS, Wiles CM, Loh L. Respiratory complications and their management in motor neurone disease. Brain 1989;112:1155.
95. Ropper AH. Guillain-Barré syndrome: management of respiratory failure. Neurology 1985;35:1662.
96. Ng KKP, Howard RS, Fish DR, et al. The management and outcome of severe Guillain Barré syndrome. QJM 1995;88:243.
97. Zifko U, Chen R, Remtulla H, et al. Respiratory electrophysiological studies in Guillain-Barré syndrome. J Neurol Neurosurg Psychiatry 1996;60:191.
98. Hughes RAC, Bihari D. Acute neuromuscular respiratory paralysis. J Neurol Neurosurg Psychiatry 1993;56:334.
99. Mulvey DA, Aquilina RJ, Eliot MW, et al. Diaphragmatic dysfunction in neuralgic amyotrophy: an electrophysiologic examination of 16 patients presenting with dyspnea. Am Rev Respir Dis 1993;147:66.
100. Chalmers RM, Howard RS, Wiles CM, et al. Respiratory insufficiency in neuronopathic and neuropathic disorders. QJM 1996;89:469.
101. Efthimiou J, Butler J, Woodham C, et al. Phrenic nerve and diaphragm function following open heart surgery: a prospective study with and without topical hypothermia. QJM 1992;85:845.
102. Chroni E, Patel RL, Taub N, et al. A comprehensive electrophysiological evaluation of phrenic nerve injury related to open-heart surgery. Acta Neurol Scand 1995;91:255.
103. Mier Jedrzejowicz AK, Brophy C, Green M. Respiratory muscle function in myasthenia gravis. Am Rev Respir Dis 1988;138:867.
104. Nicolle MW, Stewart DJ, Remtulla H, et al. Lambert-Eaton myasthenic syndrome presenting with severe respiratory failure. Muscle Nerve 1996;19:1328.
105. Smith PEM, Calverley PMA, Edwards RHT, et al. Practical problems in the respiratory care of patients with muscular dystrophy. N Engl J Med 1987;316:1197.
106. Howard RS, Wiles CM, Hirsch NP, Spencer GT. Respiratory involvement in primary muscle disorders: assessment and management. QJM 1993;86:175.
107. Trend PStJ, Wiles CM, Spencer GT, et al. Acid maltase deficiency in adults. Brain 1985;108:845.
108. Howard RS, Russell S, Losseff N, et al. Mitochondrial disease in the intensive care unit. QJM 1995;88:197.
109. Dewberry RG, Schneider BF, Cale WF, Phillips LH II. Sarcoid myopathy presenting with diaphragm weakness. Muscle Nerve 1993;16:832.
110. Spalding JMK, Opie L. Artificial respiration with the Tunnicliffe breathing jacket. Lancet 1958;1:613.
111. Russell WR, Schuster E, Smith AC, Spalding JMK. Radcliffe respiration pumps. Lancet 1956;1:539.
112. Alba A, Kahn A, Lee N. Mouth intermittent positive pressure for sleep. Rehabil Gazette 1981;24:47.
113. Meecham Jones DJ, Braid GM, Wedzicha JA. Nasal masks for domiciliary positive pressure ventilation in restrictive and obstructive disorders. Thorax 1995;50:604.
114. Drinker PA, McKhann LF. The iron lung. First practical means of respiratory support. JAMA 1986;225:1476.

115. Eve FC. Activation of the inert diaphragm by a gravity method. Lancet 1932;2:995.
116. Schuster E, Fischer-Williams M. A rocking bed for poliomyelitis. Lancet 1953;2:1074.
117. Chalmers RM, Howard RS, Wiles CM, Spencer GT. Use of the rocking bed in the treatment of neurogenic respiratory insufficiency. QJM 1994;87:423.
118. Steljes DG, Kryger MH, Kirk BW, et al. Sleep in post-polio syndrome. Chest 1990;81:133.
119. Ardran GM, Kelleher WH, Kemp FH. Cineradiographic studies of glossopharyngeal breathing. Br J Radiol 1959;254:611.
120. Dail CW, Affeldt JE, Collier CR. Clinical aspects of glossopharyngeal breathing. JAMA 1955;158:445.
121. Feigelson CI, Dickinson DG, Talner NS, Wilson JL. Glossopharyngeal breathing as an aid to coughing mechanism in the patient with chronic poliomyelitis in a respirator. N Engl J Med 1956;254:611.
122. Raphael JC, Chevre S, Bouvet F. Randomised trial of preventative nasal ventilation in Duchenne muscular dystrophy. Lancet 1994;343:1600.
123. Ellis ER, Bye PTB, Bruderer JW, Sullivan CE. Treatment of respiratory failure during sleep in patients with neuromuscular disease. Am Rev Respir Dis 1987;135:148.
124. Shneerson JM. Is chronic respiratory failure in neuromuscular diseases worth treating? J Neurol Neurosurg Psychiatry 1996;61:1.
125. Khan Y, Heckmatt JZ. Obstructive apneas in Duchenne muscular dystrophy. Thorax 1994;49:157.
126. Hill NS. Noninvasive ventilation: does it work, for whom, and how? Am Rev Respir Dis 1993;147:1050.
127. Branthwaite MA. Mechanical ventilation at home. BMJ 1989;298:1409.
128. Branthwaite MA. Noninvasive and domiciliary ventilation: positive pressure techniques. Thorax 1991;46:209.
129. Loh L. Home ventilation. Anaesthesia 1983;38:621.
130. Sawicka EH, Loh L, Branthwaite MA. Domiciliary ventilatory support: an analysis of outcome. Thorax 1988;43:31.

12
Central Nervous System Infections

Mariko Kita, Daniel T. Laskowitz, and Dennis L. Kolson

BACTERIAL MENINGITIS

Bacterial meningitis is a life-threatening illness that can be treated if detected early. Meningitis and meningoencephalitis may be clinically indistinguishable, making recognition and empiric treatment of meningitis essential.

Incidence and Pathophysiology

In the United States, the annual rate of bacterial meningitis is 0.1–10.0 cases per 100,000, with a peak incidence between late fall and early spring. The microorganisms responsible for most cases of bacterial meningitis are listed in Table 12.1 [1].

The most common cause of bacterial meningitis in adults is *Streptococcus pneumoniae*. In children, *Haemophilus influenzae* is the most common cause, although effective vaccination against *H. influenzae* type b has altered the prevalence in children [2–4]. Table 12.2 outlines the age predilection of the various causal bacteria [5,6].

Bacterial meningitis occurs when invading pathogens overcome host defense mechanisms to reach the subarachnoid space. Bacterial replication is associated with release of proinflammatory cytokines and other cellular toxins that cause inflammation and recruitment of leukocytes into the subarachnoid space [2,3,7,8]. The most important determinant of pathogenicity is the bacterial capsule (*H. influenzae* type b, *Neisseria meningitidis, S. pneumoniae*). The nasopharynx is colonized by the organisms, and in individuals who lack neutralizing antibodies to block adhesion, infection proceeds via local invasion through the nasopharyngeal epithelium [9]. During the bacteremic phase, the organism adheres to the epithelium of the choroid plexus. This is quickly followed by meningeal infection and seeding of the subarachnoid space. *H. influenzae* infection, in particular, can result in ventriculitis with subsequent thrombosis of pial veins, cortical arterioles, and venous sinuses leading to the formation of subdural effusions [10].

Table 12.1   Bacterial prevalence in meningitis in adults

Pathogen	Prevalence (%)
Haemophilus influenzae	1–3
Streptococcus pneumoniae	30–50
Neisseria meningitidis	10–35
Staphylococci	5–15
Gram-negative bacilli	1–10
Group B streptococcus *(S. agalactiae)*	5
Listeria monocytogenes	5

Source: Adapted from KL Roos. Acute Bacterial Meningitis in Children and Adults. In WM Scheld (ed), Infections of the Central Nervous System. New York: Lippincott–Raven, 1997;335–409.

Table 12.2   Age susceptibility and empiric antibiotic choices for meningitis

Age range	Most common pathogen	Empiric antibiotic choice*
<1 mo	Group B streptococcus, *Listeria monocytogenes*, *Escherichia coli*	Ceftriaxone plus ampicillin Gentamicin plus ampicillin
1 mo to 5 yrs	*Haemophilus influenzae* type b (95% are type b, others a–f)	Ceftriaxone plus ampicillin Chloramphenicol plus ampicillin plus dexamethasone
5–29 yrs	*Neisseria meningitidis*	Ceftriaxone plus ampicillin plus dexamethasone
>29 yrs	*Streptococcus pneumoniae*	Ceftriaxone plus ampicillin plus dexamethasone

*Recommended antibiotic dosages as follows. Ampicillin: younger than 1 month old, 100–200 mg/kg/day intravenously (IV); children, 300–400 mg/kg/day; adults, 2 g IV every 6 hours. Ceftriaxone: 2 g IV every 12 hours; chloramphenicol: children, 100 mg/kg/day IV; adults, 0. 5 g every 6 hours IV or orally. Gentamicin: children, 5 mg/kg/day IV; adults, load 2 mg/kg, then 5 mg/kg/day. Dexamethasone: 0.15 mg/kg IV every 6 hours × 4 days, started within 30 minutes of antibiotics.
Source: Data are summarized from JP Sanford, DN Gilbert, MA Sande (eds). The Sanford Guide to Antimicrobial Therapy. Dallas: Antimicrobial Therapy, 1996;2–3, 109–116; and JD Wenger, CV Broome. Bacterial Meningitis: Epidemiology. In HP Lambert (ed), Infections of the Central Nervous System. Philadelphia: Decker, 1991;19.

Clinical Presentation

Typically, bacterial meningitis presents with headache, photophobia, and meningismus (80%); fever (85%); and malaise and vomiting. Kernig's sign (resistance to leg extension when examiner flexes the patient's thigh on his or her abdomen and passively extends his or her leg) and Brudzinski's sign (passive flexion of the patient's neck causing flexion of his or her knees and hips) are present in only 50% of cases in adults and thus are not reliable diagnostic tools [9]. Focal neurologic signs are not common, although cranial nerve deficits, especially the eighth, may be prominent in each of the three major bacterial meningitides [10–12]. *H. influenzae* can cause ventriculitis, and *H. influenzae* meningitis may present with acute mania [2] after a several-day prodrome of fever, otitis media, and pharyngitis [10]. Pneumococcal meningitis should be suspected in patients with defective splenic function (sickle cell disease, post-splenectomy) and previous head injury with or without skull fracture [11]. Meningococcemia is associated with a rapidly developing purpuric rash within hours of infection in 50% of patients [3]. The presence of this rash demands immediate institution of antibiotic therapy [3,12]. A purpuric rash may also be seen in *H. influenzae* and *S. pneumoniae* meningitis, although rarely [12]. Clinical syndromes of central nervous system (CNS) infection with *Listeria* are remarkably variable and include diffuse encephalitis (especially in renal transplant patients), abscesses in the hemispheres, thalamus and brain stem cerebritis with focal neurologic deficits, and brain stem encephalitis [13]. Neurologic symptoms may develop precipitously and often include asymmetric cranial nerve deficits, ataxia, hemiparesis, or hemisensory loss. The early diagnosis of *Listeria* rhomboencephalitis may be elusive as only one-half of the patients show evidence of meningeal irritation or change in mental status on initial presentation.

Diagnosis

Suspicion of bacterial meningitis requires immediate examination of the cerebrospinal fluid (CSF) by lumbar puncture in all cases except cardiovascular compromise in a neonate, increased intracranial pressure, and infection in the areas where the needle would transverse. Gram's stain is 90% sensitive for *S. pneumoniae* meningitis and somewhat less sensitive for *H. influenzae* and *N. meningitidis* [11]. For bacterial antigen detection in the CSF, latex agglutination kits have replaced the counterimmunoelectrophoresis techniques because they are generally more rapid, requiring less than an hour for results [14].

Typical CSF findings in acute bacterial meningitis include an opening pressure of 200–300 mm H_2O, white blood cell count (WBC) of $1,000–5,000 \times 10^6$/liter, 80% or greater neutrophils, protein level of 100–500 mg/dl, glucose level of 40 mg/dl or less, positive Gram's stain in 60–90% (highest for *S. pneumoniae*) of patients, and positive culture in 70–85% of patients [9]. In *Listeria* meningitis the CSF profile may appear benign, and approximately 25% of patients have fewer than 4 WBC/µl (mononuclear predominance) with a normal glucose, although protein is usually modestly elevated.

Brain imaging studies are generally normal. Occasionally, *H. influenzae* meningitis leads to the formation of subdural effusions [10]. Other exceptions include cases of global cerebral edema, abscess formation (see Epidural Abscess), or *Listeria* brain stem encephalitis. In the case of *Listeria* rhomboencephalitis, magnetic resonance imaging (MRI) is much more sensitive than computed tomography, which is unrevealing in 50% of cases [13]. Figure 12.1 demonstrates MRI findings in a case of *Listeria* brain stem encephalitis. The findings improved after treatment with ceftriaxone and ampicillin [15].

Complications

Untreated bacterial meningitis often results in death, in general because of increased intracranial pressure from cerebral edema. The edema may be vaso-

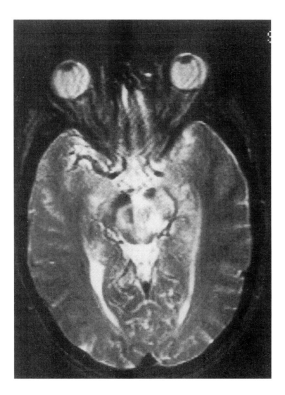

Figure 12.1   Listeria monocytogenes brain stem encephalitis. A 48-year-old man presented with a 12-day history of right facial numbness, weakness, diplopia, clumsiness, and a tendency to fall toward the right. Ten days later, this magnetic resonance image demonstrated high signal abnormality in the left cerebral peduncle and the dorsolateral aspect of the midbrain as shown. (Reprinted with permission from A Faidas, DL Shepard, J Lim, et al. Magnetic resonance imaging in listerial brain stem encephalitis. Clin Infect Dis 1993;16:187. Copyright © by University of Chicago Press.)

genic, caused by increased blood-brain barrier permeability, or cytotoxic, owing to lysis of cells by release of toxins from bacteria and polymorphonuclear leukocytes. Cerebral edema also results from obstructive hydrocephalus [6].

Treatment

Treatment of bacterial meningitis is intended to inhibit the replication of invading pathogens, prevent cerebral edema, and prevent the secondary effects of proinflammatory cytokines released within the subarachnoid space. Suspected meningitis in patients of all ages is treated empirically with third-generation cephalosporins, such as ceftriaxone, combined with ampicillin or amoxycillin for *Listeria* coverage (except in neonates up to 3 weeks of age) [9,16,17]. In neonates up to 3 weeks old, cefotaxime is preferred because of the effects of ceftriaxone on bilirubin metabolism in this age group [9]. Alternatively, ampicillin plus an aminoglycoside can be used in neonates [18]. For most cases of bacterial meningitis, the duration of treatment is 10–14 days, although 3 weeks is recommended for pneumococcal and *Listeria* infections [19].

Postoperative meningitis caused by coagulase-negative and positive stephylococis that are methicillin-sensitive can be treated with nafcillin or flucloxacillin. Methicillin-resistant infections should be treated with appropriate antibiotics when sensitivities are known (e.g., vancomycin) [17].

Dexamethasone has been recommended as adjunctive therapy for *H. influenzae* meningitis in children to decrease hearing loss from eighth nerve damage [7,10]. It is presumed to decrease proinflammatory effects of cytokines released in the subarachnoid space [7,20]. It may have some benefit for *N. meningitidis* encephalitis [21] and *S. pneumoniae* meningitis as well [22]. However, routine use of dexamethasone in acute bacterial meningitis remains controversial [23]. Dexamethasone is given at a dosage of 0.15 mg/kg every 6 hours for a total of 4 days and should be started immediately before or within 30 minutes of the institution of antibiotics [17].

Neurosurgical approaches are used for drainage of subdural empyemas and intraparenchymal abscesses and shunting of communicating hydrocephalus owing to impaired arachnoid villi reabsorption of CSF. Patients who are stuporous or comatose may benefit from intracranial pressure monitoring to maintain intracranial pressures at less than 20 mm Hg [8,9,24,25].

Increased intracranial pressure and seizures are two common and potentially life-threatening complications of bacterial meningitis and other CNS infections. Medical management of increased intracranial pressure should include

1. Elevation of the head of the bed to approximately 30 degrees.
2. Restriction of free water to 1,000 ml normal saline/m^2 body surface per day.
3. Hyperventilation to maintain P_{CO_2} at 25–30 cm H_2O.
4. Use of hyperosmolar agents, for example, mannitol, 0.25–0.50 g/kg intravenously (IV) every 4–8 hours as necessary. Steroids are not recommended in viral encephalitis.
5. (Optional) Placement of an intraventricular CSF pressure monitor can be used to keep intracranial pressure at less than 20–25 cm H_2O by drainage. This depends on the lack of clinical response to hyperosmolar agents and the severity of the mass effect as determined by neuroimaging studies.
6. Seizures can be managed by slow IV infusion of phenytoin (Dilantin) at a dose of 18 mg/kg in normal saline at a rate of less than 50 mg per minute in normal saline. Maintenance doses of approximately 300–400 mg per day are used to keep the serum level between 10 and 20 mg/ml. Alternatively, phenobarbital can be loaded at a dose of 10 mg/kg. Divided daily doses of approximately 60–120 mg are used to maintain serum levels at 20–40 mg/ml. It should be noted that this can depress the sensorium. Valproate syrup (250 mg/5 ml) can be administered via clamped rectal tube in a total volume of 30 ml with water, at a dosage of 250–500 mg every 6–8 hours to maintain blood levels of 50–100 mg/ml. This may lead to elevated blood ammonia levels and liver enzymes.

FUNGAL MENINGITIS

Incidence and Pathophysiology

The incidence of CNS fungal infections varies depending on the organism. However, the overall prevalence of life-threatening mycoses has increased as the population of immunocompromised hosts has grown. In this section, discussion is limited to infections of *Cryptococcus*, *Coccidioides*, *Candida*, and *Aspergillus*.

Cryptococcal meningoencephalitis is the most common fungal infection of the CNS. It is seen in 6–8% of all patients with acquired immunodeficiency syndrome (AIDS), and in 1994 more than 1,000 cases occurred in New York City alone [26]. Additional populations at risk include those with diabetes mellitus, a lymphoreticular malignancy, chronic renal failure, collagen vascular diseases, and organ transplants, or those receiving immunosuppressive therapy [27]. *Cryptococcus neoformans* is an encapsulated fungus and reproduces by budding. It is ubiquitous in nature and has been isolated from pigeon excrement, soil, fruits, vegetables, and dairy products [28]. *C. neoformans* presumably enters through the respiratory tract and disseminates hematogenously to the CNS. Within the CNS, *Cryptococcus* involves not only the meninges but also gray matter and basal ganglia. Histologically, lesions consist of cystic clusters of fungi surrounded by a large polysaccharide capsule with little inflammatory response. Grossly, the brain becomes swollen with the expanding foci of *Cryptococcus*. Leptomeninges are often thickened, and the subarachnoid is distended with a thick, gelatinous, white material that represents the exudative polysaccharide capsule.

Coccidioides immitis resides in the soils of the southwestern United States (southern California, Arizona, New Mexico, areas of Nevada, Utah, and southwestern Texas), northern Mexico, Pacific littoral foci, Central America (Guatemala, Honduras, and Nicaragua), and parts of Venezuela, Paraguay, Colombia, and Argentina [29–31]. In Tucson, Arizona, the incidence of coccidioidomycosis has been estimated to be 2.7%, but in the AIDS population, the infection rate is 10-fold higher [32]. In endemic regions, the prevalence of disseminated coccidioidomycosis is said to be equal to that of tuberculosis (TB) in the general population. The rate is even higher in certain subgroups with risk factors such as lymphoma, treatment with corticosteroids, and pregnancy [33].

C. immitis enters the body via the respiratory tract as an inhaled spore. At body temperature, spores are converted to tissue invasive forms. Approximately two-thirds of those infected are asymptomatic and acquire immunity [34], and an estimated 0.5% of all primary infections disseminate. Involvement of the CNS occurs primarily by hematogenous spread. *C. immitis* can invade the CNS, causing meningitis, and although this is usually preceded by a history of an obvious respiratory infection, it can occur without any evidence of prior systemic illness. It should be suspected in ill individuals who have traveled in endemic areas [35]. The basilar meninges are involved in 70–90% of cases of meningitis. Cerebral cortical sulci are also frequently involved, and cerebritis, cerebral infarction, and miliary granulomas can occur. Long-standing infections can manifest in foci of gliosis and infarction, resulting in clinically apparent neurologic signs.

Candida is part of the normal microbial flora. As such, infection can result from an alteration in host defenses or immunodeficiencies [36]. There are more than 150 species of *Candida*, but only 10 appear to be pathogenic in humans. *Candida albicans* is the most frequently isolated species in the CNS. It can colonize and locally invade mucocutaneous tissues. Gastrointestinal ulceration or cutaneous perforation with an IV needle or other instrument might be an inciting event, introducing *Candida* systemically. The CNS is involved in approximately 50% of disseminated cases. Once inside the CNS, *Candida* can infect parenchymal brain tissue and meninges, causing multiple abscesses, granulomas, or meningitis. Meningitis accounts for only 15% of *Candida* CNS disease.

Aspergillus typically enters the body via the respiratory tract. Invasion of the CNS then occurs either by direct extension or by hematogenous spread [37]. Disease may be confined to a particular organ system or become disseminated. Dissemination typically occurs in the immunocompromised host. In 60–70% of disseminated cases, evidence of CNS involvement exists [38].

Clinical Presentation

The clinical presentation of patients with CNS fungal infections may be similar to that seen with other causes of CNS infection. All of the aforementioned fungal organisms can produce a generalized meningitis or focal lesions. Fungal meningitis typically affects the basilar meninges. Focal fungal lesions include abscesses, granulomas, vasculitic lesions, and, rarely, mycotic aneurysms. *Cryptococcus*, *Coccidioides*, and *Candida* most often present with meningitis, and *Aspergillus* most frequently manifests with focal abscesses. In the immunocompetent host, fungal infections tend to take on a more indolent, chronic course, whereas in the immunocompromised individual, the course is more rapid.

Meningitis and meningoencephalitis are the most common forms of CNS cryptococcal infection. Headache, weakness, confusion, and seizures are typical presentations. Meningeal irritation is found in only approximately one-third of patients. Signs of encephalitis with agitation, irritability, change in personality, confusion, memory deficits, and psychosis may be seen in up to 45% of patients with meningitis [39]. In AIDS patients, the presentation may be nonspecific with minimal findings. Cryptococcal invasion may not be accompanied by fever.

Coccidioidomycosis infection of the CNS may not be recognized until the infection is well established and symptoms are severe. Thick proteinaceous exudates accumulate in the basal cisterns, producing increased intracranial pressure. This results in common findings of headache, fever, weakness, confusion, seizures, papilledema, visual changes, hyperreflexia, cerebellar ataxia, and multiple cranial neuropathies [31]. Nuchal rigidity may be present in up to one-third of the cases.

The clinical onset in *Candida* infections may be abrupt or subacute but is invariably associated with fever. Symptoms may include meningismus, focal neurologic signs, confusion, and lethargy. Papilledema has been recorded in 25–33% of cases [31]. CNS infections by *Aspergillus* can manifest as meningitis, meningoencephalitis, brain abscess (solitary or multiple), and granulomas [31]. Brain abscesses are most commonly found in the frontal and temporal lobes but are seen rarely in the occipital lobe or cerebellum. Frontal lobe lesions tend to be solitary, resulting from direct extension. Posterior lesions typically are a product of hematogenous spread to the posterior circulation and, hence, often result in multiple lesions [40].

Diagnosis

Because clinical presentation is relatively nonspecific, diagnosis of CNS fungal infection relies heavily on supportive laboratory data. Specifically, examination of the CSF is critical. Opening pressure may be normal or elevated. Hypoglycorrhachia is a hallmark feature although not invariably present. Generally, a modest leukocytosis is seen. Usually a lymphocytic predominance exists in the case of *C. neoformans*, but neutrophils may be present in varying numbers. In coccidioidomycosis and even cryptococcosis, neutrophilia may persist chroni-cally throughout the course of the disease [33], although there is usually a mono-cytic predominance in coccidioidomycosis. Peak CSF leukocytosis does not typically exceed 400–600/μl, except in coccidioidomycosis, in which counts can be greater than 3,000/μl. In AIDS patients, CSF cell counts may be normal in cryptococcal infection. In candidal meningitis, the pleocytosis demonstrates a neutrophilic predominance [27], and smears and cultures are often positive, but serodiagnostic testing is not reliable.

India ink smears may reveal encapsulated *C. neoformans* yeasts, and the overall diagnostic yield is approximately 50–75%. This increases to approximately 88% in the AIDS population [27]. The procedure remains useful for making a presumptive diagnosis, but positive stains must be confirmed by culture. Positive CSF culture provides the definitive diagnosis, but the yield varies according to organism. Large-volume samples (10–15 ml) and multiple samplings increase the yield. In general, *Cryptococcus* yield is fairly high. Untreated coccidioidomycosis, on the other hand, yields positive cultures in only 20–45%. Cases due to *Candida* are variably positive, and *Aspergillus* is rarely cultured.

Serodiagnostic tests can provide supplemental evidence of infection in *Cryptococcus* and *Coccidioides*. Latex agglutination testing is available for detecting the capsular antigen of *Cryptococcus*. Antigen is detected in either CSF or serum with reports of overall sensitivity and specificity nearing 100% [41]. Culture confirmation is recommended. For coccidioidomycosis, the most useful test available remains complement-fixing antibody (CFA) titer, detecting immunoglobulin (Ig) G antibody in the CSF. Although serum CFA titers greater than 1:32–1:64 suggest disseminated disease, those with coccidioidal meningitis without involvement of other organ systems may have low serum CFA titers. CSF titers seem to parallel the course of the disease and can be used for diagnosis and assessment of treatment [29]. Fewer than 5% of CSF titers have negative results. Typically, titers range between 1:2 and 1:256.

Computed tomographic (CT) scans of the brain are useful in identifying mass lesion and also in detecting hydrocephalus. Contrast-enhanced studies are recommended. Chest radiographs are also useful to identify concomitant pulmonary involvement.

Complications

The most common complication of fungal meningitis is hydrocephalus. This occurs in 5–15% of patients with cryptococcal meningitis and is associated with failed treatment and death [42]. In meningeal coccidioidomycosis, hydrocephalus occurs in 20–50% of patients and is associated with a 50–70% mortality. Variable rates have been reported with candidiasis and aspergillosis. Shunting is almost invariably required but is not without complication and may be associated with shunt infection and ventriculitis. Residual deficits are common in those who survive fungal meningitis.

Prognostic factors for CNS cryptococcal infection have been determined. These include elevated opening pressure, initial positive CSF india ink smear, initial CSF WBC count less than 20/μl, culture of *C. neoformans* from any extraneural site, initial CSF titer greater than or equal to 1:32, and coexistence of hematologic malignancy or baseline corticosteroid use [43,44]. In the AIDS population, poor prognostic signs include high CSF antigen titers (>1:10,000), altered mental status, and abnormal head CT scan [45].

Relapses of coccidioidomycosis are quite common. As such, lifelong therapy may be required. In addition to hydrocephalus, poor outcome is associated with underlying illness and nonwhite race. In candidal meningitis, increased mortality has been linked to a delay of diagnosis greater than 2 weeks after onset of symptoms, CSF glucose less than 35 mg/dl, development of increased intracranial pressure, and presence of focal neurologic deficits.

Treatment

In general, amphotericin B is the treatment of choice for the aforementioned mycoses. Treatment of meningeal coccidioidomycosis requires both IV (0.4–0.6 mg/kg/day) and intrathecal amphotericin for a total dose of at least 1 g. The usual intrathecal dosage is 0.5 mg three times a week for a total dose of 20–25 mg, but higher doses can be used if they are combined with corticosteroids [27]. Intrathecal treatment can be administered via lumbar, cisternal, or ventricular routes but is almost always associated with an arachnoiditis within the first month of therapy, often severe enough to cause paralysis. The optimal duration of intrathecal therapy remains unclear, and many continue to receive weekly injections. Patients are considered cured only after they have survived without relapse for more than 5–8 years. Because of the toxicities associated with amphotericin B, the azole antifungals are being studied. In the meantime, amphotericin B remains the mainstay of therapy.

In contrast, cryptococcal meningitis can be cured by IV amphotericin B (0.4–0.6 mg/kg/day). Amphotericin B and flucytosine are synergistic in vitro, however, and combination therapy has been examined. In one study, IV amphotericin at 0.3 mg/kg per day in combination with oral flucytosine (37.5 mg/kg every 6 hours) for 6 weeks produced fewer failures or relapses with less nephrotoxicity and more rapid clearing of CSF than a 10-week course of IV amphotericin at 0.4 mg/kg per day. The proportion of deaths in each group was equal [46]. In another study, combination therapy was used for 4 versus 6 weeks. Four-week therapy appeared to be effective in a certain subgroup: those who had no underlying illnesses, no neurologic complications, no immunosuppressive therapy, mild cryptococcal infection (serum titer <1:32), pretreatment CSF WBC greater than 20/µl, and who at 4 weeks had a negative CSF india ink smear as well as CSF titer less than 1:8 [47]. However, patients who received combination therapy were found to have a high rate (38%) of primarily hematologic flucytosine-related toxicity. It is important to monitor hematologic profiles during therapy, therefore, and the decision to use combined versus amphotericin B therapy alone must be weighed carefully in each case. When only amphotericin B is used, treatment is initiated at 0.6 mg/kg per day until weekly CSF cultures are negative, antigen titers are less than 1:8, and CSF glucose is normal. Total doses of 2–3 g are typically necessary.

Treatment in the AIDS population should be considered separately. Flucytosine doses must usually be reduced acutely in the treatment of AIDS patients. Relapses occur more frequently in this group, suggesting the need for more chronic suppressive therapy. Amphotericin B, ketoconazole, and fluconazole have been studied, and data indicate that fluconazole (200 mg/day) is the antifungal drug of choice for the prevention of relapses of cryptococcal meningitis in AIDS patients [48,49].

In the case of *Aspergillus*, higher doses of amphotericin are necessary, ranging up to 1.0–1.5 mg/kg per day. For *Candida*, amphotericin B (0.6 mg/kg/day) can be used with or without flucytosine [50,51]. The addition of flucytosine can improve outcome, especially in newborns [52].

BACTERIAL BRAIN ABSCESSES

Incidence and Pathophysiology

Brain abscesses occur with a frequency of 1.1 per 100,000 in the United States, and they can form intraparenchymally or as subdural or epidural empyemas [53]. Most commonly (50% of cases), organisms enter the CNS through the sinuses and ears, but they can also come in via hematogenous spread (20% of the time) from the mouth, lung, skin, gastrointestinal tract, and heart. Penetrating injuries of the skull account for 10% of brain abscesses [53]. The location of the abscess corresponds to the route of CNS entry. For example, the frontal lobes are seeded via the frontal, ethmoid, and sphenoid sinuses; the temporal lobes by the sphenoid and maxillary sinuses; and the cerebellum via the mastoid air cells. Epidural abscesses are more likely to form from mastoid infection, and the dura may provide an effective barrier that walls off the infection. Subdural and parenchymal abscesses can result from sinus infection, hematogenous seeding, traumatic injury, and direct infection through the cribriform plate.

The microorganisms that form most brain abscesses include aerobic and anaerobic bacteria, *Mycobacterium tuberculosis*, fungi, and parasites, including *Echinococcus*, *Toxoplasma*, and *Taenia solium*. Forty percent of brain abscesses contain streptococci (including anaerobes), and 30% contain *Bacteroides* in addition to aerobes [53]. Abscesses derived from infection within the ear usually contain gram-negative organisms, especially *Proteus*, whereas sinus infections lead to *Streptococcus* and *Pneumococcus* abscesses. Penetrating skull injuries often result in *Staphylococcus pyogenes* abscesses, while hematogenously seeded abscesses contain mixed flora. Predisposing factors for brain abscess include immunosuppression, congenital heart disease, or pulmonary arteriovenous malformations with right-to-left shunt.

Clinical Presentation

The clinical presentation of brain abscesses is nonspecific and insidious. The most common symptoms and signs include exertional headaches (50%), altered mental status (40%), fever (40%), seizures (33%), and meningismus (20%) [54]. Sinus pain or stroke syndromes secondary to cortical thrombophlebitis and ischemic infarction of the brain are sometimes seen [54]. A 1994 series of 44 infants and children with brain abscesses [55] showed the following presenting signs: papilledema (45%), hemiparesis (34%), coma (34%), cranial nerve palsies (27%), and nuchal rigidity (17%).

Diagnosis

Brain abscesses are generally diagnosed with either contrasted head CT scan or MRI scans. In bacterial brain abscesses, one typically sees a high signal ring on T1-weighted images that represents enhancement of the capsule of the abscess [57] (Figure 12.2). This capsular rim, 1–3 mm thick, is the cardinal feature of abscesses, differentiating them from tumors and granulomas, and is thought to result from increased capillary permeability and inflammation around the abscess as well as increased vascularity [53,56]. There may also be surrounding edema, which contributes to mass effect. Abscesses due to tuberculomas or fungus may appear as hypodense areas demonstrating either homogenous enhancement or thick enhancing rims with central cavities (reviewed in reference 53). Although CT scanning and MRI appear equally suitable for detection of abscesses, CT scanning is preferable for detection of subdural empyemas [56], as demonstrated in Figure 12.3 along the falx [58].

Complications

The mortality for abscesses is approximately 10%, but this depends on multiple factors, including patient age and time to diagnosis [53]. Strokes caused by abscess can result from cortical thrombophlebitis, especially after subdural empyema but also with intraparenchymal abscesses. Rupture of an abscess into a ventricle or subarachnoid space can result in meningitis and fatal ventriculitis. Increased intracranial pressure from mass effect is another cause of death [54].

Treatment

The treatment of choice for abscesses is drainage of pus by aspiration through a burr hole or open craniotomy with CT or ultrasound guidance [59]. All abscesses should be cultured for aerobes, anaerobes, fungus, and *M. tuberculosis*, but it is important to note that 20% of abscesses are "sterile," either as a result of previous antibiotic treatment or because of the fastidious growth requirements of some organisms [53]. Recommended antibiotic coverage pending culture results includes a combination of penicillin (4 million units IV every 6 hours) and metronidazole (0.5 g every 8 hours) (Table 12.3). In the case of traumatic brain injury, a penicillinase-resistant penicillin (such as flucloxacillin, nafcillin, oxacillin, cloxacillin, or dicloxacillin) is added. A third-generation cephalosporin, such as cefotaxime, should also be used. For otogenic-derived abscesses, a combination of cefotaxime and metronidazole has been used [17]. Both have good CNS penetration [60] and may provide an acceptable alternative for patients with penicillin allergies.

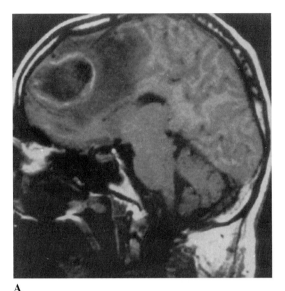

A

Figure 12.2 Magnetic resonance imaging of brain abscesses. **A.** Unenhanced T1-weighted sagittal image demonstrating frontal lobe high-intensity ring with low intensity surrounding the streptococcal abscess. **B.** T2-weighted coronal image revealing surrounding vasogenic edema. **C.** T1-weighted image showing ring enhancement with nodular inner face and smoother outer face, characteristic of abscesses (*arrows*). **D.** Multiple peptostreptococcal abscesses. (Reprinted with permission from RJ Farrell. Neuroradiology: The Requisites. In RI Grossman, DM Yousem [eds], Infectious and Noninfectious Inflammatory Diseases of the Brain. St. Louis: Mosby–Year Book, 1994;179.)

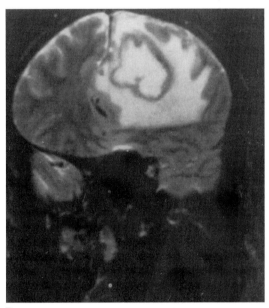

B

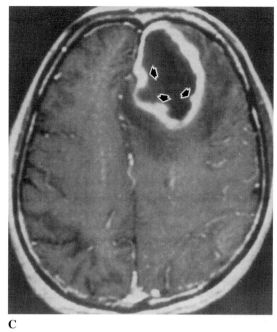

C

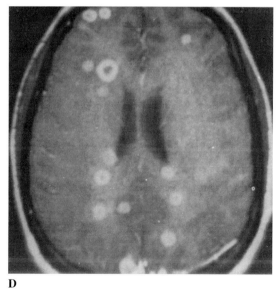

D

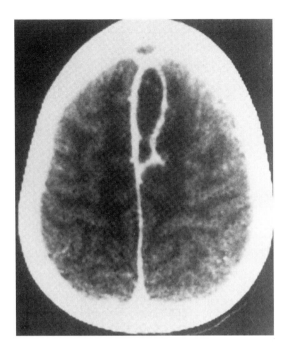

Figure 12.3   Contrast-enhanced computed tomographic scan of a subdural empyema shows a low-attenuation collection in the extra-axial space within the interhemispheric fissure. The morphologic features on the scan are similar to those of brain abscesses on magnetic resonance imaging (see Figure 12.2A). (Reprinted with permission from CA Jungreis, RI Grossman. Intracranial Infections and Inflammatory Diseases. In RE Latchaw [ed], MRI and CT Imaging of the Head, Neck, and Spine [2nd ed]. St. Louis: Mosby–Year Book, 1991;307.)

Table 12.3   Empiric treatment for brain abscesses

Modifying circumstances	Etiologies	Regimen
Otogenic (temporal, parietal, cerebellar) or unknown	*Streptococcus viridans*, anaerobic *Streptococcus*, *Bacteroides*, Enterobacteriaceae	Penicillin, 4 million units every 6 hrs, plus metronidazole plus cephalosporin (third generation)
Primary paranasal sinuses (frontal)	*Anaerobes*, *Streptococcus* spp., *Streptococcus - pneumoniae*, *Haemophilus influenzae*	Penicillin, 4 million units every 6 hrs, plus metronidazole
Young adult	*Staphylococcus aureus*	Penicillinase-resistant penicillin plus metronidazole
Postsurgical, traumatic	*S. aureus*, Enterobacteriaceae	Penicillinase-resistant penicillin plus cephalosporin (third generation) plus rifampin
Human immunodeficiency virus type 1 infected (acquired immunodeficiency syndrome)	*Toxoplasma gondii*	Pyrimethamine sulfadiazine or clindamycin

Source: Data summarized from JP Sanford, DN Gilbert, MA Sande (eds), The Sanford Guide to Antimicrobial Therapy. Dallas: Antimicrobial Therapy, 1996.

SPINAL EPIDURAL ABSCESS

Incidence and Pathophysiology

Spinal epidural abscesses often demonstrate nonspecific clinical findings, but nonetheless are highly dangerous if not treated promptly. Although it can be seen at any age, epidural abscess formation occurs most commonly in the fifth decade of life and is distinctly uncommon in children [61]. The epidural space is seeded hematogenously in 25–50% of cases and may be associated with IV drug use and infections involving the skin, oral cavity, urinary tract, or upper respiratory tract [62,63]. The epidural space may also be seeded during surgery or by vertebral osteomyelitis, paraspinal abscess, or penetrating trauma, or, rarely, after lumbar puncture or epidural anesthesia [64,65]. High-risk patients include elderly, immunocompromised, and dialysis patients, and increasing prevalence rates may reflect an aging population and high incidence of IV drug use [61].

In descending order of frequency, epidural abscesses occur in the thoracic, lumbar, and cervical spine. Infection usually tracks along the dorsal epidural space, because the dura of the ventral aspect of the spinal cord is tightly adherent to the vertebral bodies. However, the ventral epidural space may be involved in the cervical or lumbar cord, where the epidural space is widest, or when subarachnoid infection is present [62].

Clinical Presentation

Four stages of clinical signs or symptoms of epidural abscess are described [66]. Stage I is characterized by local back tenderness, fever, and leukocytosis; this is followed by stage II, which includes radicular pain, long tract signs, segmental reflex loss, nuchal rigidity, and headache. Stage III expresses progressive weakness, bowel or bladder dysfunction, and an ascending sensory level that heralds spinal cord compression. Stage IV manifests as progressive spinal cord compression with weakness and precipitous deterioration to paralysis within hours [61]. This can result from either direct compression of the spinal cord or secondary ischemia caused by venous inflammation and thrombosis.

Acute epidural abscesses (usually defined as having a symptom duration of less than 2 weeks) are most often caused by hematogenous seeding and are more apt to be associated with acute signs of systemic infection, such as fever, chills, and leukocytosis. Chronic abscesses are more likely to arise from pre-existing osteomyelitis or extension of adjacent infection [62]. A high index of suspicion is necessary in aged or immunocompromised patients with unexplained back pain [62].

Many other disease processes can mimic the symptoms of epidural abscess (Table 12.4), including disk herniation, tumors (lymphoma and metastatic prostate, lung, or breast cancer) with vertebral collapse, and progressive myelopathy. In addition, vertebral osteomyelitis progresses to chronic epidural abscess in 20% of patients [62]. Other conditions that mimic epidural abscess include transverse myelitis, epidural hematoma, psoas abscess, or intra-abdominal processes such as pyelonephritis, pancreatitis, or peptic ulcers [62]. In chronic steroid users, epidural lipomatosis can result in radicular pain and subacute myelopathy.

Table 12.4 Differential diagnosis of epidural abscess

Differential diagnosis	Associated signs, symptoms, and history	Ancillary diagnostic tests
Metastatic disease	History of lung, breast, or prostate cancer or lymphoma	Magnetic resonance imaging, plain films, cerebrospinal fluid for cytology
Intrinsic tumor or syrinx	Subacute progression of dull, poorly localized back pain over weeks or months; multiple segments often involved	Magnetic resonance imaging
	Suspended, disassociated sensory level over arms and trunk may be present	
Transverse myelitis	History of multiple sclerosis or optic neuritis; recent viral infection	Cerebrospinal fluid may show mild pleocytosis, oligoclonal bands; magnetic resonance evidence of demyelinating lesions in brain or spinal cord
Abdominal, retroperitoneal infection	History of genitourinary, pelvic infection; elevated amylase, lipase	Leukocytosis, abdominal/ spine imaging
Epidural hematoma	Acute onset of pain; myelopathic symptoms in the setting of bleeding diathesis; anticoagulation; trauma	Magnetic resonance; consider angiography if arteriovenous malformation suspected
Ischemia	Acute onset of anterior cord syndrome (loss of pain and temperature sensation, paralysis with preservation of vibration, proprioception); vascular risk factors (smoking, diabetes, peripheral vascular disease)	Absence of structural lesion on magnetic resonance imaging (may be high signal within the spinal cord)

Source: Reprinted with permission from DL Kolson, D Laskowitz. Infections and Parasitic Emergencies of the Central Nervous System. In J Cruz (ed), Neurologic and Neurosurgical Emergencies. Philadelphia: Saunders, 1998;57.

Diagnosis

Laboratory findings are rarely helpful. Elevated erythrocyte sedimentation rate and leukocytosis are inconsistent, although blood cultures are positive in two-thirds of cases and have a high correlation with organisms cultured at surgical exploration [61]. *Staphylococcus aureus* is the most common pathogen, and staphylococcal bacteremia in the setting of unexplained back pain should raise the index of suspicion for epidural abscess [67]. *Streptococcus* species are the second most common pathogens. IV drug use can increase the risk of gram-negative epidural abscess [63,68]. The possibility of atypical pathogens, including *Aspergillus*, should be considered in immunocompromised or transplant patients [69].

Lumbar puncture is not routinely performed owing to the risk of seeding the subarachnoid space. CSF glucose is usually normal, and the protein is markedly elevated, especially if complete spinal block is present. A mild pleocytosis of polymorphonuclear and mononuclear cells is commonly seen. Although chronic epidurals may have fewer than 40 cells/µl, a completely normal CSF formulation is distinctly unusual and should suggest an alternative diagnosis [70].

MRI with contrast enhancement is the initial diagnostic procedure of choice in patients suspected of having an epidural abscess [71], although myelography with spinal CT scan is acceptable when MRI is not available. Typical epidural abscess appearance on MRI is demonstrated in Figures 12.4 and 12.5 [72,73]. A typical enhancing epidural abscess in the cervical spine is demonstrated in Figure 12.4. MRI can also identify associated osteomyelitis, which may be detected on plain spinal x-rays and most other lesions that can cause a syndrome of subacute spinal cord compression. Occasionally, MRI is nondiagnostic, especially in the setting of coexistent meningitis. Radionucleotide studies rarely provide additional useful information.

Treatment

Surgical drainage and decompression represent a crucial step in the management of nontuberculous epidural abscess, and progressive neurologic deterioration mandates emergent surgical intervention. IV antibiotics that provide adequate antistaphylococcal coverage should be administered immediately. Concurrent administration of glucocorticoids in the setting of progressive neurologic deficit remains controversial, and fear of exacerbating infection remains at least a theoretic concern, although this complication has not been well documented in the setting of epidural abscess. The optimal length of treatment has not been well established. Because osteomyelitis is present in up to one-half of patients with chronic epidural abscess and 15% of patients with acute infections, however, it should be treated with an extended course (≥3 weeks) of antibiotics [5,74]. Human immunodeficiency virus type 1 (HIV-1)–associated cases may also not respond adequately to standard treatment and may require an even longer course of antibiotic therapy [5,75].

Neurologic outcome is directly related to the patient's neurologic status at the time of surgical intervention [61]. In general, patients with abscess that involves the anterior paraspinal space tend to have more complete recovery. Overall, approximately one-half of patients have complete recovery, one-fourth are left with significant neurologic deficit, and one-tenth remain paralyzed [61]. Mortality ranges from 14% to 32% in different series [61–63].

CENTRAL NERVOUS SYSTEM TUBERCULOSIS

Incidence and Pathophysiology

CNS TB is uncommon in the United States but is increasing in prevalence because of immigration from endemic areas (India, Saudi Arabia, Mexico, Korea) and the increasing incidence of AIDS. Some reports suggest that up to 18% of AIDS patients in endemic areas may have CNS TB [17]. Intracranial tuberculo-

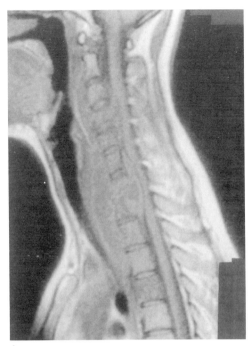

A

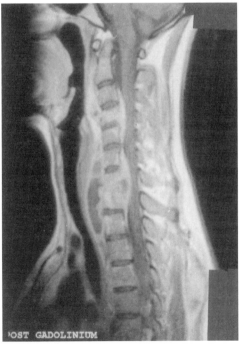

B

Figure 12.4   Magnetic resonance imaging of epidural abscesses. These are cervical cord magnetic resonance images in a 20-year-old woman presenting with gradual onset of pain and stiffness in the neck and paresthesiae in the left arm. **A.** T1-weighted sagittal image of cervical cord before contrast. **B.** Postcontrast image revealing an irregularly enhancing anterior spinal mass causing cord compression associated with bone and disk abnormalities. Note also the presence of a mass in the posterior soft tissues at the upper thoracic level. (Reprinted with permission from IM Lang, DG Hughes, JPR Jenkins, et al. MRI imaging appearances of cervical epidural abscess. Clin Radiol 1995;50:469.)

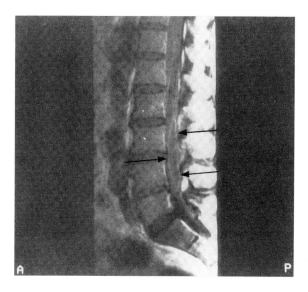

Figure 12.5 Magnetic resonance imaging of lumbosacral epidural abscess. This is a postcontrast T1-weighted sagittal image of the lumbosacral spine of a 64-year-old man taken 3 days after he received an epidural anesthetic procedure for angioplasty of the femoral arteries. The abscess is apparent in the dorsal epidural space and demonstrates a thin margin of high signal enhancement at its periphery (*arrows*). (A = anterior; P = posterior.) (Reprinted with permission from AC Mamourian, CA Dickman, BP Drayer, et al. Spinal epidural abscess: three cases following spinal epidural injection demonstrated by magnetic resonance imaging. Anesthesiology 1994;78:206.)

mas develop in 10–20% of cases of tuberculous meningitis and account for up to 20% of intracranial mass lesions in some developing countries [76]. They usually resolve with antituberculous therapy alone [76]. They can sometimes develop or increase in size despite such therapy, however, usually within 3 months, and may require neurosurgical intervention or adjunctive steroid therapy. TB meningitis is seen in 0.5% of all cases of TB.

Clinical Presentation

M. tuberculosis initially seeds the CNS via the bloodstream and forms subpial tuberculomas in the brain and spinal cord. These organisms then seed the CSF with resultant meningitis (especially at the sylvian fissure and basal cisterns) and can result in vascular occlusion at the base of the brain due to mononuclear infiltration of vessel walls. The typical clinical course involves a 2-week history of prodromal malaise, nausea, vomiting, and headache accompanied by a low-grade fever (<39°C) in 80% of cases. This is followed by neck stiffness and eventually hydrocephalus, cranial nerve palsies (one-third of patients; especially the third, fourth, sixth, and eighth nerves), and papilledema [77]. Other associated neurologic findings may include cord compression (Pott's disease), involuntary move-

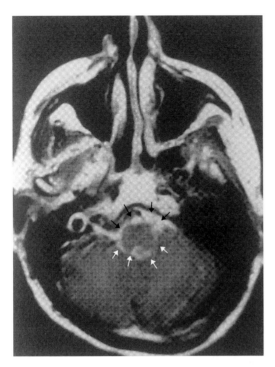

Figure 12.6   T1-weighted magnetic resonance image of tuberculous meningitis shows uniformly enhancing basilar meninges (*arrows*). (Reprinted with permission from RJ Farrell. Neuroradiology: The Requisites. In RI Grossman, DM Yousem [eds], Infectious and Noninfectious Inflammatory Diseases of the Brain. St. Louis: Mosby–Year Book, 1994;189.)

ments (approximately 13% of childhood TB cases), and, rarely, spinal cord infiltration resulting in polyradiculopathies [77]. Tuberculous meningitis often presents with multiple cranial nerve deficits because of a predilection for the basilar meninges, and it may have an insidious clinical course [77]. In cases of suspected tuberculous meningitis, one must be alert to the possible presence of tuberculomas of the brain and spinal cord [78,79] (Figures 12.6–12.9). Clinical stages of CNS TB are defined by neurologic presentation: stage I: neurologically normal; stage II: altered mental status with or without cranial nerve palsies; stage III: stupor or coma [77].

Diagnosis

Laboratory diagnosis of CNS TB depends on CSF examination [77], usually accompanied by brain imaging, and it is important to note that only approximately 50% of patients have pulmonary TB. CSF opening pressure is usually increased (40–600 mm Hg) with an increased WBC of less than 500/µl in 88% of cases. Lymphocytes predominate and may persist for months, although polymorphonuclear leukocytes predominate in the first 10 days in up to 17% of patients. CSF protein levels average 2.6 g/liter (range 0.16–41.60 g/liter), although, when examined by cisternal puncture, the protein is usually one-half to one-fourth the value obtained by lumbar puncture. Glucose levels may be low, as in bacterial meningitis [80].

Figure 12.7 Multiple intracranial tuberculomas in a 40-year-old man who was seropositive for human immunodeficiency virus. **A.** Axial contrast-enhanced, T1-weighted magnetic resonance image reveals enhancing lesions within the right temporal lobe and both cerebellar hemispheres. **B.** Axial T2-weighted magnetic resonance image reveals multiple lesions with isointense central core surrounded by a high-intensity rim. (Reprinted with permission from F Kioumehr, MR Dadsetan, SA Rooholamini, et al. Central nervous system tuberculosis: MRI. Neuroradiology 1994;36:95.)

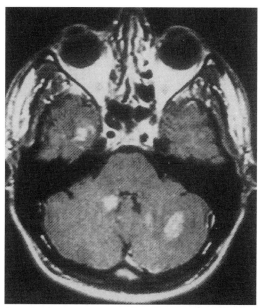

A

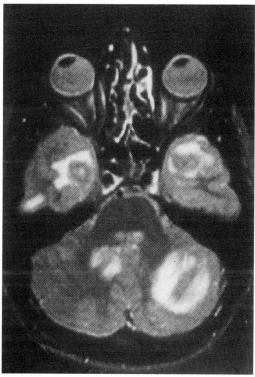

B

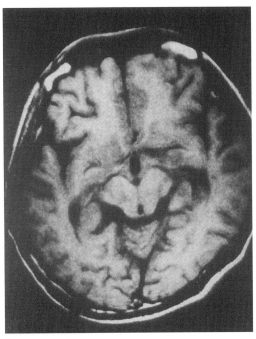

A

Figure 12.8   Multiple intracranial tuberculomas in a 30-year-old man with miliary tuberculosis and sudden onset of fever and leg weakness. **A.** Axial T1-weighted magnetic resonance image with isointense lesions within the brain that were visualized on T2-weighted images (**B**). **B.** Axial T2-weighted image reveals multiple lesions within the cerebral hemispheres and brain stem. **C.** Contrast-enhanced T1-weighted image reveals enhancement of the nodules. (Reprinted with permission from W-C Shen, T-Y Cheng, S-K Lee, et al. Disseminated tuberculomas in spinal cord and brain demonstrated by MRI with gadolinium-DPTA. Neuroradiology 1993;35:214.)

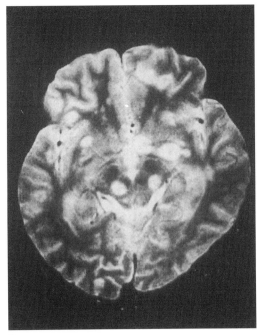

B

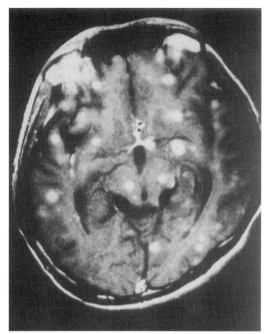

C

The acid-fast bacillus smear is essential for rapid diagnosis. It is diagnostic (positive), on average, in approximately 35% of cases at initial lumbar puncture and is positive in up to 80% of cases examined by three successive lumbar punctures, emphasizing the need for repeated examinations in suspected cases [77]. CSF cultures require prolonged incubation and are positive in 3–6 months in approximately 35% of cases even after 4 weeks of antibiotic treatment. Newer rapid techniques of latex agglutination and CSF antigen enzyme-linked immunosorbent assay (ELISA) generally are not readily available.

In CNS TB, CT scans show basilar meningeal enhancement in up to 50% of cases [17], and MRI imaging can increase this yield [17,81] (see Figure 12.6). The development of intracranial tuberculomas may be heralded by clinical deterioration 2–18 months after the start of chemotherapy [76]. It is thought to be due to a Herxheimer-like reaction [77]. Intraparenchymal tuberculomas may show low signal intensity on T2-weighted images, and nearly all show ring or nodular enhancement [81] (see Figure 12.7). Although tuberculous meningitis cannot be differentiated from other meningitides by MRI, the characteristic T2 shortening of intraparenchymal tuberculomas is not found on most other space-occupying lesions [81] (see Figure 12.7B). Immature tuberculomas may appear as scattered areas of varied intensity (see Figure 12.8), while mature tuberculomas may be seen as space-occupying lesions with a central area of low signal and surrounding edema [82] (see Figure 12.7). Calcification is rare, and approximately one-third of tuberculomas are multiple

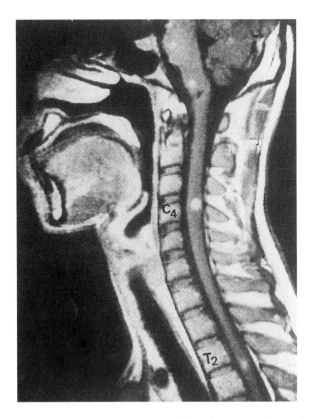

Figure 12.9   Intramedullary cervical cord tuberculoma in same patient as in Figure 12.8. Contrast-enhanced, T1-weighted magnetic resonance image reveals enhancing tuberculoma in cervical (C4) cord. (Reprinted with permission from W-C Shen, T-Y Cheng, S-K Lee, et al. Disseminated tuberculomas in spinal cord and brain demonstrated by MRI with gadolinium-DPTA. Neuroradiology 1993;35:214.)

[83]. As many as one-half attach to the dura and resemble meningiomas. Intramedullary spinal cord tuberculomas are very rare, accounting for approximately 1–5% of all CNS tuberculomas. They may appear primarily as single lesions with hyperintense T2 signals and marked gadolinium enhancement [79] (see Figure 12.9). Most intramedullary cord tuberculomas resolve with adequate chemotherapy [79,84].

The development of symptoms of increased intracranial pressure, seizures, or focal neurologic signs in treated cases of CNS TB should raise suspicion for paroxysmal enlargement of intracranial tuberculomas [76,85]. Suspicious lesions on CT or MRI scans require biopsy for definitive diagnosis in view of high false-positive radiographic findings that can mimic gliomas, cysticercosis, fungal granulomas, and metastases [82]. The positive predictive value for CT scan diagnosis is only approximately 33% [82,86].

Table 12.5   Tuberculosis therapy for adults and children

Drug	Daily dose	
	Adults	*Children*
Isoniazid	5 mg/kg PO or IM	10–20 mg/kg PO or IM
Rifampin	10 mg/kg PO or IV	10–20 mg/kg PO or IV
Pyrazinamide	15–30 mg/kg PO	15–30 mg/kg PO
Ethambutol	15–25 mg/kg PO	15–25 mg/kg PO
Streptomycin	15 mg/kg IM	20–40 mg/kg IM

Source: Adapted from LC Preheim. Tuberculosis and Other Mycobacterial Infections. In RW Carlson, MA Geheb (eds), Principles and Practice of Medical Intensive Care. Philadelphia: Saunders, 1993;425.

Treatment

The currently recommended regimen for TB in children and adults is a combination of isoniazid, rifampin, and pyrazinamide (Table 12.5), and duration of therapy should be at least 6 months or longer, depending on isolate sensitivity and clinical response [87]. In tuberculous meningitis, dexamethasone improves outcome in patients who present in stupor or with intracranial tuberculomas [77]. Tuberculomas in general are responsive to medical treatment for TB.

In cases in which clinical deterioration (to stage III) or increase in lesion size, or both, is demonstrated, corticosteroids are recommended (dexamethasone, 0.2–0.4 mg/kg every 6 hours) in addition to continued anti-TB medications for up to 6 months [76]. Surgical intervention should be considered for patients in whom this medical regimen fails.

VIRAL ENCEPHALITIS

Incidence and Pathophysiology

Of all cases of infectious encephalitis in the United States reported to the Centers for Disease Control and Prevention in 1977, 72.9% were of undetermined etiology, 10.7% were associated with arboviruses, 5.9% with exanthem viruses, 3.3% with mumps, and 7.3% with other viruses [88]. Viral encephalitis most commonly involves the cerebral hemispheres but may preferentially affect the brain stem instead. Most primary forms of encephalitis are caused by viruses, with which direct cellular damage is less commonly significant than is delayed hypersensitivity, because most viruses are recognized as foreign to their host and in many cases result in antibody formation. Clinical manifestations are diverse in severity, onset, and progression but generally share the features of fever, headache, and malaise followed by alteration of mentation. Although the diagnosis always requires a high degree of clinical suspicion, a careful history, including seasonal predominance and geography, and neurologic examination along with appropriate diagnostic tests can often identify the specific etiologic agent and suggest, in some cases, specific treatment.

Clinical Presentation

Fever, headache, neck stiffness, and altered sensorium are nearly universal, although nonspecific. In such a clinical setting, focal neurologic signs, such as aphasia, focal seizures, and cranial nerve deficits, strongly indicate infectious encephalitis and can even suggest specific viral agents. Evaluation must take into account geographic and seasonal considerations (summertime arboviruses and parainfections) and requires CSF examination as well as appropriate specific serum or CSF antibody titers (usually IgM), or both [89]. Virus isolation is possible in only a few cases.

Increased intracranial pressure is indicated by absence of spontaneous IV pulsations in the optic disk and often precedes papilledema and diffuse cerebral edema. Such findings are common in herpes simplex encephalitis (HSE), as is facial hemiparesis (seventh cranial nerve). Cutaneous vesicles in the distribution of the trigeminal nerve, especially V-1, or in the ear canal suggest varicella-zoster (zoster ophthalmicus or Ramsay Hunt syndrome, respectively). Multiple cranial nerve palsies can be seen with varicella-zoster. Hemiparesis can be seen in both herpes simplex and varicella.

Herpes Simplex Encephalitis

Epidemiology

Encephalitis infection due to herpes simplex virus type I is the most commonly occurring sporadic viral encephalitis in adults, accounting for 2–10% of all cases of encephalitis [9]. No seasonal or geographic predominance and no gender predilection exists. Only one-third of cases are preceded by a history of gingivostomatitis [91]. Untreated, HSE has a mortality of 70–90% with only 2.5% of patients surviving without neurologic sequelae.

Clinical Presentation

In HSE, one typically sees a 4- to 10-day prodromal period of fever and malaise followed by a characteristic clinical presentation that consists of alteration in consciousness (97%), fever (90%), headache (81%), and personality changes (71%) [92,93] (Table 12.6). Focal motor seizures that affect the face and upper extremities are common, indicating the predilection of herpes simplex for the temporal and frontal lobes [92]. Other focal neurologic signs, including hemiparesis and aphasia, are more common with HSE than with the other viral encephalitides.

Table 12.6   Symptoms and signs in patients with brain culture–positive herpes simplex encephalitis

Symptoms/signs	Percentage of patients
Altered consciousness	97
Fever	90
Headache	81
Dysphasia	76
Personality change	71
Seizures	67
Vomiting	47
Ataxia	40
Hemiparesis	33
Cranial nerve deficits	32
Memory loss	24
Visual field loss	14
Papilledema	14

Source: Data taken from the National Institute of Allergy and Infectious Disease Collaborative Antiviral Study Group, summarized in SM Goldsmith, RJ Whitley. Herpes Simplex Encephalitis. In HP Lambert (ed), Infections of the Central Nervous System. Philadelphia: Decker, 1991;286. They summarize clinical findings in 112 patients in whom the diagnosis of herpes simplex encephalitis was confirmed by virus culture from the brain. Ages ranged from 6 months to older than 60 years with equal distribution by decade. Men and women were equally represented; whites constituted 86% of patients.

Diagnosis

Definitive diagnosis can now be made not only by brain biopsy but also by recently developed polymerase chain reaction (PCR) techniques that are highly sensitive and specific [94–98]. Brain biopsy should be directed by neuroimaging studies to areas of suspected involvement or to the nondominant temporal lobe. Using immunofluorescence staining for viral antigens (sensitivity approximately 80%, specificity approximately 95%), a positive result can be obtained in 2–3 hours. Viral culture from the brain tissue usually requires 48 hours. Electron microscopy is approximately 98% specific but only approximately 48% sensitive and, therefore, not routinely used.

A 1995 publication from the National Institute of Allergy and Infectious Diseases Collaborative Antiviral Study Group recommends PCR detection of HSV DNA as the standard for its diagnosis [94]. Using CSF and brain tissue from 54 patients with biopsy-proven HSE, these authors demonstrated a sensitivity of 98%, specificity of 94%, positive predictive value of 95%, and negative predictive value of 98% for PCR in the CSF of patients. Furthermore, this estimate of 98% sensitivity applied to specimens collected from patients up to 7 days after initiation of antiviral therapy, after which sensitivity dramatically decreased (47% during days 8–14 of treatment). PCR assay can confirm the diagnosis as early as the first day of neurologic symptoms [99]. The CSF typically shows a lymphocytosis of 10–400 cells/µl (although 20% are normal in the first few days) along with an increased protein (80–1,000 mg/dl) and up to 1,000 red blood cells per µl (median approximately 130), indicating hemorrhagic necrosis [90]. Glucose is normal or decreased.

CT scanning with IV contrast shows gyral enhancement, temporal lobe lucencies, or mass effect in up to 65% of biopsy-proven cases by day 5 or later of clinical symptoms [100]. MRI scanning may be more sensitive, especially in earlier stages, and may allow monitoring of response to acyclovir therapy [101,102]. Figure 12.10 shows a typical T2-weighted MRI scan of a patient with HSE revealing increased signal intensity within the right temporal lobe. Electroencephalography (EEG) is often helpful, showing periodic (2- to 3-second intervals) sharp wave complexes unilaterally or bilaterally in the temporal regions as early as 2 days into the course, and is localizing in up to 81% of patients [103].

Treatment

Treatment of HSE potentially involves the management of increased intracranial pressure and seizures in addition to antiviral therapy (see Treatment under Bacterial Meningitis). Acyclovir (acycloguanosine) reduces the mortality to approximately 19% if administered early, with up to 38% survivors showing no significant sequelae [92,104]. It is administered at a dosage of 10 mg/kg IV every 8 hours for 10 days. Relapses have sometimes occurred after a 10-day course, and some authors have recommended a longer (14- to 21-day) course of acyclovir. Side effects include reversible elevation in serum creatinine (10%), local phlebitis (4%), and nausea (2%). A 1994 review of acyclovir neurotoxicity suggests that tremors, myoclonus, confusion, and lethargy secondary to acyclovir infusion occur very rarely [105]. Alternatively, adenine arabinoside can be used at a dose of 15 mg/kg IV in at least 25 ml of 5% dextrose in normal saline given over 12 hours. With this regimen, mortality is estimated at approximately 28%, with an estimated 19% of survivors being normal [106].

Varicella-Zoster Encephalitis

Epidemiology

Varicella-zoster encephalitis (VZE), like HSE, shows no seasonal or geographic predilection. Varicella-zoster infects nearly 100% of the population in temperate parts of the world [107]. VZE occurs in 0.05% of childhood chickenpox cases, typically appearing 5–6 days after the rash [108] or up to 5 weeks later [109]. It is heralded by fever, headache, and obtundation or delirium and must be distinguished from the more common acute cerebellar ataxia that develops 1 week after infection with nystagmus, dysarthria, and ataxia.

VZE is more common in adults after the age of 40 years, with an incidence of 0.5% after cutaneous zoster eruption [110]. Approximately 35–45% of patients have an antecedent cranial nerve (usually trigeminal) or mixed cranial–cervical nerve zoster dermatomal lesion, and the average time to onset of CNS symptoms

Figure 12.10 Magnetic resonance image of herpes simplex encephalitis. **A.** Sagittal T1-weighted image with low intensity in the swollen temporal lobe. **B.** T2-weighted image demonstrates high signal intensity diffusely in the left temporal lobe, along with asymmetric high signal intensity in the right temporal lobe (*arrows*). (Reprinted with permission from RJ Farrell. Neuroradiology: The Requisites. In RI Grossman, DM Yousem [eds], Infectious and Noninfectious Inflammatory Diseases of the Brain. St. Louis: Mosby–Year Book, 1994;183.)

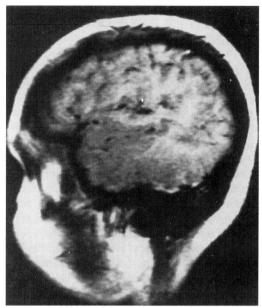

A

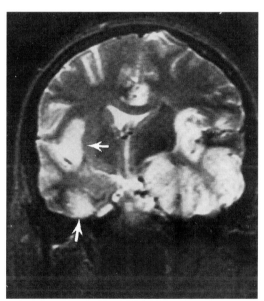

B

is 9 days but can be as long as 53 days [109]. The average duration of symptoms is 16–24 days, and average mortality is approximately 20% but is much higher in the immunosuppressed [109].

Clinical Presentation

Symptoms and signs include fever, headache, stiff neck, obtundation, delirium, or personality changes after zoster skin eruption, especially in immunocompromised patients with Hodgkin's disease and chronic lymphocytic leukemia [109]. Seizures rarely occur. An important association with necrotizing myelitis has been reported in isolated cases [111]. A clinical stroke picture of hemiparesis can develop secondary to varicella-induced vasculitis ipsilateral to ophthalmic involvement of the trigeminal nerve [112]. Although varicella infection of the CNS is not a common feature of AIDS (approximately 2–4%), VZE may occur in AIDS patients in the absence of cutaneous skin eruptions, especially later in their course [113]. Ventriculitis and necrotizing myelitis are also rare but well-recognized complications of varicella-zoster virus infection in AIDS [113,114]. Varicella-zoster that involves the seventh cranial nerve may be associated with facial paralysis and vesicles in the external auditory meatus and eardrum (Ramsay Hunt syndrome). This can progress to focal brain stem encephalitis involving the fifth, sixth, eighth, ninth, and tenth cranial nerves [115,116].

Diagnosis

The CSF usually shows fewer than 500 WBC/μl, but protein levels can vary widely [109,117]. Glucose may be low. Jemsek and associates [109] reported detection of specific antibody to varicella-zoster membrane antigen in the CSF of seven of seven patients who showed clinical encephalitis after zoster infection. In another series of 16 patients with zoster-associated encephalitis, 94% had elevated ($\geq$1:2) titers in the CSF, whereas none of 25 control subjects with other CNS pathology had positive CSF titers [118]. Using an antibody-capture ELISA technique, van Loon and colleagues [119] demonstrated varicella-zoster virus–specific IgG, IgM, and IgA in CSF patients with zoster encephalitis. In the diagnosis of VZE, brain MRI and CT scans are not generally helpful. The EEG shows diffuse slowing in nearly all cases.

Treatment

No controlled clinical trials of antiviral treatment for VZE are reported. Controlled trials of IV acyclovir in cutaneous zoster infection have demonstrated its efficacy in halting cutaneous dissemination and development of visceral zoster in immunocompromised patients [120,121]. Reports of improvement of VZE with several days of treatment with IV acyclovir suggest efficacy [122,123]. A treatment dosage similar to that used in immunocompromised patients (acyclovir, 1,500 mg/m^2/day IV) has been suggested, pending further studies [115]. The usefulness of steroids in VZE has not been demonstrated.

Enterovirus Encephalitis

Epidemiology

The enterovirus group includes the polioviruses, Coxsackie A and B echoviruses, enteroviruses, and hepatitis A, all of which infect the human alimentary tract. In patients with a clinical presentation, aseptic meningitis (see Viral Meningitis) is the most frequent neurologic manifestation (35%), followed by encephalitis (11%) and paralysis (1%). Most cases of encephalitis occur in July through September, primarily in the 10- to 29-year age group [124]. Outcome of enteroviral encephalitis is usually benign, although a mortality of 2.5% is reported.

Clinical Presentation

The clinical picture of the meningoencephalitis is nonspecific. Enterovirus 70, for example, often heralds infection with a self-limiting acute hemorrhagic conjunctivitis within 1–10 days of infection [115]. In a small number of cases, it is followed in 1–5 weeks by radicular pain with asymmetric flaccid paralysis, which may be permanent. Coxsackie viruses can cause aseptic meningitis associated with herpangina, pleurodynia, pericarditis, and rashes. Enterovirus 71 more commonly causes aseptic meningitis and encephalitis.

Diagnosis

Routine serologic screening of most enteroviral infections is impractical, requiring antibody titering against specific viruses, owing to lack of group-specific antigens. Therefore, emphasis is on viral isolation from throat swabs, stool, blood, and CSF (which was demonstrated in 41% of 111 pediatric cases of meningitis or meningoencephalitis in one report [125]). During specific outbreaks, however, a fourfold antibody rise against the specific virus is diagnostic. Routine use of CT scans and EEGs is not helpful in the diagnosis of enteroviral infections of the CNS.

Treatment

No specific antiviral therapies are available, and treatment is mainly supportive.

VIRAL MENINGITIS

Incidence and Pathophysiology

Viral meningitis is the most common cause of aseptic meningitis, an inflammatory disorder of the leptomeninges that cannot be attributed to bacterial or fungal etiology. As a group, the viral meningitides generally represent benign, self-limited illnesses. Enteroviruses (Picornaviridae family) are the most common cause of viral meningitis, and those with a particular propensity to cause meningitis include echoviruses 6, 9, and 20 and Coxsackie viruses A9, B2, B3, and B5 [126]. These viruses exist worldwide, inhabit the alimentary tract, and occur more frequently in young children, spreading by fecal-oral transmission. Enteroviral infections have an epidemic seasonal peak in summer and early fall [127].

The second most common cause of viral meningitis is the mumps virus (Paramyxoviridae family), but institution of a vaccine program has markedly decreased the number of cases in the United States. Mumps virus has a worldwide distribution with peak epidemics in winter and spring. It is spread primarily by respiratory droplets or directly through saliva, infecting glandular tissue, such as the parotid, ovaries, testes, mammary glands, and pancreas, as well as the CNS [128]. Lymphocytic choriomeningitis virus (Arenaviridae family) causes meningitis after contact with infected rodents, particularly mice and hamsters. Although disease occurs year-round, it tends to be more common in winter. Typical symptoms include fever, headache, arthralgias, and myalgias. Pneumonitis and alopecia may precede the onset of meningitis [126].

Herpes simplex virus (HSV) is a known pathogen of the central and peripheral nervous systems. Herpes simplex virus type 1 (HSV-1) and herpes simplex virus type 2 (HSV-2) are most commonly implicated in CNS disease, but both cause different diseases in adults. HSV-1 is discussed in the previous section and causes meningoencephalitis. HSV-2 is associated with aseptic meningitis in the setting of primary genital infection and also more recently with benign, recurrent lymphocytic meningitis, or so-called Mollaret's meningitis. After genital or anal transmission, the virus spreads to the CNS hematogenously to cause typical meningitic symptoms. CSF pleocytosis with lymphocytic predominance and elevated protein (approximately 110 mg/dl) is common. Thereafter, meningitic recurrences may coincide with genital recrudescence [129], but HSV-2 has also been implicated as the causal agent in Mollaret's meningitis [130–133].

Clinical Presentation

Clinical presentations of the viral meningitides are similar. Onset of illness may be relatively sudden or subacute. Most commonly, patients present with a frontal or retro-orbital headache, fever, and neck stiffness. Other symptoms include general malaise, myalgia, photophobia, nausea, and vomiting. Specific non-CNS manifestations (e.g., parotitis in mumps, genital lesions in herpes) can also occur.

Diagnosis

CSF examination should reveal clear fluid with normal or slightly elevated opening pressure. The cell count ranges from 10–1,000/μl but is usually less than 300 cells per μl [134]. Early in the course, approximately 75% of patients have a predominance of neutrophils. This is followed by a shift to a mononuclear response over the next 1–3 days. CSF glucose is usually normal (except in mumps and lymphocytic choriomeningitis), but protein is slightly elevated between 50 and 100 mg/dl. Diagnosis of mumps meningitis is typically confirmed after a history of parotitis; isolation of virus from CSF, saliva, and urine; a fourfold increase of specific antibody in serum; and the presence of antibody in CSF. In lymphocytic choriomeningitis, high CSF cell counts may be seen (>1,000 cells/μl), usually with a lymphocytic predominance and hypoglycorrhachia. Infection can be confirmed with detection of antibody in serum or, less commonly, by the presence of antibody or positive culture from CSF [129]. In the case of HSV, PCR detection in CSF is the most sensitive diagnostic tool.

Treatment

Because of the generally benign course of viral meningitides, treatment is supportive. The exception to this is HSV-2 meningitis associated with genital lesions. In this setting, acyclovir is helpful in treating the genital lesions.

CENTRAL NERVOUS SYSTEM LYME DISEASE

Incidence and Pathophysiology

Lyme disease occurs worldwide, with reported cases on every continent. In 1995, 11,603 cases of Lyme disease were reported to the Centers for Disease Control and Prevention by 43 states [135]. The majority of these cases were reported from the Northeast, Mid-Atlantic, North Central, and Pacific Coastal regions. Lyme disease is a tick-borne infection, transmitted by the tick *Ixodes* infected with the spirochete *Borrelia burgdorferi*. In the northeastern and midwestern United States, the deer tick *Ixodes dammini* is the primary vector.

Clinical Presentation

Lyme disease is a multisystem infectious disease with an estimated 10–40% of individuals having involvement of the nervous system [136]. The course of neuroborreliosis has been described as occurring in three stages. In stage 1, acute localized infection manifests as erythema migrans. During stage 2, disseminated infection takes place, and meningitis is typically seen. Stage 3 represents the late phases of rheumatologic and neurologic complications. It should be noted, however, that the clinical course of Lyme disease is variable, and these clinical manifestations do not occur in strictly chronologic sequence.

In the peripheral nervous system, Lyme disease typically causes cranial neuritis, radiculoneuritis, diffuse peripheral neuropathy, mononeuropathy multiplex, brachial or lumbosacral plexopathy, and motor neuropathy as well as a Guillain-Barré–like syndrome [137]. When Lyme disease affects the CNS, one can see meningitis (10%), encephalomyelitis (0.1%), and encephalopathy [137]. The three manifestations thought to be most "typical" for Lyme disease are lymphocytic choriomeningitis, cranial neuritis, and radiculoneuritis and are collectively generally termed *stage 2*. The lymphocytic choriomeningitis resembles an aseptic meningitis with the primary feature of headache. Fever and meningismus are less common. The meningitis is typically acute but can take on a more chronic or relapsing course if untreated. Lymphocytic meningoradiculitis is a relapsing painful mono- or polyradiculopathy with variable degrees of peripheral nerve involvement. Peripheral neuropathies may be isolated to the limb that was bitten, mimicking a mononeuropathy or brachial plexopathy, or can be widely disseminated so as to resemble Guillain-Barré syndrome. Involvement of the facial nerve, which can be bilateral in up to one-third of patients, is the most common cranial neuropathy (50%), but neuropathies of virtually all the cranial nerves have been described. When the CNS is involved, patients may develop focal deficits in relation to the site of involvement. A mild to moderate confusional state is quite common, however, and this can be seen despite normal MRI, EEG, and CSF.

In late, disseminated disease, a predominantly sensory polyneuropathy has been seen in association with the chronic skin disorder, acrodermatitis chronica atrophicans. Months to years after disease onset, a chronic encephalomyelitis may manifest. The onset is insidious with progressive worsening over months to years. Patients may present with spastic paraparesis, cranial nerve palsies, bladder dysfunction, or cognitive impairment.

Diagnosis

CSF examination typically demonstrates a lymphocytic pleocytosis, mild to moderate elevation in protein, and normal glucose. Oligoclonal bands may be present in chronic infection. Isolation of the spirochete is very difficult, and even in Lyme meningitis, *B. burgdorferi* can only be cultured from the spinal fluid in approximately 10% of patients. The key to the diagnosis of CNS Lyme disease is the demonstration of anti–*B. burgdorferi* antibodies in the CSF out of proportion to that in the serum. Indirect immunofluorescence techniques have generally been replaced. Currently, a two-test approach is recommended in the serodiagnosis of Lyme disease, consisting of an initial ELISA followed by Western blot. CSF PCR for *B. burgdorferi* genomic material is adjunctive to these studies [138,139]. Regardless of which assay is used, examination of both serum and CSF is essential. Although MRI may demonstrate evidence for meningoencephalitis, abnormalities seen on MRI are not sufficient for diagnosis.

In 1996, Halperin and associates [140] published a set of practice guidelines for the diagnosis of definite nervous system Lyme disease. Such a diagnosis requires (1) possible exposure to appropriate ticks in an area where Lyme disease occurs; (2) one or more of the following: (a) erythema migrans or histopathologically proven *Borrelia* lymphocytoma or acrodermatitis, (b) immunologic evidence of exposure to *B. burgdorferi* (e.g., positive serologic test), (c) culture, histologic, or PCR proof of the presence of *B. burgdorferi*; and (3) occurrence of one or more of the following neurologic disorders after exclusion of other potential etiologies: lymphocytic choriomeningitis, encephalomyelitis, peripheral neuropathy, and/or encephalopathy. Additional testing is indicated based on the likelihood that a given neurologic disorder is causally related to Lyme. If CNS disease is suspected, CSF should be examined for intrathecal antibody production, culture, or PCR [140].

Treatment

The optimal treatment regimen has yet to be determined. In one study, IV ceftriaxone (2 g/day IV for 2 weeks) proved superior to penicillin G (20 million units/day) [141], but other studies show similar efficacy for both and for cefotaxime [142–144]. Duration of treatment ranges from 2 to 4 weeks, depending on response to therapy. In patients who are allergic to penicillin or cephalosporins, IV chloramphenicol (250 mg every 8 hours) or oral tetracyclines (500 mg 4 times a day for 30 days) can be used. A 1994 study showed an oral regimen with doxycycline (200 mg/day for 2 weeks) to be as effective as IV penicillin [145].

CENTRAL NERVOUS SYSTEM INFECTIONS IN THE HUMAN IMMUNODEFICIENCY VIRUS POPULATION

Human Immunodeficiency Virus-1 Infection

HIV-1 infection of the CNS results in a variety of neurologic signs, symptoms, and syndromes that result either from direct effects of viral replication in the CNS (primary effects) or as a manifestation of opportunistic infections owing to generalized immunodeficiency (secondary effects). In this section, the primary effects of such infection, including meningitis and dementia, are discussed first and then the relevant opportunistic infections, including cytomegalovirus (CMV) encephalitis, toxoplasmosis, cryptococcal meningitis, and neurosyphilis.

The initial neurologic manifestation of primary HIV-1 infection is an acute, self-limited aseptic meningitis, which occurs in approximately 25–50% of patients [146–148] and which can be confused with nonsteroidal anti-inflammatory drug–induced chemical meningitis. CSF studies typically show a modest pleocytosis (approximately 5–70 lymphocytes) with elevation of protein (<90 mg/dl) and an elevated IgG index in cases of asymptomatic meningitis; such abnormalities may persist throughout the clinical course of AIDS. Notably, pleocytosis or an elevated CSF protein level may be seen in up to 59% of asymptomatic HIV-1 seropositive patients [149]. Occasionally, cranial nerve deficits are seen in patients with HIV-1 infection and may be noted at the time of seroconversion, although no specific syndrome is typical. The duration of symptoms generally does not exceed 2 weeks.

The most devastating neurologic complication of HIV-1 infection in the brain is dementia, which is seen in a clinically defined syndrome of cognitive, neuropsychological, and motor manifestations that occur in the absence of opportunistic infections and are termed the *HIV-associated dementia complex* or *AIDS dementia complex* (ADC) [150]. In general, ADC is a late manifestation of AIDS, typically appearing 2–8 years after seroconversion and ultimately affecting approximately 20% of patients. Unlike the dementia of Alzheimer's disease, ADC is characterized predominantly by early presentation of psychomotor slowing, inattentiveness, and discoordination followed later by memory deficits but with sparing of language functions [151]. It is the initial manifestation of HIV-1 infection in only approximately 1–5% of patients [151], and in suspected cases of ADC, CSF analysis is crucial to rule out other potentially treatable causes, particularly CMV encephalitis [152]. The syndrome is at least partially reversible with antiretroviral therapy according to several studies [153,154], and evidence from in vitro cell culture systems suggests that the envelope glycoprotein gp120 may be a significant factor in inducing neurotoxicity via indirect stimulation of *N*-methyl-D-aspartate receptors [155,156]. A large multicenter study using the *N*-methyl-D-aspartate receptor antagonist memantine for prevention of ADC is currently under way in the United States. This nationwide AIDS Clinical Trials Group (ACTG) study involves 120 patients with ADC ranging from mild to severe cognitive impairment and randomized either to oral memantine or placebo. The primary end point is neuropsychological performance, and, in addition, magnetic resonance spectroscopic brain imaging is being used to correlate neuropsychological performance with regional brain analysis of glial and neuronal cell metabolites. The study is scheduled to be completed in late 1999.

Cytomegalovirus Disease of the Central Nervous System

Cytomegalovirus Encephalitis

Clinical Presentation

CMV is a ubiquitous human herpesvirus that infects humans throughout life. Approximately 1% of fetuses are infected in utero, and up to 80% of adults have serologic evidence for CMV infection by age 50 years [157]. In healthy individuals, CMV infection is usually asymptomatic, although a mononucleosis-like syndrome can occur [158]. In AIDS patients, however, CMV is a major cause of morbidity and mortality, often leading to more rapid progression of disease, especially when CD4 counts are declining [159]. Systemic infection in AIDS can involve the gastrointestinal tract, lungs, adrenal glands, and eyes [157,159], and up to 44% of AIDS patients have CMV infection in the peripheral and central nervous systems [160,161] that likely is seeded hematogenously by infected monocytes [158]. Pathologic findings in the brain include microglial nodules (most common up to 100%), focal necrosis, necrotizing ventriculoencephalitis, and myelitis (approximately 10%) [161].

Arribas and associates [152] reviewed 676 cases of CMV encephalitis and found that 85% of these patients were HIV-1 seropositive, while another 12% had other causes of immunosuppression. Furthermore, autopsy-proven CMV encephalitis was present in 16% of HIV-infected patients. The most common clinical signs were confusion or lethargy or both (60%), coma (44%), cranial nerve palsies (40%), fever (37%), nystagmus (34%), leg weakness (25%), seizures (25%), ataxia (19%), headache (12%), dementia (11%), and vertigo (9%). Notably, the progression to death once clinical signs are present is rapid (weeks to months) in most cases [162,163].

Diagnosis

Diagnosis of CMV encephalitis depends on a high degree of clinical suspicion and should be considered in any HIV-1 seropositive patient with changes in mentation. The combination of encephalopathy, cranial neuropathy, and nystag-mus is often seen in patients with CMV ventriculitis [163], typically appearing as periventricular enhancement on gadolinium-enhanced MRI or contrasted CT brain images [164] (Figure 12.11).

CMV ventriculitis is associated with CSF pleocytosis (polymorphonuclear cells) and hypoglycorrhachia, but CMV encephalitis per se is often not associated with CSF pleocytosis. Therefore, attention has focused on use of PCR analysis of CSF as a more sensitive marker. In the review of Arribas and associates [152], the sensitivity of CSF PCR was 79% with a specificity of 95% in a total of 122 autopsy-proven cases of CMV encephalitis in the literature, making PCR the most useful diagnostic test. Gozlan and colleagues [165] demonstrated a sensi-tivity of 92% with a specificity of 94% in a series of 88 patients diagnosed by spe-cific clinical, histologic, and therapeutic response criteria. Alternative diagnostic methods, such as viral culture, are consistently negative [158], and CSF IgG to CMV may be detected in up to 29% of HIV-1 infected individuals with neuro-logic illnesses; whether this is useful for the diagnosis of CMV encephalitis is undetermined, however [166].

Cytomegalovirus Myelitis

CMV myelitis, or polyradiculomyelopathy, is a distinct but uncommon sub-acute syndrome of ascending motor weakness, areflexia, paresthesias, and loss of sphincter control [167–169]. Sensory deficits are highly variable, and cranial nerve deficits are occasionally seen [170,171], as well as peripheral neuropathy [172]. In cases of myelitis, the CSF typically shows a polymorpho-nuclear pleocytosis, increased protein, and hypoglycorrhachia [169]. MRI may reveal leptomeningeal enhancement of lumbar nerve roots in cases of radiculopathy. Treatment with ganciclovir or foscarnet, or both, is as outlined in Treatment.

Treatment

Treatment for CMV disease of the nervous system currently involves the use of either of two antiviral agents: ganciclovir (9-[1,3-dihydroxy-2-proposymethyl]-guanine) and foscarnet (trisodium phosphonoformate). Ganciclovir blocks viral DNA synthesis, and levels of active drug are 10 times higher in infected cells than in uninfected cells [158], making it relatively selective in vivo. It is useful for the treatment of AIDS-related CMV retinitis, colitis, and encephalitis, but treatment with ganciclovir alone may not prolong survival because of the rapid emergence of resistance [159,167]. Foscarnet resembles ganciclovir in its reversible inhibi-tion of the viral DNA polymerase but has the additional feature of activity against the reverse transcriptase of retroviruses [173]. It exhibits equivalent activity to ganciclovir against CMV retinitis, although patients may have a longer survival time as a result of its antiretroviral activity [174]. Furthermore, foscarnet may be active against ganciclovir-resistant strains of CMV [175]. Typical induction dosages of ganciclovir are 5 mg/kg IV over 1 hour every 12 hours for 14–21 days followed by maintenance therapy at 6 mg/kg per day IV for 5 days a week for an

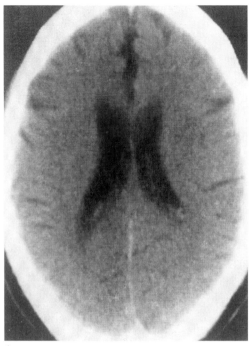

A

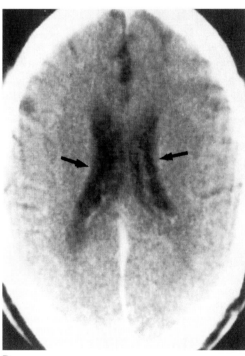

B

Figure 12.11   Cytomegalovirus ventriculitis. **A.** Axial noncontrast computed tomographic scan demonstrates cortical atrophy and ventricular enlargement in this pathologically proven case. **B.** Postcontrast study shows faint subependymal enhancement (*arrows*). (Reprinted with permission from ML Hanson Whiteman, MJ Donovan Post, EML Sklar. Neuroimaging of Acquired Immunodeficiency Syndrome. In JR Berger, RM Levy [eds], AIDS and the Nervous System. Philadelphia: Lippincott–Raven, 1997;307.)

indefinite period [5]. Alternatively, ganciclovir maintenance can be given orally at a dosage of 1 g three times a day [5]. Foscarnet induction is administered at 60 mg/kg IV over 2 hours every 8 hours for 14–21 days followed by 90 mg/kg per day for an indefinite period [5]. Some studies suggest that combination therapy with foscarnet may be superior [176].

Toxoplasmosis

Clinical Presentation

Toxoplasma gondii is a common intracellular parasite that is the most frequently seen CNS opportunistic infectious pathogen in AIDS [177]. Toxoplasmic encephalitis (TE) is the most common CNS manifestation and includes generalized or focal symptoms, or both, which often occur as part of multiple organ involvement [178]. Generalized symptoms range from headache, lethargy, apathy, and dementia to coma, while focal symptoms often include hemiparesis, ataxia, diplopia, movement disorders, tremors, seizures, and cranial nerve disorders [178,179]. Symptoms may evolve acutely with focal deficits, but more commonly generalized cerebral dysfunction develops insidiously over several weeks [180]. The varied clinical presentations reflect the multifocal nature of the infection, which pathologically involves a necrotizing encephalitis with associated edema, vasculitis, and hemorrhage and a tendency to involve the brain stem [179]. More than 95% of cases represent reactivation of a latent infection, generally when CD4 counts fall below 100/µl, and in the United States, TE can be expected to develop in approximately 10–13% of AIDS patients (one-third of all *T. gondii* seropositive patients) [179,180].

Diagnosis

Diagnosis of TE depends on clinical, serologic, and radiographic criteria, and up to 80% of patients have multiple gadolinium-enhancing lesions that are demonstrable on brain MRI imaging or contrasted CT scan [180,182,183]. These are frequently ring-enhancing and rarely homogeneous [178,184] and represent zones of hemorrhagic necrosis, commonly in the deep gray matter of the basal ganglia, the cerebellum, and also the gray-white junction [185] (Figure 12.12). Thallium-201 brain single-photon emission CT imaging can distinguish between toxoplasmosis and primary CNS lymphoma because tumor cells actively take up the thallium, whereas infectious foci do not [184,186]. CSF parameters are usually abnormal but not necessarily characteristic. In a series of 27 patients, Navia and associates [180] summarized CSF findings as follows: mean protein level of 96 mg/dl, mild mononuclear pleocytosis of 4–67 cells/µl, and, occasionally, hypoglycorrhachia (approximately 40 mg/dl). Serum IgG titers are detectable in the majority of patients but tend to vary widely (1:2–1:1,024) and rarely increase before the development of TE [179,180].

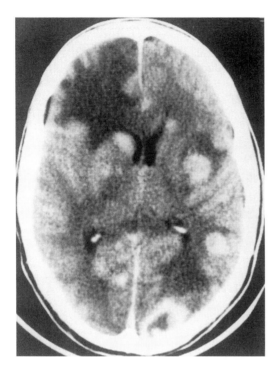

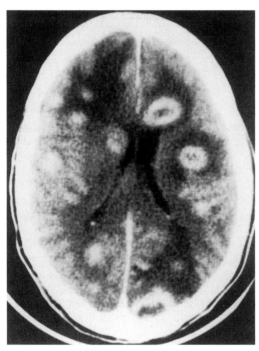

Figure 12.12   Toxoplasmic encephalitis. Postcontrast computed tomographic images of a human immunodeficiency virus–seropositive patient demonstrate multiple enhancing lesions in both hemispheres. Some lesions show nodular enhancement, whereas others demonstrate ring enhancement. (Reprinted with permission from ML Hanson Whiteman, MJ Donovan Post, EML Sklar. Neuroimaging of Acquired Immunodeficiency Syndrome. In JR Berger, RM Levy [eds], AIDS and the Nervous System. Philadelphia: Lippincott–Raven, 1997;340.)

Treatment

When treatment is begun early, the clinical outcome is often favorable. The current recommendation is for combination therapy with pyrimethamine and sulfonamides, typically sulfadiazine. Clindamycin is an acceptable alternative. Suggested dosing regimens are as follows [5]: pyrimethamine, 200 mg loading dose on day 1, then 50–75 mg per day; plus folinic acid, 10 mg orally; plus sulfadiazine, 4–8 g per day orally or IV; or clindamycin, 600 mg orally or IV every 6 hours for 3–6 weeks, then suppressive therapy.

Lifelong secondary prophylaxis with pyrimethamine and sulfadiazine against relapse of TE appears to be warranted [187]. The use of pyrimethamine for primary prophylaxis against TE in patients with advanced AIDS was studied in a randomized trial of 396 patients, which showed increased mortality in treated patients (pyrimethamine, 25 mg orally three times a day) compared to placebo control subjects (60% versus 25%, respectively, at 500 days for all patients) [188]. However, survival was increased in patients who were prophylactically treated with trimethoprim-sulfamethoxazole for *Pneumocystis carinii* pneumonia. Carr and associates [189] confirmed that low-dose trimethoprim-sulfamethoxazole (one tablet twice a day for 2 days per week) appears to be effective prophylaxis against TE in patients with *P. carinii*. Recommended lifetime prophylaxis is as follows [5]: pyrimethamine, 50 mg per day orally; plus folinic acid, 10 mg per day orally; plus sulfadiazine, 1.0–1.5 g every 6 hours orally; or clindamycin, 300 mg every 6 hours orally. Alternatively, primary prophylaxis with both dapsone (50 mg/day) and pyrimethamine (50 mg/week) may also be effective [190].

Progressive Multifocal Leukoencephalopathy

Progressive multifocal leukoencephalopathy (PML) is a progressive, usually fatal, disease caused by a ubiquitous papovavirus (JC virus) that affects approximately 5% of all AIDS patients [191–193] as well as other immunocompromised individuals, particularly those with chronic lymphocytic leukemia [192]. Up to 85% of cases occur in association with AIDS [192]. PML is characterized by focal demyelination within the CNS resulting from viral replication within oligodendrocytes, although infection has also been demonstrated in astrocytes [192]. A predilection for periventricular and occipital white matter exists [164]. JC virus is also demonstrable in peripheral blood lymphocytes in more than 90% of patients with biopsy-proven PML, and it is thought that these lymphocytes may carry the virus to the brain [194]. By adulthood, up to 90% of healthy individuals are seropositive for JC virus antibody, suggesting that clinical disease occurs as a result of reactivation of a latent infection [191,195].

Prognosis of PML remains poor. More than 80% of patients die within 1 year of the diagnosis (196–198), although prolonged survival has been documented [193]. Berger and associates [193] report personal observations of up to 7% of patients with AIDS-associated PML surviving beyond 1 year. These individuals may represent a subgroup, with PML presenting as the initial manifestation of AIDS, lack of brain stem and cerebellar involvement, generally higher CD4[+] counts, and a tendency for inflammatory infiltrates and lesion enhancement on histopathologic and radiographic studies.

Diagnosis

Definitive diagnosis of PML depends on brain biopsy; however, certain clinical and radiographic features are strongly supportive of the diagnosis. The most common presenting features include weakness, visual deficits, and cognitive dysfunction. In a pooled group of 79 patients with AIDS-associated PML, Berger and associates [193] found the most common neurologic features to be mono- or hemiparesis (66%), speech deficits (46%), sensory deficits (19%), and visual deficits (24%) such as homonymous hemianopsia and cortical blindness, in addition to cognitive disturbances (35%). The scope of cognitive disturbances is broad and includes rapidly progressive personality and behavioral changes, memory loss, dyslexia, and dyscalculia, unlike the insidious progression of global dementia without focal deficits that characterizes Alzheimer's dementia [191,193].

The radiographic appearance of PML is generally distinct, although occasionally atypical. Hypodensities of the subcortical and deep white matter on CT brain imaging may be seen [199], although MRI scans appear to be much more sensitive [164,193,200–203] (Figure 12.13).

One typically sees hyperintense lesions on T2-weighted images with no or minimal peripheral enhancement with gadolinium in 5–10% of cases [203]. The lesions are commonly seen in the frontal and parieto-occipital lobes but can occur throughout the brain, including the basal ganglia, external capsule, and posterior fossa (cerebellum and brain stem). They can be unilateral but are usually bilateral and show no mass effect [203]. Subcortical white matter lesions have a characteristic "scalloped" appearance that is presumably caused by the demyelination of the subcortical U fibers [203]. In addition, lesions may be seen in the basal ganglia where traversing myelinated axons may be affected [200,203]. Some difficulty exists in distinguishing white matter lesions in PML from HIV-1–induced demyelination, but a multifocal appearance, asymmetry, and predilection for the subcortical white matter favor the diagnosis of PML [164].

Definitive diagnosis depends on identification of papovavirus particles or DNA, or both, within plaque-like lesions in the brain. Typical virions are naked icosahedral capsids surrounding a double-stranded DNA genome (total diameter, 44 nm) and are easily identified by electron microscopy [204,205]. At the light microscopic level, enlarged oligodendrocytes with inclusion bodies are typically found at the edges of active demyelination, along with greatly hypertrophied astrocytes and lipid-laden macrophages [191,192,206]. Viral DNA can be detected within the oligodendrocytes and astrocytes by in situ hybridization, but not within neurons [207]. In addition, PCR detection of JC virus DNA in lymphocytes from the peripheral circulation can be achieved in the majority of patients with PML but also to a lesser degree in AIDS patients without PML [194]; such testing awaits further verification.

Treatment

No proven treatment for PML is available, and the low but significant survival rate makes response to therapy difficult to assess. Anecdotal reports suggest response to cytarabine, adenine arabinoside, and interferon-alpha [207–214], although a randomized, placebo-controlled study has not documented therapeutic efficacy

Figure 12.13 Progressive multifocal leukoencephalopathy. **A.** T1-weighted magnetic resonance image shows hypointense signal of the left hemisphere and posterior region of the right hemisphere. **B.** The T2-weighted image shows hyperintense signal abnormalities in the same regions. (Reprinted with permission from ML Hanson Whiteman, MJ Donovan Post, EML Sklar. Neuroimaging of Acquired Immunodeficiency Syndrome. In JR Berger, RM Levy [eds], AIDS and the Nervous System. Philadelphia: Lippincott–Raven, 1997;307.)

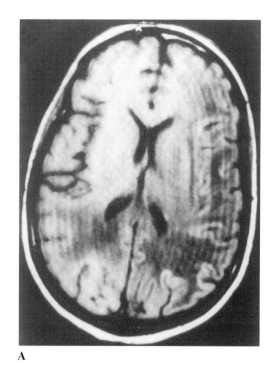

A

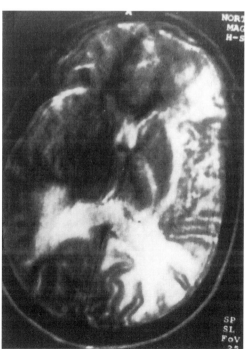

B

for any treatment to date. A randomized, double-blind, placebo-controlled study of high-dose antiretroviral therapy versus high-dose antiretroviral therapy plus either intrathecal or IV cytarabine in AIDS-associated PML was undertaken by the AIDS Clinical Trials Group (National Institute of Allergy and Infectious Disease; ACTG No. 243). Interim analysis revealed no discernible benefit from cytarabine, leading to early termination of the study. Nonetheless, considerable progress has been made in understanding JC virus replication and factors governing viral promoter activity in glial cells, with the foreseeable goal of controlling infection in vivo [215,216].

REFERENCES

1. Roos KL. Acute Bacterial Meningitis in Children and Adults. In WM Scheld (ed), Infections of the Central Nervous System. New York: Lippincott–Raven, 1997;335–409.
2. Lambert HP. Meningitis. J Neurol Neurosurg Psychiatry 1994;57:405.
3. Martin J, Tyler KL, Scheld WM. Bacterial Meningitis. In KL Tyler, JB Martin (eds), Infectious Diseases of the Central Nervous System. Philadelphia: Davis, 1993;176–187.
4. Moxon ER, Kroll JS, Kayhty MH. Haemophilus influenzae Type b Meningitis: Pathogenesis and Immunology. In HP Lambert (ed), Infections of the Central Nervous System. Philadelphia: Decker, 1991;99–104.
5. Sanford JP. The Sanford Guide to Antimicrobial Therapy. Dallas: Antimicrobial Therapy, 1997.
6. Tunkel AR, Scheld WM. Bacterial Meningitis: Pathogenic and Pathophysiologic Mechanisms. In HP Lambert (ed), Infections of the Central Nervous System. Philadelphia: Decker, 1991;1–15.
7. Lebel MH, Freij BJ, Syrogiannopoulos GA, et al. Dexamethasone therapy for bacterial meningitis. N Engl J Med 1988;319:964.
8. Roos KL, Scheld WM. The management of fulminant meningitis in the intensive care unit. Crit Care Clin 1988;4:375.
9. Tunkel AR, Scheld WM. Bacterial Meningitis. In RW Carlson, MA Geheb (ed), Principles and Practice of Medical Intensive Care. Philadelphia: Saunders, 1993;454–466.
10. Dobson SRM, Moxon ER. Haemophilus influenzae: Syndromes and Treatment. In HP Lambert (ed), Infections of the Central Nervous System. Philadelphia: Decker, 1991;105–116.
11. Conway SP. Pneumococcal and Other Gram-Positive Coccal Meningitides. In HP Lambert (ed), Infections of the Central Nervous System. Philadelphia: Decker, 1991;125–149.
12. Lambert HP. Meningitis: Diagnostic Problems. In HP Lambert (ed), Infections of the Central Nervous System. Philadelphia: Decker, 1991;32–39.
13. Armstrong WA, Fung PC. Brainstem encephalitis (rhombencephalitis) due to *Listeria* monocytogenes: case report and review. Clin Infect Dis 1993;16:689.
14. McGowan KL, Hodgkin RL. Laboratory diagnosis of fetal infections. Clin Lab Med 1992;12:523.
15. Faidas A, Shepard DL, Lim J, et al. Magnetic resonance imaging in listerial brain stem encephalitis. Clin Infect Dis 1993;16:186.
16. Bell WE, McGuinness GA. Antibacterial and Antifungal Therapy for CNS Infections. In KL Tyler, JB Martin (eds), Infectious Diseases of the Central Nervous System. Philadelphia: Davis, 1993;305–353.
17. Sanford JP. The Sanford Guide to Antimicrobial Therapy. Dallas: Antimicrobial Therapy, 1994.
18. de Louvois J. Neonatal Meningitis. In HP Lambert (ed), Infections of the Central Nervous System. Philadelphia: Decker, 1991;161–174.
19. Farrar WE, Reboli AC. Meningitis Due to *Listeria* Monocytogenes and Other Gram-Positive Bacilli. In HP Lambert (ed), Infections of the Central Nervous System. Philadelphia: Decker, 1991;175–188.
20. Tauber MG, Khayam-Bashi H, Sande MA. Effects of ampicillin and corticosteroids on brain water content, cerebrospinal fluid pressure, and cerebrospinal fluid lactate levels in experimental pneumococcal meningitis. J Infect Dis 1985;151:528.
21. Milligan NM, Newcombe R, Compson DA. A double-blind controlled trial of high dose methylprednisolone in patients with multiple sclerosis: 1. Clinical effects. J Neurol Neurosurg Psychiatry 1987;50:511.

22. Jensen K, Ranek L, Rosdahl N. Bacterial meningitis. Scand J Infect Dis 1969;1:21.
23. Prasad K, Haines T. Dexamethasone treatment for acute bacterial meningitis: how strong is the evidence for routine use? J Neurol Neurosurg Psychiatry 1995;59:31.
24. Tang L-M. Ventriculoperitoneal shunt in cryptococcal meningitis with hydrocephalus. Surg Neurol 1990;33:314.
25. Eddy VA, Vitsky JL, Rutherford EJ, Morris JA. Aggressive use of ICP monitoring is safe and alters patient care. Am Surg 1995;61:24.
26. Currie BP, Casadevall A. Estimation of the prevalence of cryptococcal infection among HIV infected individuals in New York City. Clin Infect Dis 1994;19:1029.
27. Slavoski LA, Tunkel AR. Review. Therapy of fungal meningitis. Clin Neuropharmacol 1995;18:95.
28. Levitz SM. The ecology of *Cryptococcus neoformans* and the epidemiology of cryptococcosis. Rev Infect Dis 1991;13:1163.
29. Bouza E, Dreyer JS, Hewitt WL, Meyer RD. Coccidioidal meningitis. An analysis of thirty-one cases and review of the literature. Medicine 1981;60:139.
30. Rippon JW. Medical Mycology: The Pathogenic Fungi and the Pathogenic Actinomycetes (3rd ed). Philadelphia: Saunders, 1988;297.
31. Salaki JS, Louira DB, Chmel H. Fungal and yeast infections of the central nervous system. Medicine 1984;63:108.
32. Bronnimann DA, Adam RD, Galgiani JN, et al. Coccidioidomycosis in the acquired immunodeficiency syndrome. Ann Intern Med 1987;106:372.
33. Diamond R. Fungal Meningitis. In HP Lambert (ed), Infections of the Central Nervous System. Philadelphia: Decker, 1991;229–245.
34. Winn WA. The treatment of coccidioidal meningitis. The use of amphotericin B in a group of 25 patients. Med Clin North Am 1963;47:1131.
35. Caudill RG, Smith CE, Reinarz JA. Coccidioidal meningitis: a diagnostic challenge. Am J Med 1970;49:360.
36. Young RC, Bennett JE, Geelhoed GW, Levine AS. Fungemia with compromised host resistance: a study of 70 cases. Ann Intern Med 1974;80:605.
37. Mohandas S, Ahuja GK, Sood VP, Virmani V. Aspergillosis of the central nervous system. J Neurol Sci 1978;38:229.
38. Fetter BF, Klintworth GK, Hendry WS. Mycoses of the Central Nervous System. Baltimore: Williams & Wilkins, 1967.
39. Butler WT, Alling DW, Spickard A, Uts JP. Diagnostic and prognostic value of clinical and laboratory findings in cryptococcal meningitis. N Engl J Med 1964;270:59.
40. Young RC, Bennet JE, Vogel CL, et al. Aspergillosis. The spectrum of disease in 98 patients. Medicine 1970;49:147.
41. Boom WH, Piper DJ, Ruoff KL, Ferraro MJ. New cause for false-positive results with the cryptococcal antigen test by latex agglutination. J Clin Microbiol 1985;22:856.
42. Diamond RD. Cryptococcosis. In GL Mandell, RG Douglas Jr, JE Bennett (eds), Principles and Practice of Infectious Diseases. New York: Churchill Livingstone, 1985;1460–1468.
43. Clark RA, Greer D, Atkinson W, et al. Spectrum of cryptococcus neoformans infection in 68 patients infected with human immunodeficiency virus. Rev Infect Dis 1990;12:768.
44. Diamond RD, Bennett JE. Prognostic factors in cryptococcal meningitis. A study of 111 patients. Ann Intern Med 1974;80:176.
45. Zugar A, Louie E, Holzman RS, et al. Cryptococcal disease in patients with the acquired immunodeficiency syndrome. Diagnostic features and outcome of treatment. Ann Intern Med 1986;104:234.
46. Bennett JE, Dismukes WE, Duma RJ, et al. A comparison of amphotericin B alone and combined with flucytosine in the treatment of cryptococcal meningitis. N Engl J Med 1979;301:126.
47. Dismukes WE, Cloud G, Gallis HA, et al. Treatment of cryptococcal meningitis with combination amphotericin B and flucytosine for four as compared with six weeks. N Engl J Med 1987;317:334.
48. Chuck SL, Sande MA. Infections with *Cryptococcus neoformans* in the acquired immunodeficiency syndrome. N Engl J Med 1989;321:794.
49. Powderly WG, Saag MS, Cloud G, et al. A controlled trial of fluconazole or amphotericin B to prevent relapse of cryptococcal meningitis inpatients with acquired immunodeficiency syndrome. N Engl J Med 1992;326:793.
50. Bayer AS, Edwards JE Jr, Seidel JS, Guze LB. *Candida* meningitis. Report of seven cases and review of the English literature. Medicine 1976;55:477.
51. Lipton SA, Hickey WF, Morris JH, Loscalzo J. *Candida* infection in the central nervous system. Am J Med 1984;76:101.

52. Smego RA, Perfect JR, Durack DT. Combined therapy with amphotericin B and 5-fluorocytosine for *Candida* meningitis. Rev Infect Dis 1984;6:791.
53. Bell BA, Britton JA. Brain Abscess. In HP Lambert (ed), Infections of the Central Nervous System. Philadelphia: Decker, 1991;361–373.
54. Seydoux C, Francioli P. Bacterial brain abscesses: factors influencing mortality and sequelae. Clin Infect Dis 1992;15:394.
55. Ersahin Y, Mutluer S, Guzelbag E. Brain abscess in infants and children. Childs Nerv Syst 1994;10:185.
56. Tsuchiya K, Makita K, Furui S, et al. Contrast-enhanced magnetic resonance imaging of sub- and epidural empyemas. Neuroradiology 1992;34:494.
57. Grossman RI, Yousem DM. Neuroradiology: The Requisites. St. Louis: Mosby–Year Book, 1994.
58. Jungreis CA, Grossman RI. Intracranial Infections and Inflammatory Diseases. In RE Latchaw (ed), MR and CT Imaging of the Head, Neck, and Spine. St. Louis: Mosby–Year Book, 1991;303–346.
59. Lunardi P, Acqui M, Maleci A, et al. Ultrasound-guided brain biopsy: a personal experience with emphasis on its indication. Surg Neurol 1993;39:148.
60. Sjolin J, Lilja A, Eriksson N, et al. Treatment of brain abscess with cefotaxime and metronidazole: prospective study on 15 consecutive patients. Clin Infect Dis 1993;17:857.
61. Danner RL, Hartman BJ. Update on spinal epidural abscess: thirty-five cases and a review of the literature. Rev Infect Dis 1987;9:265.
62. Verner EF, Musher DM. Spinal epidural abscess. Med Clin North Am 1985;69:375.
63. Baker AS, Ojemann RG, Swartz MN, et al. Spinal epidural abscess. N Engl J Med 1975;293:463.
64. Schemtzhard E, Aichner F, Dierck RA. New perspectives in acute spinal epidural abscess. Neurochirurgica 1986;80:105.
65. Bergman I, Wald ER, Meyer JD, et al. Epidural abscess and vertebral osteomyelitis following serial lumbar punctures. Pediatrics 1983;72:476.
66. Heusner AP. Nontuberculous spinal epidural infections. N Engl J Med 1948;239:845.
67. Schulman JA, Blumberg HM. Paraspinal and Spinal Infections. In HP Lambert (ed), Infections of the Central Nervous System. Philadelphia: Decker, 1991;374–390.
68. Kaufman DM, Kaplan JG, Litman N. Infectious agents in epidural abscesses. Neurology 1980;30:844.
69. Byrd BF, Weiner MH, McGee ZA. *Aspergillus* spinal epidural abscess. JAMA 1982;248:3138.
70. DiNubile MJ. Spinal Epidural Abscess. In D Schlossberg (ed), Infection of the Nervous System. New York: Springer–Verlag, 1990;171–178.
71. Bertino RE, Porter BA, Stimak GK, et al. Imaging spinal osteomyelitis and epidural abscess with short T1 inversion recovery. Am J Neuroradiol 1988;9:563.
72. Lang IM, Hughes DG, Jenkins JPR, et al. MR imaging appearances of cervical epidural abscess. Clin Radiol 1995;50:466.
73. Mamourian AC, Dickman CA, Drayer BP, Sonntag VKH. Spinal epidural abscess: three cases following spinal epidural injection demonstrated with magnetic resonance imaging. Anesthesiology 1994;78:204.
74. Sapico FL, Montgomerie JZ. Pyogenic vertebral osteomyelitis: report of nine cases and review of the literature. Rev Infect Dis 1979;1:754.
75. Koppel BS, Tuchman AJ, Mangiardi JR. Epidural spinal infection in intravenous drug users. Arch Neurol 1988;45:1331.
76. Afghani BN, Leiberman JM. Paradoxical enlargement or development of intracranial tuberculomas during therapy: case report and review. Clin Infect Dis 1994;19:1092.
77. Teoh R, Humphries M. Tuberculous Meningitis. In HP Lambert (ed), Infections of the Central Nervous System. Philadelphia: Decker, 1991;189–207.
78. Kioumehr F, Dadsetan MR, Rooholamini SA, et al. Central nervous system tuberculosis: MRI. Neuroradiology 1994;36:95.
79. Shen W-C, Cheng T-Y, Ho Y-J, Lee K-R. Disseminated tuberculomas in spinal cord and brain demonstrated by MRI with gadolinium-DPTA. Neuroradiology 1993;35:213.
80. Berenguer J, Moreno S, Laguna F, et al. Tuberculous meningitis in patients infected with the human immunodeficiency virus. N Engl J Med 1992;326:668.
81. Levine DP. Infections in Intravenous Drug Abusers. In RW Carlson, MA Geheb (eds), Principles and Practice of Medical Intensive Care. Philadelphia: Saunders, 1993;566–579.
82. Selvapandian S, Rajshekhar V, Chandy MJ, Idikula J. Predictive value of computed tomography–based diagnosis of intracranial tuberculomas. Neurosurgery 1994;35:845.
83. Garner CV, Baker AS. Upper Respiratory Tract Infections. In RW Carlson, MA Geheb (eds), Principles and Practice of Medical Intensive Care. Philadelphia: Saunders, 1993;474–480.

84. Eide FF, Gean AD, So YT. Clinical and radiographic findings in disseminated tuberculosis of the brain. Neurology 1993;43:1427.
85. Silman JB, Peters JI, Levine SM, Jenkinson SG. Development of intracranial tuberculomas while receiving therapy for pulmonary fibrosis. Am J Respir Crit Care Med 1994;150:1439.
86. Gupta RK, Pandey R, Khan EM, et al. Intracranial tuberculomas: MRI signal intensity correlation with histopathology and localised proton spectroscopy. Mag Res Imaging 1993;11:443.
87. Preheim LC. Tuberculosis and Other Mycobacterial Infections. In RW Carlson, MA Geheb (eds), Principles and Practice of Medical Intensive Care. Philadelphia: Saunders, 1993;422–433.
88. Downs AG. Arboviruses. In AS Evans (ed), Viral Infections of Humans: Epidemiology and Control. New York: Plenum, 1989;105–132.
89. Reiber H, Lange P. Quantification of virus specific antibodies in cerebrospinal fluid and serum: sensitive and specific detection of antibody synthesis in brain. Clin Chem 1991;37:1153.
90. Koskiniemi M, Vaheri A, Taskinen E. Cerebrospinal fluid alterations in herpes simplex virus encephalitis. Rev Infect Dis 1984;6:608.
91. Longson M. Herpes Simplex. In AJ Zuckerman, JE Banatvala, JR Pattison (eds), Principles and Practice of Clinical Virology. West Sussex, England: Wiley, 1990;2–66.
92. Whitley RJ, Soong SJ, Linneman C Jr, et al, NIAID Collaborative Antiviral Study Group. Herpes simplex encephalitis: clinical assessment. JAMA 1982;247:317.
93. Goldsmith SM, Whitley RJ. Herpes Simplex Encephalitis. In HP Lambert (ed), Infections of the Central Nervous System. Philadelphia: Decker, 1991;283–299.
94. Lakeman FC, Whitley RJ, the National Institute of Allergy and Infectious Diseases Collaborative Antiviral Study Group. Diagnosis of herpes simplex encephalitis: application of polymerase chain reaction to cerebrospinal fluid from brain-biopsied patients and correlation with disease. J Infect Dis 1995;171:857.
95. Shoji H, Koga M, Kusuhara T, et al. Differentiation of herpes simplex virus 1 and 2 in cerebrospinal fluid of patients with HSV encephalitis and meningitis by stringent hybridization of PCR-amplified DNAs. J Neurol 1994;241:526.
96. Dennett C, Klapper PE, Cleator GM, Lewis AG. CSF pretreatment and the diagnosis of herpes encephalitis using the polymerase chain reaction. J Virol Methods 1991;34:101.
97. Rowley AH, Whitley RJ, Lakeman FD, Wolinsky SM. Rapid detection of herpes-simplex-virus DNA in cerebrospinal fluid of patients with herpes simplex encephalitis. Lancet 1990;335:440.
98. Soong S-J, Watson NE, Caddell GR, et al, NIAID Collaborative Antiviral Study Group. Use of brain biopsy for diagnostic evaluation of patients with suspected herpes simplex encephalitis: a statistical model and its clinical applications. J Infect Dis 1991;163:17.
99. Aurelius D, Johansson B, Skoldenberg B, et al. Rapid diagnosis of herpes simplex encephalitis by nested polymerase chain reaction assay of cerebrospinal fluid. Lancet 1991;337:189.
100. Davis JM, Davis KR, Kleinman GM, et al. Computed tomography of herpes simplex encephalitis, with clinicopathological correlation. Radiology 1978;129:409.
101. Schroth G, Gawehn J, Thron A, et al. Early diagnosis of herpes simplex encephalitis by MRI. Neurology 1987;37:179.
102. Lester JW, Carter MP, Reynolds TL. Herpes encephalitis: MR monitoring of response to acyclovir therapy. J Comput Assist Tomogr 1988;12:941.
103. Aminoff MJ. Electroencephalography: General Principles and Clinical Applications. In MJ Aminoff (ed), Electrodiagnosis in Clinical Neurology. New York: Churchill Livingstone, 1986;21–76.
104. Whitley RJ, Soong SJ, Hirsch MS, et al, NIAID Collaborative Antiviral Study Group. Herpes simplex encephalitis: vidarabine therapy and diagnostic problems. N Engl J Med 1981;304:313.
105. Adair JC, Gold M, Bond RE. Acyclovir neurotoxicity: clinical experience and review of the literature. South Med J 1994;87:1227.
106. Whitley RJ. Herpes simplex virus infections of the central nervous system: a review. Am J Med 1988;85:61.
107. Schimdbauer M, Budka H, Pilz P, et al. Presence, distribution and spread of productive varicella zoster virus infection in nervous tissues. Brain 1992;115:383.
108. Tensor RB. Herpes Simplex and Herpes Zoster: Nervous System Involvement. In KP Johnson (ed), Neurologic Clinics: Symposium on Neurovirology. Philadelphia: Saunders, 1984;215–239.
109. Jemsek J, Greenberg SB, Taber L, et al. Herpes zoster–associated encephalitis: clinicopathologic report of 12 cases and review of the literature. Medicine 1983;62:81.
110. Ragozzino MW, Melton LJ III, Kurland LT, et al. Population-based study of herpes zoster and its sequelae. Medicine 1982;61:310.
111. Hogan EL, Krigman MR. Herpes zoster myelitis. Arch Neurol 1973;29:309.
112. Elliot KJ. Other neurological complications of herpes zoster and their management. Ann Neurol 1994;35:S57.

113. Gray F, Belec L, Lescs C, et al. Varicella-zoster virus infection of the central nervous system in the acquired immune deficiency syndrome. Brain 1994;117:987.
114. Chretien F, Gray F, Lescs MC, et al. Acute varicella-zoster virus ventriculitis and meningo-myelo-radiculitis in acquired immunodeficiency syndrome. Acta Neuropathol 1993;86:659.
115. Booss J, Esiri ME. Viral Encephalitis: Pathology, Diagnosis, and Management. Boston: Blackwell Scientific, 1986.
116. Aviel A, Marshak C. Ramsay Hunt syndrome: a cranial polyneuropathy. Am J Otolaryngol 1982;3:61.
117. McKendall RR, HI Klawans. Varicella Zoster Virus Complications. In PJ Vinken, GW Bruyn (eds), Handbook of Clinical Neurology (Vol 34), Infections in the Nervous System. New York: North Holland, 1978;161–173.
118. Gershon A, Steinberg S, Greenberg S, Taber L. Varicella zoster-associated encephalitis: detection of specific antibody in cerebrospinal fluid. J Clin Microbiol 1980;12:764.
119. van Loon AM, van der Logt JTM, Heessen FWA, et al. Antibody-capture enzyme-linked immunosorbent assays that use enzyme-labelled antigen for detection of virus-specific immunoglobulin M, A and G in patients with varicella or herpes zoster. Epidemiol Infect 1992;108:165.
120. Balfour HH, Bean B, Laskin O, et al. Acyclovir halts progression of herpes zoster in immunocompromised patients. N Engl J Med 1983;308:1448.
121. Shepp DH, Dandliker PS, Meyers JD. Treatment of varicella-zoster infection in severely immunocompromised patients. N Engl J Med 1986;314:208.
122. Steele RW, Keeney RE, Bradsher RW, et al. Treatment of varicella-zoster meningoencephalitis with acyclovir—demonstration of virus in cerebrospinal fluid by electron microscopy. Am J Clin Pathol 1983;80:57.
123. Hirsch MS, Schooley RT. Drug therapy. Treatment of herpesvirus infections. N Engl J Med 1983;309:963,1034.
124. Moore M. Enteroviral diseases in the United States. J Infect Dis 1982;146:103.
125. Chonmaitree T, Menegus MA, Powell KR. The clinical relevance of "CSF viral culture." JAMA 1982;247:1843.
126. Rubeiz H, Roos R. Viral meningitis and encephalitis. Semin Neurol 1992;12:165.
127. Wilfert CM, Lehrman SN, Katz SL. Enteroviruses and meningitis. Pediatr Infect Dis J 1983;2:333.
128. Jubelt B. Enterovirus and mumps virus infections of the nervous system. Neurol Clin 1984;2:187.
129. Ratzan KR. Viral meningitis. Med Clin North Am 1985;69:399.
130. Bergstrom T, Vahlne A, Alestig K, et al. Primary and recurrent herpes simplex virus type 2–induced meningitis. J Infect Dis 1990;162:322.
131. Tedder DG, Ashley R, Tyler K, Levin M. Herpes simplex virus infection as a cause of benign recurrent lymphocytic meningitis. Ann Intern Med 1994;121:334.
132. Bachmeyer C, de la Blanchardiere A, Lepercq J, et al. Recurring episodes of meningitis (Mollaret's meningitis) with one showing an association with herpes simplex virus type 2. J Infect Dis 1996;32:247.
133. Cohen BA, Roqley AH, Long CM. Herpes simplex type 2 in a patient with Mollaret's meningitis: demonstration by polymerase chain reaction. Ann Neurol 1994;35:112.
134. Meyers BR, Gurtman AC. The aseptic meningitis syndrome. New York: Springer–Verlag, 1990;31.
135. Centers for Disease Control and Prevention. Lyme disease: United States. JAMA 1996;276:274.
136. Garcia-Monco JC, Benach JL. Lyme neuroborreliosis. Ann Neurol 1995;37:691.
137. Halperin JJ. Neuroborreliosis. Am J Med 1995;98:52S.
138. Keller TL, Halperin JJ, Whitman M. PCR detection of *Borrelia burgdorferi* DNA in cerebrospinal fluid of Lyme neuroborreliosis patients. Neurology 1992;42:32.
139. Luft BJ, Steinman CR, Neimark HC, et al. Invasion of the central nervous system by *Borrelia burgdorferi* in acute disseminated infection. JAMA 1992;267:1364.
140. Halperin JJ, Logigian EL, Finkel MF, Pearl RA. Practice parameters for the diagnosis of patients with nervous system Lyme borreliosis (Lyme disease). Neurology 1996;46:619.
141. Dattwyler RJ, Halperin JJ, Volkman DJ, Luft BJ. Treatment of late Lyme borreliosis—randomized comparison of ceftriaxone and penicillin. Lancet 1988;1:1191.
142. Steere AC, Pachner AR, Malawista SE. Neurologic abnormalities of Lyme disease: successful treatment with high-dose intravenous penicillin. Ann Intern Med 1983;99:767.
143. Pfister HW, Preac-Mursic V, Wilske B, Einhaupl KM. Cefotaxime versus penicillin G for acute neurologic manifestations in Lyme borreliosis: a prospective randomized study. Arch Neurol 1989;46:1190.
144. Mullegger RR, Millner MM, Stanek G, Spork KD. Penicillin G sodium and ceftriaxone in the treatment of neuroborreliosis in children—a prospective study. Infection 1991;19:279.

145. Karlsson M, Hammer-Berggren S, Lindquist L, et al. Comparison of intravenous penicillin G and oral doxycycline for treatment of Lyme neuroborreliosis. Neurology 1994;44:1203.
146. McArthur JC, Cohen BA, Selnes OA, et al. Low prevalence of neurological and neuropsychological abnormalities in otherwise healthy HIV-1–infected individuals: results from the multicenter AIDS cohort study. Ann Neurol 1989;26:601.
147. McArthur JC, Cohen BA, Farzedegan H, et al. Cerebrospinal fluid abnormalities in homosexual men with and without neuropsychiatric findings. Ann Neurol 1988;23(suppl):S34.
148. McArthur JC, Cornblath DR, Welch MA, et al. Identification of mononuclear cells in CSF of patients with HIV infection. Neurology 1989;39:66.
149. Singer EJ, Syndulko K, Tourtellotte WW. Neurodiagnostic Testing in Human Immunodeficiency Virus Infection (Cerebrospinal Fluid). In JR Berger, RM Levy (eds), AIDS and the Nervous System. Philadelphia: Lippincott–Raven, 1997;255–278.
150. Janssen RS, Cornblath DR, Epstein LG, et al. Nomenclature and research case definitions for neurologic manifestations of human immunodeficiency virus–type 1 (HIV-1) infection. Neurology 1991;41:778.
151. Dal Pan GJ, McArthur JC, Harrison MJG. Neurological Symptoms in Human Immunodeficiency Virus Infection. In JR Berger, RM Levy (eds), AIDS and the Nervous System. Philadelphia: Lippincott–Raven, 1997;141–172.
152. Arribas JR, Storch GA, Clifford DB, Tselis AC. Cytomegalovirus encephalitis. Ann Intern Med 1996;125:577.
153. Pizzo PA, Eddy J, Falloon J, et al. Effect of continuous intravenous infusion of zidovudine (AZT) in children with symptomatic HIV infection. N Engl J Med 1988;319:889.
154. Sidtis JJ, Gatsonis C, Price RW, et al, AIDS Clinical Trials Group. Zidovudine treatment of the AIDS dementia complex: results of a placebo-controlled trial. Ann Neurol 1993;33:343.
155. Dreyer EB, Kaiser PK, Offermann JT, Lipton SA. HIV-1 coat protein neurotoxicity prevented by calcium channel antagonists. Science 1990;248:364.
156. Lipton SA, Sucher NJ, Kaiser PK, Dreyer EB. Synergistic effects of HIV coat protein and NMDA receptor–mediated neurotoxicity. Neuron 1991;7:111.
157. Drew WL. Cytomegalovirus infection in patients with AIDS. J Infect Dis 1988;158:449.
158. Cohen BA, Dix RD. Cytomegalovirus and Other Herpesviruses. In JR Berger, RM Levy (eds), AIDS and the Nervous System. Philadelphia: Lippincott–Raven, 1997;595–639.
159. Gallant JE, Moore RD, Richman DD, et al, the Zidovudine Epidemiology Study Group. Incidence and natural history of cytomegalovirus disease in patients with advanced human immunodeficiency virus disease treated with zidovudine. J Infect Dis 1992;166:1223.
160. Fillet AM, Katlama C, Visse B, et al. Human CMV infection of the CNS: concordance between PCR detection in CSF and pathological examination. AIDS 1993;7:1016.
161. Morgello S, Cho E-S, Nielsen S, et al. Cytomegalovirus encephalitis in patients with acquired immunodeficiency syndrome. Hum Pathol 1987;18:289.
162. Holland NR, Power C, Mathews VP, et al. Cytomegalovirus encephalitis in acquired immunodeficiency syndrome (AIDS). Neurology 1994;44:507.
163. Kalayjian RC, Cohen ML, Bonomo RA, Flanigan TP. Cytomegalovirus ventriculoencephalitis in AIDS. Medicine 1993;72:67.
164. Hanson Whiteman ML, Donovan Post MJ, Sklar EML. Neuroimaging of Acquired Immunodeficiency Syndrome. In JR Berger, RM Levy (eds), AIDS and the Nervous System. Philadelphia: Lippincott–Raven, 1997;297–381.
165. Gozlan J, El Amrani M, Baudrimont M, et al. A prospective evaluation of clinical criteria and polymerase chain reaction assay of cerebrospinal fluid for the diagnosis of cytomegalovirus-related neurological diseases during AIDS. AIDS 1995;9:253.
166. Tahseen N, Chuang EL, Berger J, Dix RD. Detection of cytomegalovirus-specific antibody within the cerebrospinal fluid of asymptomatic HIV-infected individuals is associated with intrathecal antibody synthesis (abstract). Invest Ophthalmol Vis Sci 1992;33(suppl):247.
167. Cohen BA, McArthur JC, Grohman S, et al. Neurologic prognosis of cytomegalovirus polyradiculomyelopathy in AIDS. Neurology 1993;43:493.
168. Mahieux F, Gray F, Fenelon G, et al. Acute myeloradiculitis due to cytomegalovirus as the initial manifestation of AIDS. J Neurol Neurosurg Psychiatry 1989;52:270.
169. de Gans J, Tiessens G, Poetegies P, et al. Predominance of polymorphonuclear leukocytes in cerebrospinal fluid of AIDS patients with cytomegalovirus polyradiculitis. J Acq Immune Defic Synd 1990;3:1155.
170. Small PM, McPhaul LW, Sooy DD, et al. Cytomegalovirus infection of the laryngeal nerve presenting as hoarseness in patients with acquired immunodeficiency syndrome. Am J Med 1989;86:108.

171. Behar R, Wiley C, McCutchan JA. Cytomegalovirus polyradiculoneuropathy in acquired immune deficiency syndrome. Neurology 1987;37:557.
172. Fuller GN. Cytomegalovirus and the peripheral nervous system in AIDS. J Acq Immune Defic Synd 1992;5:S33.
173. Oberg B. Antiviral effects of phosphonoformate (PFA, foscarnet sodium). Pharmacol Ther 1983;19:387.
174. AIDS Research Group, AIDS Clinical Trials Group. Mortality in patients with the acquired immunodeficiency syndrome treated with either foscarnet or ganciclovir for cytomegalovirus retinitis. N Engl J Med 1992;326:213.
175. Teich SA, Cheung TW, Friedman AH. Systemic antiviral drugs used in ophthalmology. Surv Ophthalmol 1992;37:19.
176. Enting R, de Gans J, Reiss P, et al. Ganciclovir/foscarnet for cytomegalovirus meningoencephalitis in AIDS. Lancet 1992;340:559.
177. Levy RM, Bredesen DE, Rosenblum ML. Neurological manifestations of the acquired immunodeficiency syndrome (AIDS): experience at UCSF and review of the literature. J Neurosurg 1985;62:475.
178. Mariuz P, Bosler E, Luft BJ. Toxoplasmosis. In JR Berger, RM Levy (eds), AIDS and the Nervous System. Philadelphia: Lippincott–Raven, 1997;641–659.
179. Luft BJ, Remington JS. Toxoplasmic encephalitis in AIDS. Clin Infect Dis 1992;15:211.
180. Navia BA, Petito CK, Gold JWM, et al. Cerebral toxoplasmosis complicating the acquired immune deficiency syndrome: clinical and neuropathological findings in 27 patients. Ann Neurol 1986;19:224.
181. Casado-Naranjo I, Lopez-Trigo J, Ferrandiz A, et al. Hemorrhagic abscess in a patient with the acquired immunodeficiency syndrome. Neuroradiology 1989;31:289.
182. Ciricillo SF, Rosenblum ML. Use of CT and MR imaging to distinguish intracranial lesions and to define the need for biopsy in AIDS patients. J Neurosurg 1990;73:720.
183. Post MJD, Chan JC, Hensley GT, et al. Toxoplasma encephalitis in Haitian adults with acquired immunodeficiency syndrome: a clinical-pathologic-CT correlation. AJR Am J Roentgenol 1983;140:861.
184. Jacobs LD, Cookfair DL, Rudick RA, et al, the Multiple Sclerosis Collaborative Research Group. Intramuscular interferon beta-1a for disease progression in relapsing multiple sclerosis. Ann Neurol 1996;39:285.
185. Hainfellner JA, Budka H. Neuropathology of Human Immunodeficiency Virus Related Opportunistic Infections and Neoplasms. In JR Berger, RM Levy (eds), AIDS and the Nervous System. Philadelphia: Lippincott–Raven, 1997;481–515.
186. Marra C. Distinguishing central nervous system lymphoma from *Toxoplasma* encephalitis. Ann Intern Med 1994;120:812.
187. Carr AD, Brew BJ, Cooper DA. Future Therapy of Human Immunodeficiency Virus Related Neurological Disease. In TR Berger, RM Levy (eds), AIDS and the Nervous System. Philadelphia: Lippincott–Raven, 1997;751–759.
188. Jacobson MA, Besch CL, Child C, et al, the Terry Beirn Community Programs for Clinical Research on AIDS. Primary prophylaxis with pyrimethamine for toxoplasmic encephalitis in patients with advanced human immunodeficiency virus disease: results of a randomized trial. J Infect Dis 1994;169:384.
189. Carr A, Tindall B, Brew BJ, et al. Low-dose trimethoprim-sulfamethoxazole prophylaxis for toxoplasmic encephalitis in patients with AIDS. Ann Intern Med 1992;117:106.
190. Girard P-M, Landman R, Gaudebout C, et al., the PRIO Study Group. Dapsone-pyrimethamine compared with aerosolized pentamidine as primary prophylaxis against *Pneumocystis carinii* pneumonia and toxoplasmosis in HIV infection. N Engl J Med 1993;328:1514.
191. Berger JR, Concha M. Progressive multifocal leukoencephalopathy: the evolution of a disease once considered rare. J Neurovirol 1995;1:5.
192. Major EO, Ameniya K, Tornatore CS, et al. Pathogenesis and molecular biology of progressive multifocal leukoencephalopathy, the JC virus–induced demyelinating disease of the human brain. Clin Microbiol Rev 1992;5:49.
193. Berger JR, Gallo RV, Concha M. Progressive Multifocal Leukoencephalopathy. In JR Berger, RM Levy (eds), AIDS and the Nervous System. Philadelphia: Lippincott–Raven, 1997;569–594.
194. Tornatore C, Berger JR, Houff SA, et al. Detection of JC virus DNA in peripheral lymphocytes from patients with and without progressive multifocal leukoencephalopathy. Ann Neurol 1992;31:454.
195. Walker D, Padgett BL. The Epidemiology of Human Polyomaviruses. In JL Sever, D Madden (eds), Polyomaviruses and Human Neurological Diseases. New York: Alan R. Liss, 1983;99–106.

196. von Einsiedel RW, Fife TD, Aksamit AJ, et al. Progressive multifocal leukoencephalopathy in AIDS: a clinicopathologic study and review of the literature. J Neurol 1993;240:391.

197. Kuchelmeister K, Gullotta F, Bergmann M, et al. Progressive multifocal leukoencephalopathy (PML) in the acquired immunodeficiency syndrome (AIDS). Pathol Res Pract 1993;189:163.

198. Brooks BR, Walker DL. Progressive multifocal leukoencephalopathy. Neurol Clin 1984;2:299.

199. Krupp LB, Lipton RB, Swerdlow ML, et al. Progressive multifocal leukoencephalopathy: clinical and radiographic features. Ann Neurol 1985;17:344.

200. Mark AS, Atlas SW. Progressive multifocal leukoencephalopathy in patients with AIDS: appearance on MR images. Neuroradiology 1989;173:517.

201. Karahalios D, Breit R, Dal Canto MC, Levy RM. Progressive multifocal leukoencephalopathy in patients with HIV infection: lack of impact of early diagnosis by stereotactic brain biopsy. J Acq Immune Defic Synd 1992;5:1030.

202. Post MJD, Sheldon JJ, Hensley GT, et al. Central nervous system disease in acquired immunodeficiency syndrome: prospective correlation using CT, MR imaging, and pathologic studies. Radiology 1986;158:141.

203. Whiteman MLH, Post MJD, Berger JR, et al. Progressive multifocal leukoencephalopathy in 47 HIV-seropositive patients: neuroimaging with clinical and pathologic correlation. Radiology 1993;187:233.

204. Itoyama Y, Webster H de F, Sternberger NH, et al. Distribution of papovavirus, myelin-associated glycoprotein, and myelin basic protein in progressive multifocal leukoencephalopathy lesions. Ann Neurol 1982;11:396.

205. Aksamit AJ, Major EO, Ghatak NR, et al. Diagnosis of progressive multifocal leukoencephalopathy by brain biopsy with biotin labeled DNA: DNA in situ hybridization. J Neuropath Exp Neurol 1987;46:556.

206. Rand KH, Johnson KP, Rubinstein LJ, et al. Adenine arabinoside in the treatment of progressive multifocal leukoencephalopathy: use of virus-containing cells in the urine to assess response to therapy. Ann Neurol 1977;1:458.

207. Peters ACB, Versteeg J, Bots GTAM, et al. Progressive multifocal leukoencephalopathy: immunofluorescent demonstration of simian virus 40 antigen in CSF cells and response to cytarabine therapy. Arch Neurol 1980;37:497.

208. Marriott PJ, O'Brien MD, Mackenzie CK, Janota I. Progressive multifocal leucoencephalopathy: remission with cytarabine. J Neurol Neurosurg Psychiatry 1975;38:205.

209. Steiger MJ, Tarnesby G, McLaughlin J, Schapira AHV. Successful outcome of progressive multifocal leukoencephalopathy with cytarabine and interferon. Ann Neurol 1993;33:407.

210. Portegies P, Algra PR, Hollak CEM, et al. Response to cytarabine in progressive multifocal leucoencephalopathy in AIDS. Lancet 1991;337:680.

211. Conomy JP, Beard S, Matsumoto H, Roessmann U. Cytarabine treatment of progressive multifocal leukoencephalopathy. JAMA 1974;229:1313.

212. Rauer WR, Turel AP, Johnson KP. Progressive multifocal leukoencephalopathy and cytarabine. JAMA 1973;226:174.

213. Tada H, Rappaport J, Lashgari M, et al. Trans-activation of the JC virus late promoter by the tat protein of type 1 human immunodeficiency virus in glial cells. Proc Natl Acad Sci U S A 1990;87:3479.

214. Ahmed S, Rappaport J, Tada H, et al. A nuclear protein derived from brain cells stimulates transcription of the human neurotropic virus promoter, JCVE, in vitro. J Biol Chem 1990;265:13899.

215. Ahmed S, Chowdhury M, Khalili K. Regulation of a human neurotropic virus promoter JCVE: identification of a novel activator domain located upstream from the 98 bp enhancer promoter region. Nucleic Acids Res 1990;18:7417.

216. Henson J, Saffer J, Furneaux H. The transcription factor Sp1 binds to the JC virus promoter and is selectively expressed in glial cells in human brain. Ann Neurol 1992;32:72.

13
Central Nervous System Complications of Critical Medical Illness

Barnett R. Nathan and Thomas P. Bleck

The general acceptance and understanding that neurologic disorders occur frequently in the setting of critical medical illness have emerged since the 1980s, although historically both Osler in 1892 [1] and Olsen in 1956 [2] noted weakness after sepsis and Bright described septic encephalopathy in 1827 [3]. The neurologic complications observed in critical illness fall into two major categories: central nervous system (CNS) dysfunction and dysfunction of the peripheral nervous system, including abnormalities of peripheral nerves and muscles. The etiology of these disorders is being investigated and debated and likely is multifactorial. It stands to reason, however, that the same mechanisms that contribute to multiorgan failure in sepsis also contribute to the dysfunction of the nervous system. In fact "brain failure" in sepsis conveys a similar additive mortality to sepsis as do other organ failures [4].

These neurologic disorders are quite common but tend to be under-recognized. In a 2-year prospective study of neurologic complications of critical illnesses in a combined medical intensive care unit (MICU)–coronary care unit, 217 patients of a total of 1,758 nonneurologic admissions had major CNS dysfunction [5]. Of these neurologic problems, encephalopathy was the most frequent (62 patients, or 28.6%), and among these, septic encephalopathy was the most common etiology (19 patients, or 31% of the encephalopathic group) [6]. Conversely, an easily detected encephalopathy developed in 21% of all septic patients. Because the case definition for septic encephalopathy excluded patients with severe coexisting hepatic or renal dysfunction, the actual contribution of sepsis to encephalopathy is likely greater.

Neurologic problems, particularly encephalopathies and neuromuscular disorders, which can arise during the course of an ICU stay, can impede weaning from mechanical ventilation. Kelly and Matthay [7] prospectively studied 66 consecutive adult patients who required mechanical ventilation for more than 48 hours to determine the reasons for their ventilatory problems. Neurologic problems, primarily encephalopathies, were held responsible for the continuing need for ventilatory support in 32% of the patients and contributed to this problem in another 41%. Although this study was not directed at patients who were not weaned after resolution of their presenting disease, it does highlight the role of neurologic problems early in critical illness.

Neuromuscular complications of the critically ill have a less certain epidemiology. Spitzer and associates [8] studied 21 critically ill patients who were not weaned after their presenting disease had improved to the point that their intensivists believed that mechanical ventilation should no longer have been necessary. Thirteen (62%) of these patients had a neuromuscular disorder that was either the major cause of or contributed substantially to their ventilatory problems. Only 7 of these 13 patients had critical illness polyneuropathy; other neuropathic conditions and unsuspected motor neuron disease were also uncovered. In contrast, Witt and colleagues [9], in a prospective study of 43 patients with multiorgan failure caused by sepsis, found electrophysiologic evidence of a sensorimotor axonal neuropathy in 70%. Fifteen of these patients required prolonged mechanical ventilation because of this neuropathy.

It is therefore important for the general intensivist, the neurologic intensivist, and the neurology consultant to understand and recognize these complications of critical medical illness. The cost—monetary, physical, and psychological—is significant, and although most of the syndromes discussed here are reversible if recognized early, failure to do so in an expedient manner can result in significant morbidity or death.

This chapter deals with CNS dysfunction as a complication of critical medical illness (peripheral nervous system complications are discussed in Chapter 4). CNS dysfunction in the critical care unit is most often manifested by altered mental status or coma. The differential for this includes septic encephalopathy, likely the most common cause in the MICU [10], as well as use of sedative medications, hypoxic-ischemic encephalopathy, bihemispheric or brain stem strokes, and severe metabolic (as reviewed by Chen and Young [11]) or endocrine derangements (hypoglycemia, diabetic ketoacidosis, acute uremia). In surgical units, cholesterol or fat emboli and traumatic head injury (hemorrhages or axonal shear injury) in addition to the preceding are also common.

SEPTIC ENCEPHALOPATHY

Septic encephalopathy was first described early in the nineteenth century. With increasing survival of septic patients, however, it has become more clinically relevant and a subject of research. In 1990, Young and associates [10] investigated this disorder in a prospective manner in patients admitted to a university MICU. The patients included in the study all were septic as defined by fever and positive blood cultures and were excluded if they had pre-existing brain disease, had received sedation, or had pulmonary, hepatic, or renal failure. Sixty-nine patients fit the inclusion criteria. The patients were classified as not encephalopathic, mildly encephalopathic, or severely encephalopathic. Thirty-two patients were classified as severely encephalopathic, and 53% of these died. Seventeen were mildly encephalopathic and 35% died, whereas 20 were classified as not encephalopathic, with none of these patients dying. White blood cell count, Po_2, blood urea nitrogen, creatinine, bilirubin, alkaline phosphatase, and potassium all had a linear relationship with the magnitude of the encephalopathy.

More recently, in a prospective study from Israel [12], patients with septic encephalopathy were selected according to criteria that included temperature, heart rate, respiratory rate, and hypotension or signs of systemic hypoperfusion, or both. In this study of 50 patients, encephalopathy was associated with an increase in mortality when graded by the Glasgow coma score; a score of 15 had 16% mortality, 13–14 had 20%, 9–12 had 50%, and 3–8 had 63% mortality (p <.05). Bacteremia was associated with encephalopathy (p <.001); 13% of septic patients without encephalopathy versus 59% of patients with encephalopathy had bacteremia. Similar to the previous study, patients with septic encephalopathy had elevated blood urea nitrogen and bilirubin and a higher incidence of renal failure.

The pathophysiology of septic encephalopathy is an area of intense interest. Inflammatory mediators seen in sepsis can damage the blood-brain barrier [13], and such disruption has been demonstrated in an animal model of early sepsis [14], allowing for the potential influx of cytokines and interferons into the CNS. Cytokines can affect behavior, and these effects vary with the neuroanatomic structures affected and the particular cytokine but include somnolence when injected into the locus ceruleus [15]. Interferons can also alter cortical and hippocampal neuronal activity, suggesting the potential for effects on memory and emotion [16]. The behavioral consequences of increased alertness secondary to beta-adrenergic compounds is well known. Beta-adrenergic concentrations are reduced in an experimental model of sepsis in the forebrain and brain stem [17], perhaps implicating epinephrine and norepinephrine in septic encephalopathy.

Brain dysfunction may also be a result of abnormal systemic metabolism. Mizock and associates [18] detected altered metabolism of phenylalanine in the cerebrospinal fluid (CSF) and blood in 11 patients with septic encephalopathy; in contrast, their patients with hepatic encephalopathy demonstrated elevated CSF concentrations of many other aromatic amino acids. Others have reported elevated serum concentrations of phenylalanine, ammonia, and tryptophan in encephalopathic septic patients, compared with infected patients with normal mental status, along with lower concentrations of isoleucine [19]. The significance of these studies in the pathogenesis of septic encephalopathy remains uncertain.

Recovery of CNS function appears to be complete if the patient survives, but the condition can mask other intracranial processes (e.g., hypoxic-ischemic encephalopathy, watershed infarcts, intracranial hemorrhages).

HEPATIC ENCEPHALOPATHY

In fulminant hepatic failure (FHF), malignantly increased intracranial pressure (ICP) is the major cause of death in patients awaiting transplantation [20,21]. Those whose ICP has been elevated may survive a transplant but be left with CNS deficits [22]. Development of cerebral edema in FHF is related to the stage of encephalopathy; its mechanism is uncertain [23], but it has been shown to be primarily vasogenic [24]. Autoregulation is impaired in FHF and can be demonstrated by transcranial Doppler studies [25]. This impairment of autoregulation may be a result of altered sensitivity to carbon dioxide [26], and this in turn adversely affects cerebral blood flow. The malignant cerebral edema requires aggressive treatment; steroids are not effective, but mannitol is useful [27]. Hyperventilation had previously been thought to increase mortality, but a controlled trial demonstrated its usefulness [28]. Xenon computed tomographic and positron emission tomography data, however, raise the possibility that cerebral ischemia may develop in at least some FHF patients as a result of their elevated ICP, and that this is worsened by hyperventilation [29]. At present, mannitol should be the initial treatment, with hyperventilation used if this drug fails to control ICP [30]. High-dose barbiturates may be useful if mannitol and hyperventilation do not control ICP [31]. A semiquantitative study suggests that computed tomographic scan measurement of the effects of brain edema on ventricular and cisternal dimensions can identify those at risk for elevated ICP [21]. Although it carries a small risk of intracerebral hemorrhage because of the patient's coagulopathy [32], there is no current substitute for invasive ICP monitoring in patients with FHF who are in grade 3 (stuporous) or grade 4 (comatose) states. ICP monitoring should be provided through the liver transplant operation and into the first few postoperative days [33].

Patients with FHF may also have elevated levels of apparently endogenous 1,4-benzodiazepines [34], and there are statistically significant increases in benzodiazepine receptors in the thalamus, but not the cortex, of FHF patients [35]. This may help explain stupor or coma in those FHF patients who do not have ICP elevations. Chronic hepatic encephalopathy does not appear to cause ICP elevation unless other intracranial processes occur, such as bleeding. As in FHF, endogenous benzodiazepine-like compounds (gamma-aminobutyric acid A agonists) likely play a major, if not dominant, role [36], and the use of gamma-aminobutyric acid antagonists is being actively investigated but has not yet become standard practice. Some double-blind, crossover studies of flumazenil suggest that the response rate is between 25% and 50% [37,38] in patients with chronic hepatic encephalopathy.

UREMIC ENCEPHALOPATHY

The presence of renal failure during or as a result of sepsis is a common occurrence, and therefore the encephalopathy associated with kidney failure may be masked.

The actual toxins involved in uremic encephalopathy remain debated, but several lines of evidence suggest that acute renal failure interferes with brain Na^+-K^+ adenosine triphosphatase function and that the accumulation of parathyroid hormone may also be important [39]. Other metabolic encephalopathies are common in patients with renal failure, as well as structural lesions (e.g., chronic subdural hematoma related to poor platelet function or heparinization for dialysis).

GLUCOSE DISORDERS

Hypoglycemia or hyperglycemia can produce or exacerbate focal neurologic deficits in addition to encephalopathy. This provides an important diagnostic clue as to the etiology of the encephalopathy. Nonketotic hyperglycemia is common in the critically ill patient, and treatment is primarily fluid replacement and insulin as needed. The major neurologic effects of hyperglycemic disorders are osmotic, and despite the hyperosmolar state, these patients are tremendously volume depleted. Fluid resuscitation should be given with normal saline until the blood pressure is normal. After that, one can calculate the water deficit and replace it over a day or two.

DISORDERS OF OSMOLALITY AND SODIUM

Although many hypo-osmolar states in critically ill patients are due to the syndrome of inappropriate antidiuretic hormone (SIADH), to assume this without appropriate evaluation is not only misleading but may be dangerous. Patients with subarachnoid hemorrhage or head trauma may have SIADH, but one must also consider "cerebral salt wasting" (potentially caused by an interaction between atrial natriuretic factor and antidiuretic hormone) and pseudohyponatremia from hyperglycemia or lipid disorders. Fluid-restricting hyponatremic patients with subarachnoid hemorrhage, for example, results in an increased likelihood of cerebral infarction and death [40]. Measurement of serum and urine osmolalities is crucial, along with a clinical assessment of volume status.

In most patients with CNS symptoms due to hypo-osmolality, making relatively small biochemical improvements quickly produces clinical improvement. Thus, patients with seizures related to hyponatremia (as a surrogate marker for osmolality) usually stop seizing with a modest rise in the serum sodium. This can frequently be produced by normal saline infusion along with a loop diuretic (e.g., furosemide) to lower urine osmolality. Whether central pontine myelinolysis is caused by rapid correction of hyponatremia or the severity and acuteness of the initial development of the hypo-osmolality remains hotly debated. Arieff and Ayus [41] believe that the severity of hyponatremia rather than the rate of correction is the relevant issue, and that hyponatremia should be rapidly corrected with 3% saline to prevent CNS complications.

We believe that 3% saline is only necessary for slowly developing hypo-osmolality in the setting of SIADH or cerebral salt wasting when furosemide administration is unable to lower the urine osmolality below 250 mOsm/liter. The suggestion that the serum osmolality should not be raised by more than 10 mOsm/liter per day is appropriate here as well; this represents a slower rate of correction than has been recommended previously [42].

A rare Arieff-type syndrome may exist in which very rapidly developing hypo-osmolality (<24 hours) leads to rapid brain swelling and the sequelae of ICP problems, but this is probably an uncommon occurrence. This syndrome should concentrate on reduction of ICP, using hypertonic fluids as one of the modalities but with ICP reduction as the goal, rather than a target osmolality or sodium concentration. For hyponatremia that develops over a few days to weeks, the brain appears to respond by losing solute, and ICP elevation is not the problem. In these cases, which make up the majority, rapidly correcting the serum hypo-osmolality is dangerous and is the cause of central pontine myelinolysis (as reviewed by Laureno and Karp [43]). There is no benefit to the patient in correcting the osmolality more rapidly than 10 mOsm/liter per day.

CALCIUM, MAGNESIUM, AND PHOSPHORUS DISTURBANCES

Hypercalcemia, at one time an important cause of undiagnosed coma, now seldom even reaches neurologic attention, because it is detected so early. Hypocalcemia is often blamed for a variety of CNS disturbances, including seizures, but this diagnosis may be overestimated beyond the neonatal period. Parathyroid hormone may in fact be epileptogenic and thus be responsible for some seizures that occur in patients with abnormal free calcium. The total serum calcium concentration cannot be reliably corrected for abnormalities in serum protein concentrations; therapeutic decisions should be based on ionized calcium determinations [44]. Hypermagnesemia produces stupor or coma (usually in patients with renal failure). Serum concentrations above 8 mEq/liter can produce neuromuscular junction blockade. Hypophosphatemia and phosphorus depletion have been implicated in a wide range of neurologic disorders [45].

THYROID AND ADRENAL DISORDERS

Previously undiagnosed hyperthyroidism occasionally presents in the ICU as thyroid storm and can cause coma, although the mechanism is obscure. Unsuspected hypothyroidism is much more common. One should remember to consider the possibilities of coexisting adrenal or coronary artery disease when beginning thyroid replacement. Addison's disease may go undiagnosed for some time in critically ill patients who are kept volume repleted; the CNS disturbances are frequently related to the concomitant hypoglycemia or delayed metabolism of sedative agents.

MEDICATIONS

Medications are a major confounding variable in the analysis of mental status in critically ill patients. Because renal and hepatic functions are typically impaired in the critically ill, the metabolism and clearance of hypnotic or sedative agents (e.g., benzodiazepines) are usually slowed. The long period of administration of these drugs in these patients results in accumulation of the compounds and their metabolites, resulting in large peripheral stores that must be cleared before their CNS effects will abate. This includes compounds marketed as short-acting, such as midazolam and propofol, which nevertheless can accumulate during prolonged treatment. There may, however, be useful differences among these agents in the rapidity of awakening after discontinuation of the infusion [46]. In the differential diagnosis of encephalopathy in these patients, medication effects must be considered. Although some might administer flumazenil as a diagnostic challenge in this setting [47], the possibility of triggering seizures or status epilepticus suggests that this be limited to situations in which the information to be gained outweighs the risk involved. In addition, because some cases of chronic hepatic encephalopathy also respond to flumazenil [37,38], awakening after administration of this drug is not proof that encephalopathy was due to medications.

In practice, it is difficult to distinguish medication effects from the direct cerebral effects of sepsis, metabolic disarray, hypoxia, or hypotension or the indirect effects of hepatic or renal dysfunction. Because some of the medications have predictable electroencephalographic effects, as do some of the other conditions, an electroencephalogram may be useful. Measurement of serum concentrations, however, is rarely available in an appropriate time frame. Discontinuing the potentially offending agent and observing the patient often represent the most prudent course of action.

NEUROLEPTIC MALIGNANT SYNDROME

Neuroleptic malignant syndrome (NMS) is another complication of medication administration in the ICU. It is a rare complication of treatment with dopamine antagonist drugs and is characterized by rigidity, fever, abnormal mental status, and autonomic dysfunction. Creatine kinase is usually elevated. Haloperidol is one of the most common instigators of this syndrome, but other drugs commonly used in an ICU setting, such as prochlorperazine [48] and metoclopramide [49], have been associated with NMS. NMS has been reported in a trauma patient who received haloperidol and droperidol for severe agitation and was treated successfully with dantrolene sodium [50] and in a head-injured patient [51]. In a case-controlled study of psychiatric patients with NMS, they were more likely to be agitated or dehydrated before the development of NMS [52]. The newer dopamine antagonists, such as risperidone and clozapine, have also been associated with NMS [53,54]. The incidence rate of NMS is approximately 2% of all patients who receive neuroleptics, whereas the overall mortality is in excess of 10–20%. Treatment includes discontinuation of the offending medication, hydration, supportive care (which may include mechanical ventilation), and, if symptoms are severe enough, treatment with either bromocriptine or dantrolene. The therapeutic success of plasmapheresis has been reported in a case of NMS in which conventional therapy had failed [55].

SEIZURES

The incidence of seizures in an ICU is similar to that of metabolic encephalopathies, accounting for almost 30% of all neurologic complications in an MICU, with 10% of these developing status epilepticus [5]. Similar results have been obtained in a pediatric ICU, with seizures developing in a little more than 20% of ventilator-dependent patients [56]. Conversely, in a Mayo Clinic study over a 9-year period, 213 of more than 27,000 (0.8%) patients admitted to the ICU had at least one episode of a generalized seizure. Almost 50% (103) of these patients had a previous seizure history [57]. Drug toxicity and drug withdrawal (i.e., alcohol, narcotics) can incite seizures in a patient with no known seizure history. Additionally, seizures can occur in the face of new cerebrovascular disease or as the result of metabolic derangements as discussed in Disorders of Osmolality and Sodium and Calcium, Magnesium, and Phosphorus

Disturbances. In treating seizures in the ICU, we recommend first evaluating for metabolic derangements or drug withdrawal and treating these conditions, and then, if the seizures are still a clinical concern, treating with anticonvulsants. Continuous electroencephalographic monitoring in the ICU setting may also be of value.

CONCLUSIONS

CNS problems and complications in critically ill patients are relatively common and can have a negative impact on the patient's outcome and length of hospital stay. The ability to recognize, diagnose, and treat these entities is important in the care and prognosis of these patients. Research is moving forward in our understanding of the neurologic complications of severe illness, and the hope is that in the future better diagnostic and treatment options will be available.

REFERENCES

1. Osler W. The Principles and Practice of Medicine, Designed for the Use of Practitioners and Students of Medicine. New York: D. Appleton, 1892;14.
2. Olsen C. Lesions of peripheral nerves developing during coma. JAMA 1956;160:39.
3. Bright R. Reports of Medical Cases Selected with a View of Illustrating the Symptoms and Cure of Diseases, with a Reference to Morbid Anatomy. London: Longman, Rees, Orme, Brown and Green, 1827;178.
4. Knaus W, Wagner D, Draper E: APACHE III prognostic system. Risk prediction of hospital mortality for critically ill patients. Chest 1991;100:1619.
5. Bleck T, Smith M, Pierre-Louis J, et al. Neurologic complications of critical medical illnesses. Crit Care Med 1993;21:98.
6. Bleck T. Neurologic Complications of Critical Illness. In A Ropper (ed), Neurological and Neurosurgical Intensive Care. New York: Raven, 1993;193–201.
7. Kelly B, Matthay M. Prevalence and severity of neurologic dysfunction in critically ill patients. Influence on need for continued mechanical ventilation. Chest 1993;104:1818.
8. Spitzer A, Giancarlo T, Maher L, et al. Neuromuscular causes of prolonged ventilator dependency. Muscle Nerve 1992;15:682.
9. Witt N, Zochodne D, Bolton C. Peripheral nerve function in sepsis and multiple organ failure. Chest 1991;99:176.
10. Young G, Bolton C, Austin T, et al. The encephalopathy associated with septic illness. Clin Invest Med 1990;13:297.
11. Chen R, Young GB. Metabolic encephalopathies. Baillieres Clin Neurol 1996;5:577.
12. Eidelman LA, Putterman D, Putterman C, Sprung CL. The spectrum of septic encephalopathy. Definitions, etiologies, and mortalities. JAMA 1996;275:470.
13. Quagliarello V, Wispelwey B, Long WJ, Scheld W. Recombinant human interleukin-1 induces meningitis and blood-brain barrier injury in the rat. Characterization and comparison with tumor necrosis factor. J Clin Invest 1991;87:1360.
14. du Moulin GC, Paterson D, Hedley-White J, Broitman SA. E. coli peritonitis and bacteremia cause increased blood-brain barrier permeability. Brain Res 1985;340:261.
15. De Sarro G, Masuda Y, Ascioti C, et al. Behavioural and ECoG spectrum changes induced by intracerebral infusion of interferons and interleukin 2 in rats are antagonized by naloxone. Neuropharmacology 1990;29:167.
16. Reyes-Vazquez C, Prieto-Gomez B, Georgiades J, Dafny N. Alpha and gamma interferons' effects on cortical and hippocampal neurons: microiontophoretic application and single cell recording. Int J Neurosci 1984;25:113.

17. Kadoi Y, Saito S, Kunimoto F, et al. Impairment of the brain beta-adrenergic system during experimental endotoxemia. J Surg Res 1996;61:496.
18. Mizock B, Sabelli H, Dubin A. Septic encephalopathy. Evidence for altered phenylalanine metabolism and comparison with hepatic encephalopathy. Arch Intern Med 1990;150:443.
19. Sprung C, Cerra F, Freund H. Amino acid alterations and encephalopathy in the sepsis syndrome. Crit Care Med 1991;19:753.
20. Nora L, Bleck T. Increased intracranial pressure complicating hepatic failure. J Crit Illness 1989;4:87.
21. Wijdicks EFM, Plevak D, Rakela J, Wiesner R. Clinical and radiologic features of brain edema in fulminant hepatic failure. Mayo Clin Proc 1995;70:119.
22. O'Brien C, Wise R, O'Grady J, Williams R. Neurological sequelae in patients recovered from fulminant hepatic failure. Gut 1987;28:93.
23. Zaki A, Ede R, Davis M. Experimental studies of blood brain barrier permeability in acute hepatic failure. Hepatology 1984;4:359.
24. Kato M, Hughes R, Keays R, Williams R. Electron microscopic study of brain capillaries in cerebral edema from fulminant hepatic failure. Hepatology 1992;15:1060.
25. Strauss G, Adel Hansen B, Kirkegaard P, et al. Liver function, cerebral blood flow autoregulation, and hepatic encephalopathy in fulminant hepatic failure. Hepatology 1997;25:837.
26. Gazzard B, Portmann B, Murray-Lyon I, Williams R. Causes of death in fulminant hepatic failure and the relationship to quantitative histological assessment of parenchymal damage. QJM 1975;44:615.
27. Canalese J, Gimson A, Davis C. Controlled trial of dexamethasone and mannitol for the cerebral oedema of fulminant hepatic failure. Gut 1982;23:625.
28. Ede R, Gimson A, Bihari D, Williams R. Controlled hyperventilation in the prevention of cerebral oedema in fulminant hepatic failure. J Hepatol 1986;2:43.
29. Wendon J, Harrison P, Keays R, Williams R. Cerebral blood flow and metabolism in fulminant hepatic failure. Hepatology 1994;19:1407.
30. Bleck T. Neurologic consequences of fulminant hepatic failure. Mayo Clin Proc 1995;70:195.
31. Forbes A, Alexander G, O'Grady J. Thiopental infusion in the treatment of intracranial hypertension complicating fulminant hepatic failure. Hepatology 1989;10:306.
32. Blei A, Olafsson S, Webster S, Levy R. Complications of intracranial pressure monitoring in fulminant hepatic failure. Lancet 1993;341:157.
33. Keays R, Potter D, O'Grady J. Intracranial and cerebral perfusion pressure changes before, during and immediately after orthotopic liver transplantation for fulminant hepatic failure. QJM 1991;79:425.
34. Basile A, Hughes R, Harrison P. Elevated brain concentrations of 1,4-benzodiazepines in fulminant hepatic failure. N Engl J Med 1991;325:473.
35. Macdonald GA, Frey KA, Agranoff BW, et al. Cerebral benzodiazepine receptor binding in vivo in patients with recurrent hepatic encephalopathy. Hepatology 1997;26:277.
36. Jones E, Skolnick P, Gamal S. The gamma-amino-butyric acid A (GABAA) receptor complex and hepatic encephalopathy. Ann Intern Med 1989;110:532.
37. Gyr K, Meier R, Haussler J, et al. Evaluation of the efficacy and safety of flumazenil in the treatment of portal systemic encephalopathy: a double blind, randomised, placebo controlled multicentre study. Gut 1996;39:319.
38. Pomier-Layrargues G, Giguere J, Lavoie J. Flumazenil in cirrhotic patients in hepatic coma: a randomized double-blind placebo-controlled crossover trial. Hepatology 1994;19:32.
39. Fraser C. Neurologic Manifestations of the Uremic State. In A Arieff, R Griggs (eds), Metabolic Dysfunction in Systemic Disorders. Boston: Little, Brown, 1992;139–166.
40. Wijdicks EFM, Vermeulen M, ten Haaf J. Volume depletion and natriuresis in patients with a ruptured intracranial aneurysm. Ann Neurol 1985;18:211.
41. Arieff A, Ayus J. Treatment of symptomatic hyponatremia: neither haste nor waste. Crit Care Med 1991;19:748.
42. Bleck T. Metabolic Encephalopathy. In W Weiner (ed), Emergent and Urgent Neurology. Philadelphia: Lippincott, 1991;27–57.
43. Laureno R, Karp BI. Myelinolysis after correction of hyponatremia [see comments]. Ann Intern Med 1997;126:57.
44. Zaloga G, Chernow B. Hypocalcemia in critical illness. JAMA 1986;256:1924.
45. Knochel J, Montanari A. Central Nervous System Manifestations of Hypophosphatemia and Phosphorus Depletion. In A Arieff, R Griggs (eds), Metabolic Dysfunction in Systemic Disorders. Boston: Little, Brown, 1992;183–204.
46. Ronan K, Gallagher T, George B, Hamby B. Comparison of propofol and midazolam for sedation in intensive care unit patients. Crit Care Med 1995;23:286.

47. Bauer T, Ritz R, Haberthur C. Prolonged sedation due to accumulation of conjugated metabolites of midazolam. Lancet 1995;346:145.
48. Pesola GR, Quinto C. Prochlorperazine-induced neuroleptic malignant syndrome. J Emerg Med 1996;14:727.
49. Friedman L, Weinrauch L, D'Elia J. Metoclopramide-induced neuroleptic malignant syndrome. Arch Intern Med 1987;147:1495.
50. Burke C, Fulda GJ, Castellano J. Neuroleptic malignant syndrome in a trauma patient [see comments]. J Trauma 1995;39:796.
51. Perez-Vela JL, Sanchez Casado M, Sanchez–Izquierdo Riera JA, et al. Neuroleptic malignant syndrome in a patient with head injury. Intensive Care Med 1996;22:593.
52. Sachdev P, Mason C, Hadzi–Pavlovic D. Case-control study of neuroleptic malignant syndrome. Am J Psychiatry 1997;154:1156.
53. Meterissian GB. Risperidone-induced neuroleptic malignant syndrome: a case report and review. Can J Psychiatry—Revue Canadienne de Psychiatrie 1996;41:52.
54. Chatterton R, Cardy S, Schramm TM. Neuroleptic malignant syndrome and clozapine monotherapy [see comments]. Aust N Z J Psychiatry 1996;30:692.
55. Gaitini L, Fradis M, Vaida S, et al. Plasmapheresis in neuroleptic malignant syndrome [see comments]. Anaesthesia 1997;52:165.
56. Tasker R, Boyd S, Harden A, et al. The clinical significance of seizures in critically ill young infants requiring intensive care. Neuropediatrics 1991;22:129.
57. Wijdicks EFM, Sharbrough F. New onset seizures in critically ill patients. Neurology 1993;43:1042.

14
Pediatric Neurologic Critical Care

Fenella Kirkham

SIMILARITIES AND DIFFERENCES FROM ADULT NEUROLOGIC INTENSIVE CARE

Many conditions commonly seen in pediatric neurointensive care are very similar to adult diseases, with an adjustment in dosage being the only difference in management. However, a number of diseases present with acute neurologic manifestations that are unique to children or are very uncommon in adults. In addition, in a number of children with systemic conditions, such as congenital heart disease or renal problems, neurologic disorders develop as a complication, and management may have to be modified because of the underlying disease process. This chapter provides an overview of the diagnostic and therapeutic approach to children with neurologic disorders that are potentially fatal and that also may have profound long-term effects on the quality of life for the child and his or her family.

NEONATAL NEUROLOGIC INTENSIVE CARE

Birth Asphyxia

Term, preterm, and particularly post-term babies are at risk of birth asphyxia if they experience significant hypoxia or ischemia, or both, although many neonates born after apparently equally difficult deliveries have no short- or long-term sequelae. A low Apgar score at 5 minutes and a low umbilical cord pH are more likely to be abnormal in those infants who have had a significant insult, but in term babies, the most useful guide to the severity of the asphyxial insult, which often occurs pre- or intrapartum rather than at the time of delivery, is the severity of the postnatal encephalopathy and, in particular, whether seizures occur [1]. Severe birth asphyxia leads to multiorgan failure, and death often occurs from renal failure or severe respiratory difficulties. The main long-term sequela is cerebral palsy, either spastic quadriparesis (usually with cognitive and visual difficulties), which is closely but not perfectly associated with severe encephalopathy, or dystonia (with which intellect may be preserved), which appears to result from a short but profound period of asphyxia with mild or moderate encephalopathy only. A number of techniques have been shown to be useful in predicting long-term neurologic outcome in asphyxiated neonates very soon after the insult and might be used in the future to predict those patients who are unlikely to benefit from intensive care or who might conceivably be suitable for trials of resuscitative agents. Electroencephalogram (EEG) and cerebral function monitoring [2] and magnetic resonance (MR) techniques, including phosphorus [3] and proton-MR spectroscopy [4] and T2-weighted [5] and diffusion-weighted [6] imaging, may all be useful but at present are only available in centers that undertake research projects. Management is at present supportive—that is, management of associated organ failure and of the seizures [7]. Hypothermia is a candidate for brain resuscitation [8], but other possible agents require considerable further investigation before trials can be considered in humans, as the mechanisms that lead to cell death after severe asphyxia are complex and are akin to the normal processes of development.

Birth Trauma

Birth may be associated with injuries to the head (skull fracture and intracranial hemorrhage), spinal cord, and brachial plexus. The evidence for an association of facial palsy with traumatic forceps delivery is rather tenuous. Management is usually conservative, although surgery may be useful in improving functional outcome in babies with brachial plexus injuries that persist beyond the age of 4 months.

Neonatal Seizures

Neonatal seizures have a number of causes, including birth asphyxia, birth trauma, meningitis, cerebral malformations, metabolic conditions, and venous sinus thrombosis. The seizures may be very subtle clinically, and continuous EEG or cerebral function monitoring has been used in high-risk neonates (e.g., those with birth asphyxia or with abnormalities of the brain on ultrasound). There may be clinical clues to diagnosis, such as the abnormal "kinky" hair in a boy with Menkes' disease or the typical facies and extreme hypotonia of a child with a peroxisomal disorder. Pyridoxine deficiency may also present in the neonatal period, and all seizing infants should be given a dose of intravenous pyridoxine during a diagnostic EEG; because there is a risk of acute hypotonia and collapse, resuscitation equipment should be available. In unexplained neonatal convulsions, biotin should be given as well until the biotinidase assay result is obtained. The workup should also include lumbar puncture (to exclude infection and to look for glycine and lactate), neuroimaging (initially ultrasound and later computed tomographic [CT] scan [e.g., to exclude calcification in congenital infection]) and/or magnetic resonance imaging (MRI) (e.g., to look for structural malformation), and blood and urine samples (to exclude specific metabolic conditions [e.g., sulfite oxidase deficiency]). A number of cases remain idiopathic despite very extensive investigation; follow-up should include a repeat MRI at the age of 1–2 years, because some structural malformations cannot be diagnosed until this stage.

The first-line anticonvulsant is usually phenobarbital in this age group, as it is often effective and well tolerated, and it is relatively easy to achieve therapeutic levels. Phenytoin can be used in the neonatal period, but drug levels must be measured regularly, particularly if treatment is continued into infancy, at which time the pharmacokinetics change. Benzodiazepine infusions are often used in intractable cases.

Neonatal Meningitis

Meningitis can present in a number of subtle ways in neonates, and those who care for them should have a low threshold for performing a lumbar puncture. The common organisms are group B streptococcus, *Listeria monocytogenes,* and *Escherichia coli*, and commonly used antibiotics when the organism is unknown are ampicillin plus gentamicin or a cephalosporin; the prognosis is worst for the third of these organisms, but many patients with the first two do well. Unusual organisms may become opportunistically pathogenic in the severely ill neonate, and there should be very close liaison with the microbiology department over appropriate antibiotic cover, as resistance is an ever-increasing problem.

Hypoglycemia

Those at risk for hypoglycemia include babies who are of low birth weight for gestational age, infants of diabetic mothers, and neonates with serious illnesses, for example, septicemia or necrotizing enterocolitis; other rare causes, such as nesidioblastosis, exist [9]. Because the outcome for symptomatic hypoglycemia is very poor, monitoring of blood sugar is mandatory in those at risk; glucose infusions are commenced in those with a blood sugar of less than 2.5 mmol/liter.

Kernicterus

With the improvement in detection and treatment (with phototherapy and exchange transfusion) of hyperbilirubinemia, frank kernicterus, which is associated with dystonic cerebral palsy and deafness with relatively preserved cognition in the long term, is now extremely rare. Premature infants are at risk, however, and the threshold for treatment of hyperbilirubinemia is set much lower in this group [10]; despite this, isolated high tone deafness continues to occur.

The Floppy Infant

A large number of causes of hypotonia in infancy exist, but although many babies require prolonged hospital care, usually because of poor feeding, relatively few need prolonged ventilation and intensive care. Diagnosis is often made clinically, even if the child is ventilated. Essential investigations include creatine phosphokinase, DNA testing for dystrophia myotonica, and electromyography and nerve conduction studies. These usually guide the next investigations, which might include imaging of the brain or spinal cord, or both; chromosomal analysis; an edrophonium test; or a muscle biopsy. Most conditions are not treatable, but it is important that those that are, such as myasthenia, are diagnosed and managed appropriately. On the whole, the prognosis is poor for independent function in those who are ventilator dependent, but it is very important to make a diagnosis, if possible, because of the genetic implications, and it is often difficult to withdraw support after it is started.

Prematurity

Premature birth is defined as birth before a gestational age of 37 weeks, but the majority of systemic and neurologic problems occur in those born before 35 weeks. Babies born before 25 weeks have a very high mortality and morbidity at the present time. The two main brain pathologies in the premature infant are hemorrhage into the germinal matrix or ventricles, associated in some with posthemorrhagic hydrocephalus, and periventricular leukomalacia. The lesions can be demonstrated on ultrasound scanning of the infant brain through the anterior fontanel and are risk factors for cerebral palsy in this group [11]. Whereas germinal matrix/intraventricular hemorrhage is classically associated with diplegia, periventricular leukomalacia may be associated with quadriparesis, vision problems, and cognitive deficits; the two pathologies, however, sometimes coexist. As the risk factors and management protocols are somewhat different, strategies for prevention and treatment are considered separately.

Intraventricular Hemorrhage

Antenatal steroids have been convincingly shown to reduce the risk of intraventricular hemorrhage with or without prolonged rupture of membranes and independently of the additional reduction in respiratory distress syndrome [12]. Trials of vitamin K, phenobarbital, ethamsylate, and allopurinol have not shown convincing benefit, but postnatal indomethacin appears to prevent intraventricular hemorrhage [13]. Management of posthemorrhagic hydrocephalus is fraught with difficulty because ventriculoperitoneal shunts commonly become blocked or infected, repeated tapping does not improve outcome, and medical treatment, such as acetazolamide, is not effective [14]. Attempts at prevention of hydrocephalus using agents that encourage clot lysis have not been particularly successful. Ventriculosubgaleal shunting may be a short-term alternative to the ventriculoperitoneal route.

Periventricular Leukomalacia

Periventricular leukomalacia has long been thought to be a lesion caused by ischemia, with evidence for abruptio placentae and neonatal hypotension and hypocapnia as risk factors. One of the most important antenatal risk factors is pro-longed rupture of the membranes, with the associated risk of infection, and it is possible that the pathogenesis is inflammatory [15]. Antenatal antibiotics may play a part in reducing incidence; although the use of antenatal steroids in this sit-uation has long been controversial, the balance is probably now in favor of their use. Hypotension does occur in premature neonates and should be avoided wher-ever possible, although this is probably a less important risk factor for periven-tricular leukomalacia than hypocapnia. The latter may explain the possible association of high-frequency jet ventilation with periventricular leukomalacia, although this has not been borne out in all studies [16].

Retinopathy of Prematurity

The main risk factor for retinopathy of prematurity is high oxygen tension, although a number of other influences play a role in high-risk premature infants [17]. Pulse oximetry monitoring is inadequate in this group, and frequent moni-toring of blood gases is mandatory.

NEUROLOGIC PROBLEMS AFTER CARDIOPULMONARY BYPASS

Open heart surgery for children has been in use since the 1950s, and great advances in techniques have resulted in reduced mortality. Current pediatric sur-gical practice is to repair at an earlier age, often in a single-stage complex pro-cedure. More attention is now being paid to assessing and preventing morbidity, especially neurologic, incurred as a consequence of the operating technique. While in the intensive care unit in the immediate postoperative phase, an esti-mated 1–25% of children have significant events; the incidence of acute neuro-logic events in a single unit over a 1-year period was 6% [18]. One series of consecutive children, operated on in 1987–89, reported that 22% had cerebral palsy and the same proportion had an IQ below 70 at follow-up [19]. In the gen-esis of acute and long-term neurologic sequelae, the relative importance of pre-morbid neurologic status, intraoperative factors, such as the duration of cardiopulmonary bypass and the use of deep hypothermic ischemic arrest, and postoperative events, such as hypotension, all remain controversial [20].

In the acute postoperative period, a variety of clinical syndromes have been reported. These include convulsions; coma; movement disorders, including gen-eralized hypotonia; chorea; hemiparesis, monoparesis, and paraparesis; visual field defects; gaze palsies; and behavioral problems. Neuroimaging may reveal intracranial hemorrhage or infarction, even in asymptomatic patients [21], and electromyography and nerve conduction studies may reveal evidence for ante-rior horn cell damage secondary to spinal cord infarction or generalized or local neuropathies.

It is important that good working relationships are established between the members of the team who undertake the operation and those who are responsi-ble for postoperative care so that unexpected but recognized complications of car-diopulmonary bypass, such as air embolus or poor cardiac output, are found and dealt with promptly. Poor cardiac output can be managed with inotropes and by splinting the chest open; ultrafiltration and extracorporeal membrane oxygenation (ECMO) may be useful. If available, hyperbaric oxygen is the treatment of choice for air embolus [22]; because the severity of the cardiac insult can determine outcome, an alternative is to support the circulation temporarily using ECMO. As with a number of situations in the cardiac intensive care unit, neurophysiology is very important in assessing the severity of the neurologic insult, because these children are always sedated and often paralyzed for ventilation. Moving the patient for neuroimaging may sometimes be impossible, although in-hospital transport has improved and some intensive care units are located very close to neuroimaging suites. Noninvasive imaging is occasionally useful in excluding specific conditions, but MRI is usually more sensitive to infarction than B-scan ultrasound, which can only be performed in infants. Some of the most obvious acute neurologic problems have a relatively good long-term prognosis, and it is essential that the person who discusses outcome with families is appropriately experienced.

Seizures are the most common acute neurologic problem after pediatric cardiopulmonary bypass, occurring in approximately 3% of patients. Children who are undergoing repairs of the aortic arch, including simple coarctation as well as more complex lesions, such as interrupted arch, are particularly at risk [18], perhaps because air can enter along the suture lines. In many children, the seizures are idiopathic; possible etiologies include venous sinus thrombosis and arterial ischemic stroke as well as fluid balance shifts and electrolyte abnormalities such as hyponatremia. An EEG is useful in demonstrating discharges, particularly if there are alternative possibilities for the clinical manifestations, such as an extrapyramidal movement disorder; the underlying diagnosis is occasionally suggested, for example, in venous sinus thrombosis. An anticonvulsant, such as intravenous phenytoin (given slowly using a syringe pump), is usually required in the acute phase, but the long-term outcome is often good, and if the child is seizure-free and without neurologic signs in the early follow-up period, he or she can be weaned off the anticonvulsant.

Postoperative chorea has been recognized since the introduction of cardiopulmonary bypass surgery, with an incidence of 0.6–3.0% [23]. The onset is characteristically delayed by 2–7 days, and most patients have a clear period of normality between the operation and the presentation with choreiform movements. Facial choreiform movements are characteristic, and an oculomotor apraxia is common, although difficult to diagnose and not necessarily universal. This appears to resolve, leaving, in some cases, milder problems (e.g., coarse saccadic eye movement). The diagnosis is clinical, and neuroimaging is often noncontributory, although single-photon emission CT scanning may show focal perfusion abnormalities in the basal ganglia and deep gray matter [24]. No specific treatment exists, but children may require sedation for prolonged periods. Although transient choreiform movements seen in infants undergoing cardiopulmonary bypass usually resolve, sequelae, including persistent choreiform movements, mild pyramidal signs, dysarthria, expressive language difficulties, and other developmental problems, are the rule in older children who have a severe extrapyramidal movement disorder after bypass. A significant mortality exists in the latter group.

SEIZURES AND STATUS EPILEPTICUS
IN NEONATES AND CHILDREN

Prolonged and multiple seizures have long been associated with brain damage in humans, and an abundance of experimental evidence exists to show that seizures can cause neuronal loss, but the mechanisms are controversial, and the relative importance of the underlying etiology remains uncertain. Status epilepticus can occur in the context of febrile convulsions in previously normal young children, in which case epilepsy and neurologic handicap are rare long-term outcomes, even for prolonged seizures [25]. On the other hand, in patients with neurologic handicap or chronic epilepsy, or both, the underlying brain damage is assumed to be responsible, and it may be difficult to demonstrate any additional effect of the status on cognitive or neurologic function. Acute encephalopathy caused by infection [26], as well as hypoxia-ischemia [27], is the third most common scenario in which status occurs. It has become clear that, even with a high standard of nursing care on an intensive care unit, insults secondary to hypoxia, hypotension, intracranial hypertension, and hyperpyrexia can occur.

Widespread use of intravenous and rectal diazepam, both by medical professionals and by the families of those with chronic epilepsy, has substantially reduced the mortality and morbidity for status epilepticus in childhood [28]. Bolus doses of intravenous diazepam (0.2–0.3 mg/kg) can be used to control individual seizures; the drug can be given rectally in an emergency if intravenous access cannot be established, but it is very important that the dose not be exceeded in unventilated patients because of the risk of respiratory depression. Lorazepam has theoretic advantages and is replacing diazepam in some institutions. Rectal paraldehyde (0.3 ml/kg in an equal volume of arachis oil) is a useful alternative if available, as it is cheap, effective, and nonsedating. If the seizures continue, intravenous phenobarbital (loading dose of 20 mg/kg, then 5–10 mg/kg/day) or phenytoin (loading infusion of 20 mg/kg over 30 minutes, then 8–10 mg/kg/day) can then be given; precise dosage must be guided by daily plasma levels. If these anticonvulsants are not effective, midazolam or lorazepam can be given by infusion. Chlormethiazole by infusion (1 ml/kg/hour) has a useful role, provided that the patient is not in renal failure, as a large volume of fluid must be given. Many patients who require these infusions also need ventilating; one-to-one nursing care is mandatory because of the risk of respiratory complications associated with sedation and with excessive secretions. Barbiturate coma (loading dose of 5–8 mg/kg, followed by an infusion of 2–10 mg/kg/hour, guided by plasma levels) can be used in intractable status epilepticus [29] in ventilated patients. Pyridoxine dependency has been described as presenting at up to 2 years of age and should always be considered as a possible cause of status epilepticus in a child [30]; the response to intravenous pyridoxine may not be as dramatic as in neonates, and an oral trial of at least 100 mg per day should be continued if any doubt exists. Biotinidase deficiency has also been described as presenting as epilepsy in infancy [31], without the characteristic rash or hair abnormality, and a trial of biotin should always be given in suspected cases until the level of enzyme has been measured.

Intracranial pressure (ICP) rises during generalized tonic-clonic, absence, adversive, and myoclonic seizures in childhood and may remain high for some time after the electrical activity has ceased. Children who do not recover consciousness within an hour of the termination of a prolonged seizure should receive a single dose of mannitol, and most then wake up. If this does not happen or status is continuing, the child should be ventilated and carefully monitored. Electroencephalographic monitoring, using a compressed spectral array or a cerebral function analyzing monitor, may be helpful [32], but it is important to have expert support from the neurophysiology department, including intermittent 8- or 16-lead EEGs as confirmation of potentially important findings [33]. Subtle and electroencephalographic seizures may be documented [26,32], although their importance remains controversial.

Although the routine use of anticonvulsants is not indicated after febrile status, it is important to look at the effectiveness of and compliance with the previously prescribed anticonvulsant in those who have epilepsy, particularly if they also have neurologic damage, because recurrent status occurs particularly in this group.

COMA

The general approach to the management of unconscious children and adults is similar, but important differences in etiology and in the frequency of potential secondary insults exist, as well as in physiologic measurements, which mean that there are advantages in admitting these children to specialty units. In addition, many patients on pediatric wards and intensive care units become unconscious during the management of their underlying disease, and several teams with expertise in a single organ system may be involved, in addition to the pediatric intensivists and neurologists.

Principles of Management

Clinical Assessment

A useful pediatric coma scale should be able to be administered easily, be consistent between observers, and be sufficiently discriminating to identify levels of coma that require specific interventions. The unmodified Glasgow scale has been used in several pediatric series of traumatic coma, but considerable difficulties with application in this age group exist. In particular, the verbal scale is inappropriate in very young children, who often do not speak because they cannot or are too frightened rather than because they are unconscious. In addition, children younger than the age of 10 months cannot localize pain, and those younger than 18 months do not obey commands because their receptive language is not sufficiently developed.

Several alternative pediatric scales have been designed, but as yet none has been universally adopted. Although interobserver variation is least for the Seshia scale [34], probably because it is made up of only four levels, advantages exist in using a scale that is as close as possible to the widely accepted adult Glasgow Coma Scale, as observations and decisions must often be made quickly by relatively inexperienced emergency staff. Some scales have only five categories for

Table 14.1   Examination of the unconscious child (modified Glasgow Coma Scale)

Score	Eye opening	Verbal skills	Motor skills
6	—	—	>5 yrs: obeys commands; <5 yrs: normal spontaneous movements
5	—	>5 yrs: orientated; <5 yrs: alert, babbles, coos, words or sentences normal	Localizes to supraocular pain (>9/12)
4	Spontaneous	>5 yrs: confused; <5 yrs: less than usual ability, irritable cry	Withdraws from nailbed pressure
3	To voice	>5 yrs: inappropriate words; <5 yrs: cries to pain	Flexion to supraocular pain (diencephalic stage)
2	To pain	>5 yrs: incomprehensible sounds; <5 yrs: moans to pain	Extension to supraocular pain (midbrain or upper pontine stage)
1	None	No response to pain	No response to supraocular pain (lower pontine stage)

the motor scale, leaving out withdrawal because of the possibility of confusion with spinal withdrawal reflexes in brain stem death. The advantages of the six-point scale are that it has been widely adopted by units that care for adults and that there is some evidence that withdrawal has a better prognosis than abnormal flexion (e.g., in children after head injury). Awake infants usually move all four limbs either spontaneously or in response to voice or touch. The modification suggested by James and Trauner [35] (Table 14.1), which includes withdrawal to touch and to pain as well as normal spontaneous movements, is probably preferable to that of the Adelaide scale, in which these levels are deleted, thus reducing the total number of categories in very young children. The other advantages of this scale are that the number of categories is the same over the full age range, and expressive rather than receptive language is used for the verbal scale. Training is very important, and it is useful to have clear descriptions of the different levels on the form, particularly if they vary with age. Parental concerns about level of consciousness must always be taken seriously, because the subtle abnormalities of language function that distinguish between a normal child with a Glasgow score of 15 and one with a score of 11, who, for example, requires immediate drainage of an extradural hematoma, are often recognized only by those who know the child well. It is also worth remembering that motor restlessness suggests deep coma and the possibility of imminent deterioration.

For the unconscious child, the recognition and management of impending transtentorial herniation may well make all the difference between potentially useful life versus death or severe handicap. In addition, the assessment of brain stem function has been shown to improve prognostic power in several studies of traumatic and nontraumatic coma in children [36,37]. Because recovery is extremely unlikely if the patient has reached the lower pontine or medullary stage, if children are seen with some or all of the signs, either at the diencephalic

Table 14.2   Herniation syndromes

Stage	Characteristics
Uncal	Unilateral, fixed, dilatated pupil
	Unilateral ptosis
	Minimal deviation of eyes on oculocephalic or oculovestibular testing
	Hemiparesis
Diencephalic	Small or midpoint pupils reactive to light
	Full deviation of eyes on oculocephalic or oculovestibular testing
	Flexor response to pain or decorticate posturing, or both
	Hypertonia or hyperreflexia, or both, with extensor plantars
	Cheyne-Stokes respiration
Midbrain or	Midpoint pupils, fixed to light
upper	Minimal deviation of eyes on oculocephalic or oculovestibular testing
pontine	Extensor response to pain or decerebrate posturing, or both
	Hyperventilation
Lower pontine	Midpoint pupils, fixed to light
	No response on oculocephalic or oculovestibular testing
	No response to pain or flexion of legs only
	Flaccidity with extensor plantars
	Shallow or ataxic respiration
Medullary	Pupils dilatated and fixed to light
	Slow, irregular, or gasping respiration
	Respiratory arrest with adequate cardiac output

or midbrain and upper pontine phases (Table 14.2), emergency management should be instituted at once.

Emergency Management

It is essential to maintain an airway, and if the patient is deeply unconscious (Glasgow coma score less than 9 or any signs of impending transtentorial herniation), intubation and ventilation are mandatory; great care must be taken to stabilize the patient's neck first in trauma victims. Hypoxia and hypotension must be avoided if at all possible. Maintenance of the systemic circulation is a priority, with plasma (20 ml/kg) and inotropic agents (e.g., dopamine, 2.5–20.0 µg/kg/minute), particularly in children who are shocked. Adrenaline is relatively contraindicated as there is evidence for an associated lactic acidosis, at least in patients with septic shock [38]. Crystalloid fluids should be restricted to approximately 60% of the age-appropriate requirements during the initial resuscitation, and hyposmolar fluids must be avoided. Presumed intracranial hypertension can be managed with a bolus dose of 20% mannitol (0.25–1.00 g/kg), provided that no established renal failure or evidence of a space-occupying intracranial hemorrhage exists. If the patient has become unconscious in a peripheral unit, he or she should be transferred with preliminary treatment in progress to a center with full facilities for neurologic intensive care.

All unconscious patients need a CT scan on admission to exclude surgically treatable etiologies (e.g., extradural or intracerebral hemorrhage, hydrocephalus, or tumor) and to look for evidence of cerebral edema, although a normal CT scan does not exclude intracranial hypertension [39]. It is potentially dangerous to perform lumbar puncture on an unconscious patient, even if meningitis is the most likely diagnosis, unless a CT scan has excluded a mass lesion and ICP can be appropriately managed if the patient shows clinical signs of coning [40]. Broad-spectrum antibiotics, either a third-generation cephalosporin such as ceftriaxone or cefotaxime (30–100 mg/kg/day in two to three divided doses), or, alternatively, in the developing world, chloramphenicol (100 mg/kg/day in four divided doses) and penicillin (300 mg/kg/day in six divided doses) should be commenced after a septic screen but before cerebrospinal fluid (CSF) is obtained. Even when the CT scan is reported as normal, lumbar puncture must be undertaken with caution and can be deferred, particularly if the patient is afebrile. If lumbar puncture is performed, the procedure should take place in the intensive care unit, with a nondisplacement transducer available to record the pressure; if the patient's condition deteriorates, he or she should be treated with mannitol 20% (1g/kg) and immediate ventilation. The timing of other investigations (e.g., blood tests, EEG, and MRI scan) is governed by the clinical situation, and an experienced physician should always be involved in these decisions and in those concerned with appropriate management of the underlying etiology. An EEG can give prognostic information and assist in the diagnosis of diverse conditions, including subtle status epilepticus, herpes simplex encephalitis, and cerebral venous thrombosis. If no obvious cause for coma exists, the child should receive acyclovir (750–1,500 mg/m^2/day intravenously in three divided doses) to cover the possibility of herpes simplex encephalitis.

Diagnosis and Management of the Common Causes of Coma in Childhood

Trauma

Nonaccidental Injury

Nonaccidental injury is an extremely important cause of seizures, focal neurology, and coma in the first year of life and should not be forgotten as a potential etiology in the older child. Impact and shaking can cause severe brain damage [41,42]. Every infant who presents with these neurologic syndromes should be carefully examined for retinal hemorrhages and should undergo skull x-ray (and, if there is any doubt, CT scan of the bony skull) to exclude fractures and CT scan of the brain to exclude intracranial hemorrhage and subdural effusion; head ultrasound is not sufficient. MRI may be helpful in certain circumstances (e.g., in revealing subdural hemorrhages that are isodense with brain on CT scan and therefore in disclosing whether serial abuse has occurred); MR spectroscopy has also been used on a research basis [43]. Pitfalls for the unwary exist, however (e.g., arterial dissection in trivial accidental trauma and subdural effusion in association with an acute neurologic presentation in glutamic aciduria type I); it is wise to obtain an experienced opinion [42]. Prognosis is poor if the patient presents in coma or if cerebral edema is present on neuroimaging.

Accidental Trauma

Extradural hematomas are less common in children than in adults but account for some of the patients whose conditions deteriorate secondarily; prognosis in this subgroup appears to be better in younger patients. Rapid decompression is recommended by many and is always indicated in those whose conditions are deteriorating, although conservative management may be appropriate for small hematomas in fully conscious patients [44]. Prognosis appears to be related to the level of consciousness at the time of craniotomy [45], and it is therefore important that children are referred for CT scan at a stage before eye closure and obvious abnormal motor posturing. A Glasgow coma score of 13–15 does not exclude a surgically treatable hematoma [46], and clinicians should have a very low threshold for performing a CT scan in children who have sustained a head injury; clinical symptoms and signs are not predictive in this age group. A case has been made for emergency CT scan in all young patients with apparently trivial head injury as a cost-effective alternative to hospital admission [47], and because significant intracranial injury, which sometimes requires neurosurgical intervention, is not entirely predictable by any other means.

Alternative causes of deep coma after a lucid interval following an apparently minor head injury are seizures and the syndrome of diffuse cerebral edema [48]. Early clinical seizures after head injury are common occurrences in deeply unconscious children; subclinical seizures can occur [49], and treatment may be associated with an improvement in level of consciousness. Phenytoin is the drug of choice for the prevention of early post-traumatic seizures in the pediatric age group, but the dosage may need to be adjusted upward, and levels should be measured frequently. Diffuse brain edema, originally described by Bruce and associates [50] in children, appears to be equally common but more serious in adults [51]. No evidence for an association with hyperemia exists [52], but diffuse axonal injury, subarachnoid hemorrhage, and early hypotension appear to be risk factors [51]. As in adults, hypotension is associated with poor outcome in children with head injury, particularly if associated with hypoxemia; the latter does not appear to be predictive in isolation [53].

Other important associations with head injury in childhood exist. Cervical spine injury should be excluded in all preverbal and unconscious patients and in any children who present with neck pain; the patient's neck should be immobilized in the neutral position before he or she is moved and an x-ray is obtained, although cord injury can occur without evidence of bony injury in young children, and high-dose methylprednisolone (30 mg/kg as a bolus, followed by an infusion of 5.4 mg/kg/hour for 23 hours) should be given as soon as possible if any doubt exists [54]. Cervical injury is sometimes associated with carotid or vertebrobasilar dissection and can be demonstrated using MRI, with fine cuts in the axial and coronal planes and fat suppression. If a very high index of suspicion exists (e.g., evidence of vascular disease in a distribution that suggests posterior circulation disturbance), formal angiography should be considered. Carotid dissection can also occur after minor head injury and should be considered in any patient who presents with focal neurologic signs; MRI and MR angiography are usually diagnostic provided that the relevant sequences are requested. Acute hemiparesis after apparently trivial head injury may also be associated with basal ganglia hypodensity on neuroimaging of uncertain etiology [55]. Although spontaneous subarachnoid hemorrhage is rare in childhood, this complication can occur after severe pediatric head trauma [56] in association with vasospasm (Apparicio and Kirkham, unpublished observations); treatment with nimodipine is a controversial issue in adults and is not recommended in children at present. Traumatic aneurysms may require surgery or interventional neuroradiology [57]. Cerebral venous thrombosis also occurs in pediatric head trauma [58], but anti-coagulation is controversial.

Management of associated injuries, including fractures and abdominal trauma, may be fraught with difficulty; operation may need to be timed very carefully and in some cases is not necessary. Secondary problems, such as stress ulceration and pancreatitis, are not uncommon, and a high risk of infection exists. Nutrition, either parenteral or jejunal, is important for all severely injured patients; intra-gastric feeding is contraindicated because of the risk of aspiration.

Management strategies are similar to those proposed for adults. Emergency treatment of shock, with plasma expanders, and prevention of hypoxia and hypotension at the scene of the accident and during intensive care are most important. ICP monitoring appears to be safe and to guide management, although the ideal cerebral perfusion pressure in children remains controversial. Mannitol and ventricular or lumbar drainage [59] are the mainstays of the management of intracranial hypertension at present; hyperventilation is best avoided except during brief bagging for sudden spikes. Results of controlled trials of hypothermia in adults have been encouraging, although complications, such as neutropenia, infection, and pancreatitis, continue to be a problem. Use of steroids in head injury has long been controversial; meta-analysis of the controlled trials suggests a small benefit, but no studies have been performed in children. Surgical decom-pression may be lifesaving in very severe intractable hypertension [60]. Serial neuroimaging is essential, as potentially treatable complications develop in approximately 40% of severely head-injured children [61].

Central Nervous System Infections

Meningitis and Meningococcal Shock

Introduction of an effective vaccine for *Haemophilus influenzae* has led to a very substantial reduction in, but not eradication of, this disease, which is com-monly complicated by subdural effusion; ventricular dilation secondary to obstruction of CSF absorption pathways; and basal cerebral artery spasm, steno-sis, and occlusion. Meningococcal disease appears to be on the increase and is now the most common cause of meningitis in preschool-aged children. Pneu-mococcal infection, including meningitis, often occurs in "at-risk" populations (e.g., those who have had a splenectomy or who have sickle cell disease, a group that is usually taking penicillin prophylaxis long term); the increasing incidence of severe *Streptococcus pneumoniae* infections and the emergence of resistance to this antibiotic and others are worrisome. Meningococcal shock has a high mor-tality, despite increased public and medical awareness, which have led to earlier antibiotic prescription. Tuberculous meningitis can present acutely, with seizures and coma, in young children, and a number of organisms are pathogens in the immunocompromised, including those with acquired immunodeficiency syndrome. Although full recovery is the rule, particularly in those who survive meningitis caused by *Neisseria meningitidis* or *H. influenzae*, even children with neurologic signs initially [62] still have a significant morbidity and mortality in meningitis, particularly those whose level of consciousness deteriorates during the course of the illness.

Primary care physicians and general practitioners are increasingly encouraged to give parenteral penicillin if they suspect meningitis or meningococcal shock. The third-generation cephalosporins, such as ceftriaxone, should be used as first-line empiric therapy in most situations at the present time, although local policies may vary, often depending on the prevalence of drug-resistant pneumococci, and should be followed. Vancomycin or meropenem may be required for drug-resistant pneumococcal meningitis. Whether steroids improve outcome in terms of survival or neurologic morbidity in meningitis is still very controversial. Clinical (fever) and laboratory (CSF glucose, lactate, and protein) parameters appeared to improve more rapidly with steroids, and the incidence of deafness and neurologic sequelae was apparently reduced in controlled trials [63] despite considerable concerns about methodology. The evidence for efficacy is best in meningitis caused by *H. influenzae,* which is now rare, but steroids may have benefit in pneumococcal disease [64]; no data have been obtained on meningococcal meningitis, and some concern about detrimental effects exists. Some studies have shown an excess mortality in the steroid-treated group but no apparent benefit in terms of morbidity [65]. Many, but not all, pediatricians in the developed world give a dose of dexamethasone before the antibiotics in suspected meningitis and continue the regime for 48 hours. Whether this is appropriate for the developing world, where the bulk of the morbidity is seen, remains uncertain.

Brain herniation may be found at postmortem and may be apparent clinically in some cases of meningitis [66]. When measured by the lumbar route, mean resting CSF pressure has been shown to be increased in the acute phase of the illness in most patients [67]. Delaying lumbar puncture is reasonable in seriously ill, unconscious children with fever, particularly if focal signs are present, especially as meningitis can be confirmed by rapid antigen screening or using the polymerase chain reaction. Antibiotic therapy should certainly never be delayed. Meningitis is sometimes associated with meningococcal shock, but lumbar puncture is not the main priority in this situation.

It is probably more important to be aware of the possibility of cerebral herniation, particularly after the diagnostic lumbar puncture and probably after seizures, than to monitor ICP, as in most cases this complication occurs soon after admission. ICP monitoring is relatively contraindicated, as the inflamed brain may bleed. Intracranial hypertension is thought to be caused by a combination of cerebral edema and communicating hydrocephalus. With due care, CSF drainage can be achieved by the lumbar route, although many clinicians prefer to treat with regular small doses of mannitol or glycerol [68]. Autoregulation and carbon dioxide reactivity are preserved in most patients, and ventilating patients to hypocapnia can reduce cerebral blood flow below the ischemic threshold [69]. Hyponatremia appears to be related to hypovolemia rather than to the syndrome of inappropriate antidiuretic hormone release in the majority of patients, and patients should be given replacement for their dehydration as well as maintenance, at least initially [70]. Electrolytes should be measured frequently, and an occasional patient may require fluid restriction for the syndrome of inappropriate antidiuretic hormone release. Subdural effusions do not appear to affect morbidity and usually do not require drainage, although empyema, which may be difficult to distinguish, does. Vasospasm, stenosis, and occlusion of the basal cerebral arteries are important, but as yet untreatable, causes of morbidity and can be diagnosed using transcranial Doppler ultrasound.

Encephalitis

Coma is a poor prognostic sign in all forms of encephalitis, including that caused by herpes simplex infection, for which the prognosis has undoubtedly improved since the advent of effective antiviral agents [71]. Seizures are characteristic of this infection but are not universal. All children who present with an undiagnosed encephalopathy should be treated with acyclovir until an alternative diagnosis is made. It is now possible to make a positive diagnosis using the polymerase chain reaction, although there are problems with oversensitivity, and the test is not universally available. The treatment of choice is high-dose acyclovir for at least 10 days, because the relapse rate is unacceptably high with a lower dose or a 5-day course [72]. Human herpesvirus type 6 causes encephalitis and roseola infantum in children [73]. Enteroviruses are a common cause of encephalitis in children, although physicians are often reluctant to perform a comprehensive virologic screen, as these illnesses are usually self-limiting and treatment is not available. Central nervous system involvement in *Mycoplasma pneumoniae* can take a number of forms [74], including coma and seizures; is not necessarily associated with chest disease; and is probably more common than has previously been recognized. The roles of erythromycin and steroids in altering the course of what is usually a self-limiting disease remain controversial. Postinfectious encephalitis occurs several weeks after a number of childhood exanthemas, including measles and chickenpox. Even after a very extensive microbiologic workup, the cause of an apparent encephalitis may remain obscure and may not be infectious. Intracranial hypertension is associated with encephalitis, particularly in those who present in coma [75]. Supportive management should therefore be directed to the maintenance of cerebral perfusion pressure and the treatment of seizures.

Cerebral Malaria

Cerebral malaria, usually caused by *Plasmodium falciparum*, is the most common cause of pediatric coma in the world and is increasingly seen in the West [76], usually after travel to endemic areas without adequate prophylaxis. Both quinine and artemether are effective in achieving parasite clearance and clinical cure at the present time [77], although there are concerns about the emergence of resistance, and considerable evidence has been found that the neurologic morbidity and mortality are not directly related to the parasite. Pathologically, parasite sequestration and endovascular adhesion take place in the venules of the major organs, including the brain.

Seizures are a prominent feature, occurring in 60–80% of patients, either before or during admission, with status epilepticus in a significant proportion [26]. Manifestations may be very subtle, including eye deviation and slight unilateral clonic twitching of the mouth or limbs. In the developing world, the only anticonvulsant available may be phenobarbital, which may not prevent recurrent convulsions. Whenever possible, strenuous efforts should be made to control seizures and status epilepticus (see Seizures and Status Epilepticus in Neonates and Children), as they contribute substantially to morbidity. Cerebral edema is a common postmortem finding in children, and some evidence suggests that intracranial hypertension is a feature in pediatric cerebral malaria and is an important association with death and severe handicap [37,78]. In the developing world, the only practical treatment at present is an osmotic diuretic, for which efficacy is unproven [78]. In the West, ICP monitoring and management, as well as ventilation, are indicated in patients who remain unconscious despite control of seizures. Steroids have been shown to be deleterious. Exchange transfusion is associated with rapid parasite clearance and has been used in developed countries [79], although controlled trials are not available.

Diabetic Ketoacidosis

Diabetic coma is a common emergency in children, and the majority of patients improve within 12 hours of rehydration and insulin therapy. Deterioration of consciousness level despite treatment is a well-recognized phenomenon and appears to be associated with raised CSF pressure and with cerebral edema at postmortem in those who die. Subclinical cerebral edema may be quite common [80], and it is important to realize that, paradoxically, brain swelling is maximal at a time when the patient's biochemistry is improving. The role of rapid fluid administration in precipitating brain herniation is controversial, but a significant inverse relationship exists between the timing of herniation and the rate of fluid administration in the published cases, with excessive secretion of antidiuretic hormone as a probable additional factor. Careful calculation of the rate of rehydration is important, with an emphasis on slow, steady correction of fluid and electrolyte imbalance [81]. Failure to regain consciousness in parallel with biochemical improvement or clinical signs of incipient brain herniation are indications for urgent management of presumed cerebral edema with mannitol, ventilation, and a reduction in the rate of fluid administration. Associated shock and pulmonary edema have been described and must be managed appropriately.

Hypoxic-Ischemic Encephalopathy

Cardiac Arrest

Hypoxic-ischemic encephalopathy after cardiac arrest is not uncommon in children, and prognosis is poor [27]. An additional ischemic insult worsens the prognosis for other encephalopathies such as those that occur after head injury. Some experimental and clinical evidence for secondary deterioration after ischemia exist [27,82]. Intracranial hypertension is associated [83], but whether this is a preventable cause of secondary deterioration is controversial [84]. For both in-hospital and out-of-hospital cardiac arrest in childhood, immediate cardiopulmonary resuscitation, ventilation, and correction of hypotension with adequate doses of epinephrine are the mainstays of management. A case can be made for

ICP monitoring in an individual child who has been well resuscitated using modern cardiopulmonary resuscitation techniques in whom the EEG has recovered to diffuse slowing or better but who remains unconscious or sedated for ventilation, provided that cerebral perfusion pressure (CPP) is also frequently recorded and is managed appropriately. No neuroprotective agents can be recommended for children at the present time.

Near Drowning

The prognosis for the child pulled from the water apparently dead is excellent, provided that cardiopulmonary resuscitation is commenced immediately and that the child gasps within minutes of rescue and regains consciousness soon afterward [85]. The prognosis is much worse for the child admitted to the emergency room deeply unconscious with fixed, dilatated pupils and without a detectable pulse, therefore requiring continuing cardiopulmonary resuscitation, and with an arterial pH of less than 7.00 and a high plasma glucose, especially if consciousness is not recovered by the time of admission to the intensive care unit [86,87]. None of these poor prognostic indicators precludes a good outcome, however, and apparently miraculous recoveries have occurred, mainly in children who have nearly drowned in very cold water.

Intracranial hypertension is a common but not universal feature of the encephalopathy that follows serious near-drowning incidents [88], although, again, whether measurement of ICP is of prognostic use or treatment prevents secondary deterioration is controversial. A controlled trial showed that thiopental did not improve outcome [89], and although continuing hypothermia might be a therapeutic approach, the risks of infection apparently outweigh any benefits [90]. In children who have had a cardiac arrest, a more aggressive approach may occasionally be justified for 24–48 hours; prognosis can then be determined using neurophysiologic or MR [91] techniques. It is important to remember that drowning, particularly in bathtubs, may be a manifestation of child abuse.

Electrocution

Electrocution is an unusual event in childhood but can be devastating in its consequences. Small children are most at risk for electrocution in the home, whereas older boys are more commonly involved in high-tension electrical injuries. Neurologic problems can be directly caused by the electrical injury or the associated cardiac arrest. Atonic and myoclonic seizures are not uncommon in the long term, and there is a very high incidence of emotional disorders. Children occasionally recover after prolonged coma [92].

Lightning Injuries

Lightning injuries can occur at any age; the pathology, which can affect any part of the neuraxis, including the spinal cord, results either directly from the injury or as a consequence of cardiac arrest. The prognosis is poor with a 30% mortality and sequelae (not necessarily neurologic) in the majority of survivors; cardiopulmonary arrest, loss of consciousness at the scene, and leg or cranial burns suggest a poor prognosis [93]. Acutely, the neurologic manifestations in children can include coma, seizures, and ataxia; changes in memory and mood can persist for long periods [94].

Burns

Encephalopathy with seizures or coma, or both, is well recognized after major and relatively minor burns and scalds in children, with a reported incidence of 5–14% in published series [95]. Cerebral edema with cerebellar herniation has been described at postmortem, and the condition may also be associated with significant neurologic morbidity. The etiology appears to be multifactorial, with hyponatremia, hypocalcemia, and sepsis often implicated. It is possible that the incidence and severity may be decreasing with improved management of fluid and electrolyte balance, although encephalopathy is still a significant problem in children with major burns, particularly if they are exacerbated by hypoxia caused by smoke inhalation. Intracranial hypertension has been described and should be monitored in those who are unconscious. Sepsis, including meningitis, is always a potential cause of mortality and morbidity. The other serious neurologic complication of burns is central pontine myelinolysis, which may be associated with high serum osmolality.

Reye's Syndrome

Reye's syndrome, a life-threatening encephalopathy characterized by cerebral edema and fatty infiltration of the liver, has been reported since the 1960s [96], mainly in children with recent infections such as influenza and varicella. It has become very rare, at least in part in parallel with the withdrawal of aspirin in the mid-1980s [97]. Those cases that are seen now are usually caused by metabolic abnormalities, such as ornithine carbamoyltransferase deficiency [98]. The most common cause of death is cerebral herniation secondary to cerebral edema, and the management is that of intracranial hypertension, with the aim of maintaining cerebral perfusion pressure.

Hepatic Encephalopathy

In children, the most common cause of hepatic encephalopathy is severe viral hepatitis; paracetamol overdose is rare, although decompensation of chronic liver disease can occur. Cerebral edema has been found at postmortem in a large number of patients dying from fulminant hepatic failure and can be demonstrated on CT scan in those in grade III or IV hepatic coma [99]. Flumazenil may produce transient improvement in consciousness level, although this is controversial [100], but the treatment of choice for fulminant hepatic failure in children is transplantation, because the outcome in conservatively managed cases that have reached grade III or IV of the staging system is so poor at the present time. Alternative therapies, initially for those who are not suitable for transplantation, include interferon and cyclosporin A [101].

Hemolytic-Uremic Syndrome

Hemolytic-uremic syndrome is not uncommon in childhood and is often associated with *E. coli* O157 gastrointestinal infections; the related thrombotic thrombocytopenic purpura occurs more rarely. Coma occurring as a complication of hemolytic-uremic syndrome is of grave prognostic significance [102], particularly if the patient's respiratory pattern is abnormal [103]. Generalized cerebral edema [104] and major cerebral vessel thrombosis [105] in association with stroke have been described; both may be associated with intracranial hypertension acutely but are compatible with good long-term outcome if they are managed appropriately [106]. Repeated plasma infusions are the mainstay of treatment, but plasma exchange may be beneficial in those with severe disease.

Hypertensive Encephalopathy

The prognosis for hypertensive encephalopathy in children is usually good [107]. Visual symptoms may precede deterioration in consciousness, and seizures are a common feature; neuroimaging may show low density in the white matter, particularly in the parieto-occipital regions [108], but may be normal. Deep coma, presumably caused by cerebral ischemia, occasionally follows rapid reduction of blood pressure. A particular risk exists if the patient is hypovolemic. Raised ICP may be a management problem in this group and can lead to brain herniation [109].

Management of uncomplicated hypertensive encephalopathy is straightforward, and a variety of antihypertensive agents can be used safely, provided that hypovolemia is corrected and that blood pressure is not reduced precipitously. Diazoxide can produce a precipitous fall in blood pressure to below the lower limit of autoregulation and is contraindicated. Nifedipine is often effective, and captopril has some theoretic advantages, as it acutely shifts the whole autoregulatory curve to the left [110], possibly secondary to a direct vasodilatory effect on the large cerebral arteries. If blood pressure is very high, the alpha/beta blocker labetalol can be used, as it is easy to titrate and can reduce sympathetic vasoconstriction of the larger cerebral arteries. After shock and coma have supervened, a very small therapeutic margin exists between the benefits of reducing blood pressure and the risks of increasing intracranial hypertension and worsening ischemia. Drugs that are cerebral vasodilators, such as hydralazine and sodium nitroprusside, are definitely contraindicated because they increase ICP [110]. Blood pressure may have to be reduced over a period of days to weeks, while cerebral perfusion pressure is maintained appropriately.

Shock

Coma is a feature of shock syndromes (e.g., septic shock caused by meningococcus or phage group I staphylococcal infection). Hemorrhagic shock and encephalopathy occurs in infants, and hyperthermia may play a role, in part because of overwrapping [111]; cerebral edema has been demonstrated on CT scan and at postmortem. The prognosis for neurologic function in hemorrhagic shock and encephalopathy has been uniformly poor, despite aggressive management of cerebral edema and convulsions.

The main priorities in septic shock are to ensure that the patient has an adequate intravenous dose of antibiotics as quickly as possible and that the circulation is maintained, initially with plasma and then with inotropic support. Epinephrine (adrenaline) is relatively contraindicated because of the evidence of an associated lactic acidosis [38]. Adequate ventilation is important, and ECMO has a place in intractable shock [112]. Plasma or whole blood exchange may also be beneficial. Trials of therapies that directly target endotoxins are in progress, but despite apparent benefit in adults (e.g., in meningococcal disease), the preliminary results have been disappointing in children, and none can be recommended at present except in the context of a controlled trial; at the time of this writing, one ongoing study is of recombinant bactericidal permeability increasing factor.

Toxins

Accidental ingestion of drugs and toxins is common in childhood; occasionally, drugs are deliberately administered by a caregiver. The majority of incidents are not serious, and the prognosis for those that are can be determined by the cardiac manifestations rather than by the neurologic condition. Nevertheless, some drugs and toxins cause coma, seizures, or stroke. Alcohol intoxication can cause severe hypoglycemia in children, and therapy must be specifically directed toward this complication. Severe lead encephalopathy occurs occasionally, usually in children with pica who live in unmodernized accommodations. Intracranial hypertension is characteristic and may be so severe as to require surgical decompression [113]. Outcome is determined by the serum lead level and by the severity of the encephalopathy. Iron poisoning is commonly fatal because of the associated reduction in cardiac output, but intact survival has been reported with the use of deferoxamine infusions, together with meticulous attention to cardiovascular status with the aid of a Swan-Ganz catheter [114]. Aspirin and ibuprofen can cause shock, metabolic acidosis, and coma when taken in overdose by young children; treatment is supportive.

Focal Lesions with Failure of Volume Compensation

Children with focal lesions, including intracerebral hemorrhage, ischemic stroke, tumor, and abscess, may present acutely in coma. The management is of the underlying condition, but immediate surgical decompression is usually required in hemorrhage, tumor, and abscess and may be the treatment of choice in hemispheric stroke [115].

Monitoring

Intracranial Pressure and Cerebral Perfusion Pressure

Monitoring of ICP is controversial; it is certainly more important to maintain the airway, correct hypovolemia and/or hypotension, and treat urgently any underlying cause, such as meningitis, than to insert an ICP monitor. Increased awareness of potential cerebral problems complicating life-threatening diseases in children may mean that intracranial hypertension can be prevented by careful management of, for example, fluid and electrolyte balance and ventilation. Persistent intracranial hypertension is a potentially treatable feature of all pediatric encephalopathies, however, and ICP monitoring should be considered in children in deep coma (Glasgow coma score less than 9) once rapidly reversible causes (e.g., seizures) have been treated. As the child's condition may be very unstable at the time a decision to monitor ICP is made, he or she should be in the intensive care unit. An intraparenchymal fiberoptic device can be used in most situations and has been shown to reliably reflect intraventricular pressure; an intraventricular version of the same device can be inserted if the ventricles can be located, as this allows CSF drainage. Often, an associated coagulation disorder exists, particularly in hepatic failure and sometimes in severe infections, so that the potential benefits of monitoring must be weighed against the additional risks.

A minimum CPP of less than 30 mm Hg for more than a few minutes does not appear to be compatible with intact survival, whatever the etiology [83,116,117]. Outcome is also related to mean CPP [83], but not to opening, maximum, or mean ICP. Controversy exits over the optimal CPP for an unconscious child, and more research is needed in this area.

It has proved difficult to show that treating raised ICP improves outcome. Despite early optimism, little evidence exists to show that the prognosis for the nearly drowned comatose child has been improved by brain resuscitation protocols. Similarly, the prognosis for most children with hypoxic-ischemic encephalopathy can be determined at the time of the original arrest. Early treatment of bacterial meningitis with adequate doses of antibiotics is more important than management of late cerebral edema in this condition. It is, however, important to be aware of the potential for intracranial hypertension and poor cerebral perfusion in nontraumatic coma, as anticipation and early treatment can prevent secondary ischemia and deterioration in those patients who were originally predicted to do well.

Neurophysiology

Tasker and his colleagues [33] have suggested that serial eight-channel EEG recording might be useful in addition to ICP and CPP monitoring as, in their series, prognosis was accurately predicted by EEG in the group with poor outcome in whom minimum CPP overlapped with the good outcome group. EEG within 24 hours of the insult appears to be useful in predicting outcome in children in coma caused by cardiac arrest or near drowning [17]. High-amplitude diffuse slowing is a pattern commonly seen in children in coma and does not appear to be useful in discriminating outcome groups. Somatosensory evoked potentials are particularly helpful in outcome prediction.

The main use of continuous EEG is to follow changes over long periods. After a cardiac arrest, the length of time taken for continuous electroencephalographic activity to return gives very useful prognostic information, and the effects of various medical interventions on this recovery can be observed. Deterioration of the electroencephalographic pattern may be followed (e.g., by loss of the faster frequencies, decrease in amplitude of the compressed trace, or a change to a pattern of graver prognostic significance). Seizures, which are often subclinical in the unconscious patient paralyzed for ventilation, may also be seen as changes in the trace and can be treated [29]. Whether such monitoring and management make any difference to outcome remains controversial, but EEG is undoubtedly a useful prognostic tool.

Monitoring of Cerebral Hemodynamics and Metabolism

Transcranial Doppler and near infrared spectroscopy have been used to monitor cerebral hemodynamics, in addition to the Kety-Schmidt technique to measure cerebral blood flow. Jugular venous saturation and brain tissue oxygen can be monitored as a measure of metabolism. All of these are research rather than routine techniques at present.

Management of Prolonged Coma

Patients should be nursed flat or with head elevation to 30 degrees, depending on the optimal CPP. The patient's head should be in the midline so that the jugular venous drainage is not obstructed. Adequate paralysis and sedation are essential. Great care must be taken with endotracheal suction, and transport to the operating room or the radiology department must be very carefully supervised. Clinical seizures must be managed appropriately (see Seizures and Status Epilepticus in Neonates and Children), and a case can be made for detecting and managing subclinical seizures in ventilated unconscious patients. Because the association of hypocapnia with cerebral ischemia in head injury and in meningitis is a concern, it is preferable to ventilate at normo- or slight hypocapnia.

If the child remains unconscious for several days, arterial and central venous pressures and core and peripheral temperatures must be monitored, a careful fluid balance chart should be kept, the child should be weighed frequently using bed scales, and plasma electrolytes and osmolality should be measured at least twice a day. Hyponatremia can be associated with deterioration in level of consciousness caused by cerebral edema and with poor outcome. Rapid correction may be associated with central pontine myelinolysis, and hyponatremia should therefore always be corrected slowly. Low serum sodium is more likely to be caused by salt loss than by inappropriate antidiuretic hormone secretion. Severe dehydration must be avoided, and patients should not be given large volumes of hyposmolar fluids, such as 10% dextrose; evidence is accumulating that the widespread practice of fluid restriction is potentially detrimental. Fluid prescriptions must be very regularly reviewed and revised according to the data from measurements of blood pressure, central venous pressure, core-peripheral temperature gap, plasma electrolytes and osmolality, body weight, and fluid balance. Infusions of colloid may be required if central venous pressure is low or biochemical parameters indicate prerenal failure. If central venous pressure is normal or high, inotropes may be required to maintain blood pressure. Low-dose dopamine can be useful in improving renal perfusion and preventing anuria. Therapy with other vasodilating drugs, such as sodium nitroprusside, is usually contraindicated, as these drugs also have an effect on the cerebral circulation, increasing ICP and altering the autoregulatory range. If a bleeding diathesis is present, infusions of platelets or fresh frozen plasma, or both, may be required. Careful attention must be paid to nutrition; intracranial hypertension is not affected by parenteral feeding. Acute renal failure may be a particular problem in hypoxic-ischemic encephalopathy, which is often accompanied by acute tubular necrosis of the kidneys. Early peritoneal dialysis or hemofiltration enables fine control of fluid balance if renal failure becomes established.

Steroids are probably indicated in bacterial meningitis but not in other encephalopathies. It is probably reasonable to give a single dose of mannitol immediately after resuscitation from cardiac arrest or during the early phase after stroke, provided that blood pressure is adequate, to decrease the osmotic gradient between blood and brain during the reperfusion period and therefore perhaps to reduce cerebral edema. Rapid administration of osmotic agents is beneficial in the short term in coma caused by meningitis, encephalitis, cerebral malaria, status epilepticus, and metabolic conditions, and many previously unrousable children regain consciousness after a single dose of 0.5–1.0 g/kg mannitol. Prolonged use (more than 48 hours) may be associated with rebound intracranial hypertension, and it is better to give an occasional small (0.25 g/kg) dose of mannitol in response to acutely raised ICP in this situation than to administer regular doses without guidance from an ICP monitor. Serum osmolality should not be allowed to rise above 300 mOsm, and mannitol should not be administered to children with established renal failure unless hemofiltration is in progress.

Barbiturate coma is occasionally useful in the unconscious patient with intractable intracranial hypertension or status epilepticus provided that the systemic circulation can be maintained. The pharmacokinetics of thiopental can make the clinical diagnosis of brain stem death impossible, as plasma levels may remain high for some time after an infusion has been discontinued. From animal data and clinical experience in cardiac surgery, no doubt exists that hypothermia is protective if it is commenced before ischemia occurs. Core temperature at the time of the insult is an important variable in determining neurologic and pathologic outcome in animal models of global ischemia and in human stroke. Cerebral metabolic rate increases directly with temperature, and considerable experimental evidence exists of deranged metabolism if ischemic brain is also subjected to hyperthermia. It is likely that the rate of potentially damaging processes, including, for example, excitotoxic damage, is much faster at higher body and brain temperatures. No controlled trials of the use of hypothermia in nontraumatic coma have been performed, but a good case can be made for the strict maintenance of normothermia or very mild (34°–37°C) hypothermia. At lower temperatures, the potential benefits may be outweighed by side effects, such as neutropenia and susceptibility to sepsis, myocardial depression, and hematologic dysfunction. If a cooling turban or blanket is available, hypothermia can be initiated quickly during resuscitation. One practical advantage of hypothermia over barbiturate coma for reducing cerebral metabolic rate is that the former is easily reversible for neurologic examination.

If an intraventricular catheter is inserted, CSF can be drained either in response to ICP peaks or continuously to maintain ICP below a certain level, predetermined by the height of the valve chamber. Risk of infection exists, but continuous drainage of CSF may be an alternative to the side effects and problems with rebound intracranial hypertension that are associated with prolonged drug therapy and hyperventilation. Surgical decompression has been successfully used for the encephalopathies associated with lead poisoning [113], Reye's syndrome [118], and encephalitis [119], as well as large middle cerebral artery infarction [115] and head trauma [60]. Craniectomy may offer an alternative to prolonged and eventually unsuccessful medical management of intracranial hypertension in certain circumstances; indications are required in the light of modern monitoring methods, and controlled trials are warranted.

Outcome and Outcome Prediction

Outcome

The outcome for coma varies considerably, mainly depending on the etiology, although duration of coma is also an important predictor. For some conditions, such as cerebral malaria, although mortality may be high, the overall outcome for survivors is excellent, although subtle deficits may go unrecognized. Despite the fact that the outcome for meningitis is good in the majority of patients, with only a few going on to have significant hearing loss or recurrent seizures, the prognosis for the child who presents in coma is much more guarded; many of the long-standing deficits in this situation appear to be related to the vascular complications of the disease. The outcome for severe head injury is very mixed, with some children being left with a severe movement disorder while others make an apparently good recovery, although behavioral difficulties and personality change may be common in this group [120].

Prognosis is undoubtedly worse if a global hypoxic-ischemic event occurs, whatever the underlying etiology. The outcome for cardiac arrest varies greatly from series to series, depending on the selection of patients. For pediatric inpatients, up to 64% may be resuscitated [121]. Survival drops rapidly so that long-term mortality reaches 60–90%, even in children. The proportion of those resuscitated from out-of-hospital arrest tends to be lower. Overall, the prognosis for hypoxic-ischemic encephalopathy in children is poor. Survivors of near drowning in childhood either make an excellent recovery, sometimes with minor motor problems, or are left in a vegetative state. Moderate and severe handicaps are seen after cardiac arrest, as well as the vegetative state, but good outcome, with no obvious deficit, is more common in survivors.

Patterns of Neurologic Damage in Survivors

Very few long-term follow-up data on children who have survived encephalopathies exist. In addition, it may be difficult to document specific neurologic handicaps in a young child, and these may change with time in the developing brain. Occasionally, considerable recovery takes place in the first year after injury, although this is more likely in the cognitive and visual spheres; a severe mixed motor disorder that is apparent soon after an encephalopathy usually persists and sometimes can mask improvement in intellectual function.

Persistent Vegetative State

Persistent vegetative state (PVS) can be defined as a state of consciousness without awareness and is well recognized in children after head injury and severe ischemic insults; recovery of consciousness, but usually not independent function, is more commonly seen in the former group [122]. The patient can open his or her eyes, and sleep may be distinguished from wakefulness, but he or she has no contact with the environment. Early development of motor posturing, spontaneous blinking, and roving conjugate eye movements may be associated with eventual PVS, but prognosis at this stage can be misleading, and a significant proportion of patients apparently in a PVS at 1 month after the insult eventually regain consciousness. Most patients whose best outcome is no better than PVS die fairly soon after the original insult, but those who survive for prolonged periods pose enormous social and economic problems. Although PVS is a common outcome after intensive therapy for pediatric near drowning, the overall incidence appears to be lower in children with hypoxic-ischemic encephalopathy than in adults.

Neurologic Sequelae

Blindness is a common consequence of coma in children. The occipital cortex is particularly vulnerable to ischemic damage either because the posterior cerebral circulation is compromised directly or because border zone ischemia occurs between the posterior and middle cerebral arteries. Vision recovers to some extent in the majority of patients, and some children who are apparently blind for months after the insult eventually make a good recovery [123].

Hemiparesis occurs after cerebral malaria, perhaps as a result of the prolonged unilateral clonic seizures in this disorder. Quadriparesis (often mixed dystonic and spastic) is a relatively common consequence of hypoxic-ischemic encephalopathy in infants and young children [124]. Patients who have experienced traumatic brain stem injury or spontaneous brain stem or cerebellar hemorrhage may appear to be "locked-in" for considerable periods, although often slow progress is made over months to years with some degree of motor recovery. A similar situation has been reported in nontraumatic coma, probably secondary to incomplete cerebral herniation with vascular injury to the brain stem [125]. An almost normal EEG can occur in the locked-in state and may help to distinguish it from the vegetative state, which is important because the former benefits from a very intensive rehabilitation program, including communication aids. Bibrachial paresis is well recognized in adults after cardiac arrest and appears to be secondary to border zone ischemia in the territories between the middle and anterior cerebral arteries; a similar pattern is occasionally seen in children. Dystonia with a delay in onset (mean delay, 12.9 years) has been well described after traumatic and hypoxic-ischemic insults in children [126] and may respond to treatment with anticholinergics. A transient dystonic syndrome with onset a few days after the insult has also been recognized. Action myoclonus occasionally develops and sometimes responds to sodium valproate, clonazepam, or a serotonin precursor. Spinal cord damage can occur after head injury, cardiac arrest, or cardiopulmonary bypass surgery. Critical care polyneuropathy occurs in pediatric intensive care [127], often in association with sepsis. A characteristic amnestic syndrome has been described after cardiac arrest and encephalitis in adults and children and may be temporary or permanent. Other cognitive and behavioral problems commonly occur.

Brain Death

The clinical criteria for brain death may be used in young children, provided that they are very strictly followed, particularly with regard to the precondition of establishing a cause. Thus, relatively few problems with traumatic coma exist, even in infants who have been nonaccidentally injured, although legal questions may arise in the latter cases that require resolution. The problems concern nontraumatic coma, which is commonly idiopathic in children. Attention has therefore been drawn to those cases of brain stem encephalitis or polyneuropathy that have "mimicked" brain death [128]; they are important as a reminder that patients in intensive care require thorough investigation if no obvious etiology is present. Difficulties also arise in patients who have been ventilated for multiorgan failure for prolonged periods in cases in which the etiology of coma may be multifactorial; this is a particular problem in the neonatal period [129]. Guidelines have evolved in units with extensive experience in diagnosing pediatric brain death and include the use of neurophysiologic and imaging techniques, which may be particularly useful in infants younger than 1 year old [130].

Prediction of Outcome

Clinical signs appear to be useful predictors of outcome in adults in nontraumatic coma and may have some predictive power in previously well children who present in coma. The situation is very different in children who become unconscious in the context of another illness. As part of their management, they are often already paralyzed on the intensive care unit and are thus not accessible for clinical examination. Considerable literature is available concerning the prediction of outcome using conventional EEG in pediatric coma. Several centers have also used either the original cerebral function monitor, which records an amplitude trace only; the cerebral function analyzing monitor; or the compressed spectral array, both of which display amplitude and frequency. Using the cerebral function analyzing monitor, the traces can be graded, although subtle features may not be recognized. With the compressed spectral array, an unchanging trace is usually associated with poor outcome. Deterioration of the pattern is also a poor prognostic sign, but this may be more distressing for relatives and nursing staff than serial EEGs. Electroencephalographic monitoring may be useful in the management of status epilepticus but should assist in the interpretation of, rather than replace, serial EEGs. Visual, auditory brain stem, and somatosensory evoked potentials can be elicited in children in nontraumatic coma. They have a role in the prediction of outcome, particularly if the EEG is in an intermediate group. Somatosensory evoked potentials appear to be the most useful, but predictive value is greater if the data from all three modalities are combined.

Neuroimaging can be used to look for evidence of focal or global brain damage. A CT scan performed soon after cardiac arrest may show cerebral swelling with effacement of the sulci or widespread loss of gray-white differentiation or low density in the basal ganglia [131]. The "reversal sign," with low density in the cerebral hemispheres and relatively higher densities in the basal ganglia, is not uncommon [132]. All of these patterns are associated with poor prognosis, but a normal CT scan does not guarantee a good outcome. T2-weighted MRIs have been shown to be sensitive to ischemic damage in animal studies, but no large-scale clinical investigations have been attempted because of the practical difficulties. Diffusion-weighted imaging and proton spectroscopy may eventually be useful but are in the early stages of clinical development.

Counseling Parents about Outcome

Parents should only be counseled by a doctor with extensive experience in outcome prediction who is in full possession of all the available data. No need exists for a junior doctor to "prepare the family for the worst," because this will be the uppermost thought in the parents' minds. If an outcome of moderate or severe handicap is certain, the exact meaning of this should be spelled out very clearly, but if continuing doubt over prognosis exists, it is better to admit this, while acknowledging the family's fears. Ideally, the family should be met with intermittently by an experienced pediatric neurologist, so that secondary problems can be detected easily and managed appropriately.

ACUTE FOCAL WEAKNESS

Stroke

Stroke is a rare presentation in children, with an incidence of at least 2.6 and 3.1 per 100,000 white and black children, respectively [133]. Half of the strokes are hemorrhagic, requiring immediate transfer to a neurosurgical unit in case decompression is required. Ischemic strokes have traditionally been considered to be idiopathic and to have a good prognosis with a low recurrence risk and good recovery of motor function and school performance. Conventionally, they have not been extensively investigated, on the belief that management would not be altered. A significant mortality exists, however, as well as considerable morbidity and a risk of recurrence, none of which have been adequately defined epidemiologically. In addition, evidence exists that neurologic outcome can be improved, at least in some subgroups, by appropriate emergency management, and, particularly, that recurrence may be preventable.

A focal neurologic deficit that lasts for more than 24 hours is defined as a stroke, while a similar episode that lasts for a shorter period is considered to be a transient ischemic neurologic deficit. The term *reversible ischemic neurologic deficit* has been coined to cover those instances in which the deficit lasts for more than 24 hours but the patient eventually recovers fully. This is an important concept in the context of treatment trials but is difficult to predict when the patient first presents. In children, it is always tempting to assume that the deficit will recover fully, although the evidence suggests that that is rarely the case. Modern imaging techniques are challenging these traditional clinical concepts. MRI is more sensitive than CT scanning for the diagnosis of infarction within 24 hours and is comparable for the diagnosis of hemorrhage. It is now clear that, although the majority of patients with prolonged clinical deficits eventually have infarction on neuroimaging, similar but clinically and radiologically reversible syndromes can occur (e.g., in severe hemiplegic migraine) in which contralateral EEG slowing and a scan that shows edema without infarction are clues to the diagnosis [134]. On the other hand, patients with short-lasting neurologic syndromes or even with no clinical symptoms at all may have experienced infarction, sometimes quite extensive (e.g., in sickle cell disease).

A large number of chronic pediatric conditions, including congenital heart disease and sickle cell anemia, predispose to stroke [135], although at least one-half of these patients have no previous medical history. Venous thrombosis (associated with cyanosis and polycythemia) and embolus are the common mechanisms in cardiac disease, but primary arterial cerebrovascular disease occurs in a number of syndromes (e.g., Down and Williams) associated with cardiac disease and may be more common than has previously been assumed. Unexpected cerebrovascular pathologies, such as arterial dissection, may also be associated with stroke in children with cardiac disease [136], and MRI and angiography should be performed in all. The pathology in sickle cell disease is usually large vessel disease [137], which commonly presents as hemiparesis, but seizures or headaches may not be benign in this condition, and MRI, including venography, should be considered. In previously well children, a history of trauma, however minor, may suggest arterial dissection [138,139]; injuries to the carotid while carrying a sharp object (e.g., a pencil) in the mouth are also characteristic in this age group. Infections, including varicella [140], human immunodeficiency virus [141], and meningitis, can cause cerebrovascular disease, but the presentation with stroke may be remote from the original illness. Sudden onset may indicate an embolic origin, usually presumed to be cardiogenic in children, while a slowly evolving or stuttering neurologic deficit suggests thrombosis and, therefore, cerebrovascular disease as the most likely underlying pathology. Such clinical clues to stroke syndromes and subtypes have been worked out in adult populations, but more prospective data are needed in children.

Most children who have experienced a stroke present with a hemiparesis, sometimes accompanied by hemisensory signs or visual field defect. Gaze palsy or head turning suggests a large supratentorial infarct [142]. If headache is present, arterial dissection or venous thrombosis [143] should be considered; migraine is common, and, although stroke can occur in adults, this is a rare association in the young, and other causes must be excluded [139]. Seizures, with or without an associated focal neurologic deficit, are a common presentation of cerebral venous thrombosis, particularly in neonates [143]. A deterioration in level of consciousness is common in cerebral hemorrhage, large middle cerebral artery territory infarcts, and, occasionally, in posterior fossa strokes and is an indication for immediate transfer to an intensive care unit with pediatric neurology and neurosurgery available.

More than 80% of children with ischemic stroke have cerebrovascular disease. In the past, this required demonstration by invasive angiography, but the increasing sensitivity of MR angiography (MRA) [144] and transcranial Doppler ultrasound [145] means that large vessel disease can be diagnosed acutely using these techniques. Because carotid dissection is now diagnosable by MRA in the majority of cases, a good case exists for urgent MRA in young patients, but the radiologist should be informed of this possibility so that the appropriate sequences can be obtained; similar consideration should be given to the exclusion of venous thrombosis. MRA is therefore the preliminary investigation of choice, but when this is not available, CT scanning to exclude hemorrhage is mandatory. After an interval, conventional angiography is usually required to exclude arteriovenous malformation or aneurysm in cerebral hemorrhage, unless an obvious clotting derangement is present, and may be needed in ischemic stroke to resolve diagnostic issues, particularly if small vessel disease (e.g., isolated cerebral angiitis [146]) is a possibility, although the decision to proceed should be made in the knowledge that the risk of stroke is 1%.

The diagnostic rate for conventional echocardiography is disappointingly low, but considerable evidence is available from the young adult population that otherwise insignificant cardiac anomalies, particularly patent foramen ovale, are associated with stroke; the role of transesophageal echocardiography and contrast transcranial Doppler sonography has not yet been defined in childhood stroke. It is important to exclude cervical instability if the distribution of infarction is compatible with posterior circulation disease. Most pediatricians investigating a child with stroke undertake a prothrombotic screen. In fact, the prevalence of the inherited prothrombotic disorders that can be documented at present is probably not higher in pediatric ischemic stroke than in the background population, except perhaps for the factor V Leiden [147]. The role of other potentially treatable abnormalities, such as hyperhomocystinemia [148], requires investigation.

In adults, the main focus of studies in the 1990s has been in investigating the possibility of thrombolysis for internal carotid or middle cerebral artery thrombosis or embolus and in looking for neuroprotective agents. Because the trials in adults have produced conflicting results and the risk of hemorrhage is substantial, the use of thrombolysis in the pediatric age group cannot be justified. No neuroprotective agent is currently available that could be recommended for use in children. Nevertheless, a number of management strategies exist for individual patient groups that may make a difference, in addition to the need for clot removal in hemorrhage. Stroke units have clearly been shown to improve outcome in adults, and the organization of care in the pediatric age group should be addressed. A case can be made for surgical decompression in children who present in coma with large ischemic middle cerebral infarcts, which are almost always fatal if managed conservatively. In children with sickle cell disease, exchange transfusion to reduce the percentage of sickle cells is recommended acutely, although this must be conducted slowly and cautiously in view of the association with neurologic deterioration.

The question of anticoagulation in acute stroke remains a difficult one. Some large trials in adults have suggested benefit, whereas others have demonstrated increased morbidity and mortality with subcutaneous low-molecular-weight heparin; one disadvantage, compared with the use of conventional heparin, is that it is not possible to monitor the anticoagulant effect. Despite the risk of hemorrhage, patient groups exist, including those with vessel dissection, venous sinus thrombosis, and known prothrombotic abnormalities, who should be anticoagulated acutely. Aspirin seems to present a lower risk and appears to be beneficial in acute stroke in adults; however, the risk of Reye's syndrome means that this medication cannot be recommended for children at the present time.

At least 10% of children who have a first ischemic stroke have recurrences, but consensus over prevention has not been reached. Considerable uncertainty exists over the appropriate dosage and duration of aspirin treatment in all patient groups with cerebrovascular disease, including children, mainly because of the risks of cerebral hemorrhage and gastrointestinal complications. No evidence has been found of an association between Reye's syndrome and low-dose aspirin, but studies are needed to assess the risk-benefit ratio in the long term. In the meantime, it seems reasonable to use low-dose aspirin (1 mg/kg) when documented cerebrovascular disease is present; because the lesions often disappear in the long term, repeat MR angiography might allow discontinuation of treatment. Low-dose aspirin does not prevent painful crises in sickle cell disease; currently, no data exist on its use in stroke prophylaxis in this disorder, and it is therefore not recommended. The relative risk between further stroke and life-threatening hemorrhage with long-term warfarin use has not been assessed for patients with inherited thrombophilias, such as factor V Leiden, but a case has been made for cautious anticoagulation, particularly if ongoing symptoms are present; otherwise, it is difficult to justify this treatment strategy in the young, particularly in view of the need for frequent blood tests. Although patent foramen ovale can be closed at catheterization, the long-term risk-benefit ratio is impossible to determine at present, particularly when the natural history is uncertain. Patients with moyamoya disease can benefit from revascularization, in terms of both cognitive and motor performance [149]. This may also apply to some patients with sickle cell disease [150], for whom the present recommendation of long-term transfusion remains unsatisfactory because of the inevitable iron overload and the difficulties in ensuring adequate chelation. Bone marrow or cord blood stem cell transplantation is an option if a suitable sibling donor is available, although severe cerebrovascular disease is a relative contraindication because of the risk of further ischemic or hemorrhagic stroke, and great care is needed around the time of transplantation to avoid neurologic complications.

Other Causes of Acute Focal Weakness

Tumor is usually distinguished on CT scan. Brain abscess that presents with focal signs or seizures, rather than coma, can often be treated conservatively with intravenous antibiotics, including cover for anaerobic organisms. Acute disseminated encephalomyelitis may present with focal signs that mimic stroke, and a recent infection or vaccination is often implicated. Serial MRI is useful in making the diagnosis and distinguishing this entity from multiple sclerosis and ischemic stroke [151]. Steroids are almost certainly of benefit, although there has not been an adequately controlled trial. Immunoglobulin may also be helpful [152], and plasmapheresis may be useful in fulminant cases that present in coma or in those with a prolonged course [153].

ACUTE GENERALIZED WEAKNESS

The differential diagnosis of acute weakness in childhood includes Guillain-Barré syndrome, poliomyelitis, botulism, myasthenia gravis, transverse myelitis, cord tumors, and discitis. Unsteadiness of gait followed by ascending weakness and areflexia is the characteristic presentation of Guillain-Barré syndrome [154], with bulbar weakness, bilateral facial palsy, and paralytic squint in some; the Miller-Fisher variant also occurs in children, and descending weakness is occasionally seen. In the classic form, the finding of bulbar or facial weakness is helpful in excluding a high cervical lesion as the cause of the flaccid weakness but is usually an indication to ventilate. Sensory testing is extremely difficult in young children so that poliomyelitis (e.g., after oral vaccination [155] or in unvaccinated populations) is usually distinguished by the meningeal irritation and the asymmetric weakness. Diagnosis of infantile botulism requires a high index of suspicion, but in a child younger than 1 year old with acute weakness, the diagnosis should be suggested by a history of poor feeding and constipation and by prominent cranial nerve signs, including poor gag, bilateral facial weakness, absent doll's eye, ptosis, and fixed pupils [156]. Compressing lesions of the spinal cord, transverse myelitis and discitis are usually distinguishable clinically, and an emergency MRI of the spine is essential if there is bladder or bowel involvement or if the child is not areflexic; careful testing may be helpful in demonstrating a sensory level in the older child. The MRI should be performed in a unit with a neurosurgeon available to undertake emergency decompression if necessary. The young child may not complain of pain, but limb discomfort suggests Guillain-Barré syndrome, whereas back pain might be caused by discitis. Occasionally, chronic metabolic or degenerative conditions, such as tyrosinemia [157], Leigh's disease [158], or metachromatic leukodystrophy, may present in very similar fashion to Guillain-Barré syndrome; simple blood (lactate) for Leigh's disease and urine (succinyl acetone to exclude tyrosinemia and metachromatic granules for metachromatic leukodystrophy) testing are usually sufficient to exclude these conditions. If MRI is undertaken in Guillain-Barré syndrome, involvement of the cauda equina may be demonstrated. Nerve conduction studies may be normal in the early stages of Guillain-Barré, but they are more likely to be positive in confirming this diagnosis than is lumbar puncture, as a high protein is rarely seen before the second week, although the latter is helpful in pointing toward an alternate diagnosis of poliomyelitis or transverse myelitis if the cell count is high. Neurophysiology is also very useful in distinguishing poliomyelitis and infantile botulism.

Immunoglobulin appears to be effective in nonambulant children with Guillain-Barré syndrome [159], although no controlled trials have been performed to date. Milder cases do not need this expensive treatment unless they continue to deteriorate, and less evidence exists for benefit in patients who require ventilation; some of these may need plasmapheresis. The prognosis for long-term functional recovery in childhood Guillain-Barré syndrome is excellent. High-dose steroids probably shorten the course in transverse myelitis [160]. Antibiotics are often used in discitis, although no evidence exists for benefit; a plaster spica cast may be required to reduce pain.

Myasthenia may present as acute generalized weakness in the neonatal period (transient neonatal and congenital forms), in infancy (usually congenital or possibly secondary to undiagnosed maternal myasthenia), and in childhood (juvenile antibody-positive or -negative myasthenia gravis or congenital forms) [161]. Repeated apneas, frequent chest infections, or unexplained respiratory failure should suggest the diagnosis, which has probably been underdiagnosed in the past; arthrogryposis, which may be subtle and affect only the hands, may also be a clinical clue [162]. Any child with myasthenia and significant respiratory compromise should be ventilated. Edrophonium testing must be done with the greatest of care, with full resuscitation equipment, as well as atropine, available and only after giving a test dose. Even with the use of video, results may be inconclusive, and all children should have an electromyogram, including single-fiber studies [163], as well as antibody testing of child and mother. Doubt may persist, in which case a trial of pyridostigmine or neostigmine is indicated. In the juvenile form of myasthenia gravis, plasmapheresis may be required [164] but may be technically difficult in toddlers; the use of steroids and thymectomy is controversial but may have benefit in an otherwise serious situation.

NEONATAL TETANUS

Neonatal tetanus is a common problem in developing countries and occasionally occurs in the West, usually in infants born in unhygienic conditions to unimmunized mothers. The spasms tend to present around day 6 of life and respond to diazepam; very large doses may be necessary. Sedation with phenobarbital or chlorpromazine is also beneficial. Tube feeding is required, and, if available, paralysis and ventilation should be considered for severe cases. The mortality continues to be high, particularly in developing countries.

SUMMARY

Although considerable overlap with adult practice exists, some conditions that require neurologic intensive care are either exclusive to pediatrics or much more common in children. In addition, important distinctions in differential diagnosis and in management of children with coma, stroke, and acute weakness exist. This chapter highlights the specific problems that face those who care for children with acute neurologic problems.

REFERENCES

1. Sarnat HB, Sarnat MS. Neonatal encephalopathy following fetal distress. A clinical and electroencephalographic study. Arch Neurol 1976;33:696.
2. Hellstrom-Westas L, Rosen I, Svenningsen NW. Predictive value of early continuous amplitude integrated EEG recordings on outcome after severe birth asphyxia in full term infants. Arch Dis Child Fetal Neonatal Ed 1995;72:F34.
3. Martin E, Buchli R, Ritter S, et al. Diagnostic and prognostic value of cerebral 31P magnetic resonance spectroscopy in neonates with perinatal asphyxia. Pediatr Res 1996;40:749.

4. Penrice J, Cady EB, Lorek A, et al. Proton magnetic resonance spectroscopy of the brain in normal preterm and term infants, and early changes after perinatal hypoxia-ischemia. Pediatr Res 1996;40:6.
5. Barkovich AJ, Westmark K, Partridge C, et al. Perinatal asphyxia: MR findings in the first 10 days. AJNR Am J Neuroradiol 1995;16:427.
6. Cowan FM, Pennock JM, Hanrahan JD, et al. Early detection of cerebral infarction and hypoxic ischemic encephalopathy in neonates using diffusion-weighted magnetic resonance imaging. Neuropediatrics 1994;25:172.
7. Levene MI. Management of the asphyxiated full term infant. Arch Dis Child 1993;68:612.
8. Wyatt JS, Thoresen M. Hypothermia treatment and the newborn. Pediatrics 1997;100:1028.
9. Hawdon JM, Ward Platt MP, Aynsley-Green A. Prevention and management of neonatal hypoglycaemia. Arch Dis Child Fetal Neonatal Ed 1994;70:F60, F65.
10. Watchko JF, Claassen D. Kernicterus in premature infants: current prevalence and relationship to NICHD Phototherapy Study exchange criteria. Pediatrics 1994;93:996.
11. Whitaker AH, Feldman JF, Van Rossem R, et al. Neonatal cranial ultrasound abnormalities in low birth weight infants: relation to cognitive outcomes at six years of age. Pediatrics 1996;98:719.
12. Garland JS, Buck R, Leviton A. Effect of maternal glucocorticoid exposure on risk of severe intraventricular hemorrhage in surfactant-treated preterm infants. J Pediatr 1995;126:272.
13. Fowlie PW. Prophylactic indomethacin: systematic review and meta-analysis. Arch Dis Child Fetal Neonatal Ed 1996;74:F81.
14. International PHVD Drug Trial Group. International randomised controlled trial of acetazolamide and furosemide in post-haemorrhagic ventricular dilatation in infancy. Lancet 1998;352:433.
15. Perlman JM, Risser R, Broyles RS. Bilateral cystic periventricular leukomalacia in the premature infant: associated risk factors. Pediatrics 1996;97:822.
16. Clark RH, Dykes FD, Bachman TE, Ashurst JT. Intraventricular hemorrhage and high-frequency ventilation: a meta-analysis of prospective clinical trials. Pediatrics 1996;98:1058.
17. Cunningham S, Fleck BW, Elton RA, McIntosh N. Transcutaneous oxygen levels in retinopathy of prematurity. Lancet 1995;346:1464.
18. Fallon P, Aparicio JM, Elliott MJ, Kirkham FJ. Incidence of neurological complications of surgery for congenital heart disease. Arch Dis Child 1995;72:418.
19. Miller G, Tesman JR, Ramer JC, et al. Outcome after open-heart surgery in infants and children. J Child Neurol 1996;11:49.
20. Kirkham FJ. Prevention of neurological complications after cardiopulmonary bypass. Pediatr Cardiol 1998;19:331.
21. McConnell JR, Fleming WH, Chu WK, et al. Magnetic resonance imaging of the brain in infants and children before and after cardiac surgery. A prospective study. Am J Dis Child 1990;144:374.
22. Kol S, Ammar R, Weisz G, Melamed Y. Hyperbaric oxygenation for arterial air embolism during cardiopulmonary bypass. Ann Thorac Surg 1993;55:401.
23. Medlock MD, Cruse RS, Winek SJ, et al. A 10-year experience with postpump chorea. Ann Neurol 1993;34:820.
24. du Plessis AJ, Treves ST, Hickey PR, et al. Regional cerebral perfusion abnormalities after cardiac operations. Single photon emission computed tomography (SPECT) findings in children with postoperative movement disorders. J Thorac Cardiovasc Surg 1994;107:1036.
25. Verity CM, Greenwood R, Golding J. Long-term intellectual and behavioral outcomes of children with febrile convulsions. N Engl J Med 1998;338:1723.
26. Crawley J, Smith S, Kirkham F, et al. Seizures and status epilepticus in childhood cerebral malaria. QJM 1996;89:591.
27. Kirkham FJ. Coma after Cardiac Arrest. In JA Eyre (ed), Coma in Childhood. London: Baillaire Tindall, 1994;1–40.
28. Aicardi J, Chevrie JJ. Convulsive status epilepticus in infants and children. A study of 239 cases. Epilepsia 1970;11:187.
29. Tasker RC, Boyd SG, Harden A, Matthew DJ. EEG monitoring of prolonged thiopentone administration for intractable seizures and status epilepticus in infants and young children. Neuropediatrics 1989;20:147.
30. Baxter P, Griffiths P, Kelly T, Gardner-Medwin D. Pyridoxine-dependent seizures: demographic, clinical, MRI and psychometric features, and effect of dose on intelligence quotient. Dev Med Child Neurol 1996;38:998.
31. Collins JE, Nicholson NS, Dalton N, Leonard JV. Biotinidase deficiency: early neurological presentation. Dev Med Child Neurol 1994;36:268.
32. Tasker RC, Boyd SG, Harden A, Matthew DJ. The cerebral function analysing monitor in paediatric medical intensive care: applications and limitations. Intensive Care Med 1990;16:60.

33. Tasker RC, Boyd S, Harden A, Matthew DJ. Monitoring in non-traumatic coma. Part II: electroencephalography. Arch Dis Child 1988;63:895.
34. Newton CR, Kirkham FJ, Johnston B, Marsh K. Inter-observer agreement of the assessment of coma scales and brainstem signs in non-traumatic coma. Dev Med Child Neurol 1995;37:807.
35. James HE, Trauner DA. The Glasgow Coma Scale. In HE James, NG Anas, RM Perkin (eds), Brain Insults in Infants and Children. New York: Grune & Stratton, 1985;179–182.
36. Seshia SS, Johnston B, Kasian G. Non-traumatic coma in childhood: clinical variables in prediction of outcome. Dev Med Child Neurol 1983;25:493.
37. Newton CR, Kirkham FJ, Winstanley PA, et al. Intracranial pressure in African children with cerebral malaria. Lancet 1991;337:573.
38. Day NP, Phu NH, Bethell DP, et al. The effects of dopamine and adrenaline infusions on acid-base balance and systemic haemodynamics in severe infection. Lancet 1996;348:219.
39. Tasker RC, Matthew DJ, Kendall B. Computed tomography in the assessment of raised intracranial pressure in non-traumatic coma. Neuropediatrics 1990;21:91.
40. Mellor DH. The place of computed tomography and lumbar puncture in suspected bacterial meningitis. Arch Dis Child 1992;67:1417.
41. Brown JK, Minns RA. Non-accidental head injury, with particular reference to whiplash shaking injury and medico-legal aspects. Dev Med Child Neurol 1993;35:849.
42. Wilkins B. Head injury—abuse or accident? Arch Dis Child 1997;76:393.
43. Haseler LJ, Arcinue E, Danielsen ER, et al. Evidence from proton magnetic resonance spectroscopy for a metabolic cascade of neuronal damage in shaken baby syndrome. Pediatrics 1997;99:4.
44. Lahat E, Livne M, Barr J, et al. The management of epidural haematomas—surgical versus conservative treatment. Eur J Pediatr 1994;153:198.
45. Dhellemmes P, Lejeune JP, Christiaens JL, Combelles G. Traumatic extradural hematomas in infancy and childhood. Experience with 144 cases. J Neurosurg 1985;62:861.
46. Rivara F, Tanaguchi D, Parish RA, et al. Poor prediction of positive computed tomographic scans by clinical criteria in symptomatic pediatric head trauma. Pediatrics 1987;80:579.
47. Davis RL, Hughes M, Gubler KD, et al. The use of cranial CT scans in the triage of pediatric patients with mild head injury. Pediatrics 1995;95:345.
48. Snoek JW, Minderhoud JM, Wilmink JT. Delayed deterioration following mild head injury in children. Brain 1984;107:15.
49. Beni L, Constantini S, Matoth I, Pomeranz S. Subclinical status epilepticus in a child after closed head injury. J Trauma 1996;40:449.
50. Bruce DA, Alavi A, Bilaniuk L, et al. Diffuse cerebral swelling following head injuries in children: the syndrome of "malignant brain edema." J Neurosurg 1981;54:170.
51. Lang DA, Teasdale GM, McPherson P, Lawrence A. Diffuse brain swelling after head injury: more often malignant in adults than children? J Neurosurg 1994;80:675.
52. Sharples PM, Stuart AG, Matthews DS, et al. Cerebral blood flow and metabolism in children with severe head injury. Part 1. Relation to age, Glasgow coma score, outcome, intracranial pressure, and time after injury. J Neurol Neurosurg Psychiatry 1995;58:145.
53. Pigula FA, Wald SL, Shackford SR, Vane DW. The effect of hypotension and hypoxia on children with severe head injuries. J Pediatr Surg 1993;28:310, 315.
54. Bracken MB, Shepard MJ, Collins WF, et al. A randomized, controlled trial of methylprednisolone or naloxone in the treatment of acute spinal-cord injury. Results of the Second National Acute Spinal Cord Injury Study. N Engl J Med 1990;322:1405.
55. Dharker SR, Mittal RS, Bhargava N. Ischemic lesions in basal ganglia in children after minor head injury. Neurosurgery 1993;33:863.
56. Dolinskas CA, Zimmerman RA, Bilaniuk LT. A sign of subarachnoid bleeding on cranial computed tomograms of pediatric head trauma patients. Radiology 1978;126:409.
57. Ventureyra EC, Higgins MJ. Traumatic intracranial aneurysms in childhood and adolescence. Case reports and review of the literature. Childs Nerv Syst 1994;10:361.
58. Taha JM, Crone KR, Berger TS, et al. Sigmoid sinus thrombosis after closed head injury in children. Neurosurgery 1993;32:541, 545.
59. Levy DI, Rekate HL, Cherny WB, et al. Controlled lumbar drainage in pediatric head injury. J Neurosurg 1995;83:453.
60. Morgalla MH, Krasznai L, Buchholz R, et al. Repeated decompressive craniectomy after head injury in children: two successful cases as result of improved neuromonitoring. Surg Neurol 1995;43:583, 589.
61. Stein SC, Spettell CM. Delayed and progressive brain injury in children and adolescents with head trauma. Pediatr Neurosurg 1995;23:299.

62. Pomeroy SL, Holmes SJ, Dodge PR, Feigin RD. Seizures and other neurologic sequelae of bacterial meningitis in children. N Engl J Med 1990;323:1651.
63. Odio CM, Faingezicht I, Paris M, et al. The beneficial effects of early dexamethasone administration in infants and children with bacterial meningitis. N Engl J Med 1991;324:1525.
64. Kanra GY, Ozen H, Secmeer G, et al. Beneficial effects of dexamethasone in children with pneumococcal meningitis. Pediatr Infect Dis J 1995;14:490.
65. Qazi SA, Khan MA, Mughal N, et al. Dexamethasone and bacterial meningitis in Pakistan. Arch Dis Child 1996;75:482.
66. Rennick G, Shann F, de Campo J. Cerebral herniation during bacterial meningitis in children. BMJ 1993;306:953.
67. Minns RA, Engleman HM, Stirling H. Cerebrospinal fluid pressure in pyogenic meningitis. Arch Dis Child 1989;64:814.
68. Kilpi T, Peltola H, Jauhiainen T, Kallio MJ. Oral glycerol and intravenous dexamethasone in preventing neurologic and audiologic sequelae of childhood bacterial meningitis. The Finnish Study Group. Pediatr Infect Dis J 1995;14:270.
69. Ashwal S, Stringer W, Tomasi L, et al. Cerebral blood flow and carbon dioxide reactivity in children with bacterial meningitis. J Pediatr 1990;117:523.
70. Powell KR, Sugarman LI, Eskenazi AE, et al. Normalization of plasma arginine vasopressin concentrations when children with meningitis are given maintenance plus replacement fluid therapy. J Pediatr 1990;117:515.
71. Whitley RJ. Viral encephalitis. N Engl J Med 1990;323:242.
72. Barthez-Carpentier MA, Rozenberg F, Dussaix E, et al. Relapse of herpes simplex encephalitis. J Child Neurol 1995;10:363.
73. Jones CA, Isaacs D. Human herpesvirus-6 infections. Arch Dis Child 1996;74:98.
74. Thomas NH, Collins JE, Robb SA, Robinson RO. Mycoplasma pneumoniae infection and neurological disease. Arch Dis Child 1993;69:573.
75. Rebaud P, Berthier JC, Hartemann E, Floret D. Intracranial pressure in childhood central nervous system infections. Intensive Care Med 1988;14:522.
76. McCaslin, RI, Pikis A, Rodriguez WJ. Pediatric Plasmodium falciparum malaria: a ten-year experience from Washington, DC. Pediatr Infect Dis J 1994;13:709.
77. van Hensbroek MB, Onyiorah E, Jaffar S, et al. A trial of artemether or quinine in children with cerebral malaria. N Engl J Med 1996;335:69.
78. Newton CRJC, Crawley J, Sowumni A, et al. Intracranial hypertension in Kenyan children with cerebral malaria. Arch Dis Child 1997;76:219.
79. Looareesuwan S, Phillips RE, Karbwang J, et al. Plasmodium falciparum hyperparasitaemia: use of exchange transfusion in seven patients and a review of the literature. QJM 1990;75:471.
80. Krane EJ, Rockoff MA, Wallman JK, Wolfsdorf JI. Subclinical brain swelling in children during treatment of diabetic ketoacidosis. N Engl J Med 1985;312:1147.
81. Harris GD, Fiordalisi I, Harris WL, et al. Minimizing the risk of brain herniation during treatment of diabetic ketoacidemia: a retrospective and prospective study. J Pediatr 1990;117:22.
82. Constantinou JE, Gillis J, Ouvrier RA, Rahilly PM. Hypoxic-ischaemic encephalopathy after near miss sudden infant death syndrome. Arch Dis Child 1989;64:703.
83. Kirkham FJ. Intracranial pressure and cerebral blood flow in non-traumatic coma in childhood. In RA Minns (ed), Measurement of intracranial pressure and cerebral blood flow in children. Clin Developmental Med 1991;113–114:283–338.
84. Le Roux PD, Jardine DS, Kanev PM, Loeser JD. Pediatric intracranial pressure monitoring in hypoxic and nonhypoxic brain injury. Childs Nerv Syst 1991;7:34.
85. Pearn J. The management of near drowning. BMJ 1985;291:1447.
86. Ashwal S, Schneider S, Tomasi L, Thompson J. Prognostic implications of hyperglycemia and reduced cerebral blood flow in childhood near-drowning. Neurology 1990;40:820.
87. Habib DM, Tecklenburg FW, Webb SA, et al. Prediction of childhood drowning and near-drowning morbidity and mortality. Pediatr Emerg Care 1996;12:255.
88. Nussbaum E, Galant SP. Intracranial pressure monitoring as a guide to prognosis in the nearly drowned, severely comatose child. J Pediatr 1983;102:215.
89. Nussbaum E, Maggi JC. Pentobarbital therapy does not improve neurologic outcome in nearly drowned, flaccid-comatose children. Pediatrics 1988;81:630.
90. Bohn DJ, Biggar WD, Smith CR, et al. Influence of hypothermia, barbiturate therapy, and intracranial pressure monitoring on morbidity and mortality after near-drowning. Crit Care Med 1986;14:529.
91. Kreis R, Arcinue E, Ernst T, et al. Hypoxic encephalopathy after near-drowning studied by quantitative 1H-magnetic resonance spectroscopy. J Clin Invest 1996;97:1142.

92. Horsfield P, Williams AJ. Recovery after electrical injury. Dev Med Child Neurol 1977;19:224.
93. Cooper MA. Lightning injuries: prognostic signs for death. Ann Emerg Med 1980;9:134.
94. Kotagal S, Rawlings CA, Chen SC, et al. Neurologic, psychiatric, and cardiovascular complications in children struck by lightning. Pediatrics 1982;70:190.
95. Mohnot D, Snead OC 3d, Benton JW Jr. Burn encephalopathy in children. Ann Neurol 1982;12:42.
96. Glasgow JF, Moore R. Reye's syndrome 30 years on. BMJ 1993;307:950.
97. Hardie RM, Newton LH, Bruce JC, et al. The changing clinical pattern of Reye's syndrome 1982–1990. Arch Dis Child 1996;74:400.
98. Yoshida I, Yoshino M, Watanabe J, Yamashita F. Sudden onset of ornithine carbamoyltransferase deficiency after aspirin ingestion. J Inherit Metab Dis 1993;16:917.
99. Wijdicks EFM, Plevak DJ, Rakela J, Wiesner RH. Clinical and radiologic features of cerebral edema in fulminant hepatic failure. Mayo Clin Proc 1995;70:119.
100. Devictor D, Tahiri C, Lanchier C, et al. Flumazenil in the treatment of hepatic encephalopathy in children with fulminant liver failure. Intensive Care Med 1995;21:253.
101. Yoshiba M, Sekiyama K, Inoue K, Fujita R. Interferon and cyclosporin A in the treatment of fulminant viral hepatitis. J Gastroenterol 1995;30:67.
102. Crisp DE, Siegler RL, Bale JF, Thompson JA. Hemorrhagic cerebral infarction in the hemolytic-uremic syndrome. J Pediatr 1981;99:273.
103. Bos AP, Donckerwolcke RA, van Vught AJ. The hemolytic-uremic syndrome: prognostic significance of neurological abnormalities. Helv Paediatr Acta 1985;40:381.
104. Rooney JC, Anderson RM, Hopkins IJ. Clinical and pathological aspects of central nervous system involvement in the haemolytic uraemic syndrome. Proc Aust Assoc Neurol 1971;7:28.
105. Trevathan E, Dooling EC. Large thrombotic strokes in hemolytic-uremic syndrome. J Pediatr 1987;111:863.
106. Qamar IU, Ohali M, MacGregor DL, et al. Long-term neurological sequelae of hemolytic-uremic syndrome: a preliminary report. Pediatr Nephrol 1996;10:504.
107. Wright RR, Mathews KD. Hypertensive encephalopathy in childhood. J Child Neurol 1996;11:193.
108. Kandt RS, Caoili AQ, Lorentz WB, Elster AD. Hypertensive encephalopathy in children: neuroimaging and treatment. J Child Neurol 1995;10:236.
109. Griswold WR, Viney J, Mendoza SA, James HE. Intracranial pressure monitoring in severe hypertensive encephalopathy. Crit Care Med 1981;9:573.
110. Barry DI, Lassen NA. Cerebral blood flow autoregulation in hypertension and effects of antihypertensive drugs. J Hypertens 1984;2(suppl):S519.
111. Sofer S, Yerushalmi B, Shahak E, et al. Possible aetiology of haemorrhagic shock and encephalopathy syndrome in the Negev area of Israel. Arch Dis Child 1996;75:332.
112. Goldman AP, Kerr SJ, Butt W, et al. Extracorporeal support for intractable cardiorespiratory failure due to meningococcal disease. Lancet 1997;349:466.
113. McLaurin RL, Nichols JBJ. Extensive cranial decompression in the treatment of severe lead encephalopathy. Pediatrics 1957;39:653.
114. Cheney K, Gumbiner C, Benson B, Tenenbein M. Survival after a severe iron poisoning treated with intermittent infusions of deferoxamine. J Toxicol Clin Toxicol 1995;33:61.
115. Rieke K, Schwab S, Krieger D, et al. Decompressive surgery in space-occupying hemispheric infarction: results of an open, prospective trial. Crit Care Med 1995;23:1576.
116. Goitein KJ, Amit Y, Mussaffi H. Intracranial pressure in central nervous system infections and cerebral ischaemia of infancy. Arch Dis Child 1983;58:184.
117. Tasker RC, Matthew DJ, Helms P, et al. Monitoring in non-traumatic coma. Part I. Invasive intracranial measurements. Arch Dis Child 1988;63:888.
118. Ausman JI, Rogers C, Sharp HL. Decompressive craniectomy for the encephalopathy of Reye's syndrome. Surg Neurol 1976;6:97.
119. Kirkham FJ, Neville BGR. Successful management of severe intracranial hypertension by surgical decompression. Dev Med Child Neurol 1986;28:506.
120. Berryhill P, Lilly MA, Levin HS, et al. Frontal lobe changes after severe diffuse closed head injury in children: a volumetric study of magnetic resonance imaging. Neurosurgery 1995;37:392,399.
121. Von Seggern K, Egar M, Fuhrman BP. Cardiopulmonary resuscitation in a pediatric ICU. Crit Care Med 1986;14:275.
122. Heindl UT, Laub MC. Outcome of persistent vegetative state following hypoxic or traumatic brain injury in children and adolescents. Neuropediatrics 1996;27:94.
123. Weinberger HA, van der Woude R, Maier HC. Prognosis of cortical blindness following cardiac arrest in children. JAMA 1962;179:126.
124. Kriel RL, Krach LE, Luxenberg MG, et al. Outcome of severe anoxic/ischemic brain injury in children. Pediatr Neurol 1994;10:207.

125. Kotagal S, Rolfe U, Schwarz KB, Escober W. "Locked-in" state following Reye's syndrome. Ann Neurol 1984;15:599.
126. Saint Hilaire MH, Burke RE, Bressman SB, et al. Delayed-onset dystonia due to perinatal or early childhood asphyxia. Neurology 1991;41:216.
127. Heckmatt JZ, Pitt MC, Kirkham F. Peripheral neuropathy and neuromuscular blockade presenting as prolonged respiratory paralysis following critical illness. Neuropediatrics 1997;24:123.
128. Ragosta K. Miller Fisher syndrome, a brainstem encephalitis, mimics brain death [letter]. Clin Pediatr 1993;32:685.
129. Okamoto K, Sugimoto T. Return of spontaneous respiration in an infant who fulfilled current criteria to determine brain death. Pediatrics 1995;96:518.
130. Fishman MA. Validity of brain death criteria in infants. Pediatrics 1995;96:513.
131. Kjos BO, Brant–Zawadzki M, Young RG. Early CT findings of global central nervous system hypoperfusion. AJR Am J Roentgenol 1983;141:1227.
132. Han BK, Towbin RB, De Courten-Myers G, et al. Reversal sign on CT: effect of anoxic/ischemic cerebral injury in children. AJR Am J Roentgenol 1990;154:361.
133. Broderick J, Talbot GT, Prenger E, et al. Stroke in children within a major metropolitan area: the surprising importance of intracerebral hemorrhage. J Child Neurol 1993;8:250.
134. Lai CW, Ziegler DK, Lansky LL, Torres F. Hemiplegic migraine in childhood: diagnostic and therapeutic aspects. J Pediatr 1982;101:696.
135. Roach ES, Riela AR. Pediatric Cerebrovascular Disorders (2nd ed). Armonk, NY: Futura, 1995.
136. Ganesan V, Kirkham FJ. Stroke secondary to carotid dissection in a child with cardiac disease. Arch Dis Child 1997;76:175.
137. Adams RJ, Nicols FT, McVie V, et al. Cerebral infarction in sickle cell anemia: mechanism based on CT and MRI. Neurology 1988;38:1012.
138. Schievink WI, Mokri B, Piepgras DG. Spontaneous dissections of cervicocephalic arteries in childhood and adolescence. Neurology 1994;44:1607.
139. Ganesan V, Kirkham FJ. Carotid dissection causing stroke in a child with migraine. BMJ 1997;314:291.
140. Ganesan V, Kirkham FJ. Mechanisms of childhood stroke following chickenpox. Arch Dis Child 1997;76:523.
141. Park YD, Belman AL, Kim T-S, et al. Stroke in pediatric acquired immunodeficiency syndrome. Ann Neurol 1990;28:303.
142. Hacke W, Schwab S, Horn M, et al. "Malignant" middle cerebral artery territory infarction: clinical course and prognostic signs. Arch Neurol 1996;53:309.
143. Barron TF, Gusnard DA, Zimmerman RA, Clancy RR. Cerebral venous thrombosis in neonates and children. Pediatr Neurol 1992;8:112.
144. Wiznitzer M, Masaryk TJ. Cerebrovascular abnormalities in pediatric stroke: assessment using parenchymal and angiographic magnetic resonance imaging. Ann Neurol 1991;29:585.
145. Adams R, McKie V, Nichols F, et al. The use of transcranial ultrasonography to predict stroke in sickle cell disease. N Engl J Med 1992;326:605.
146. Matsell DG, Keene DL, Jimenez C, Humphreys P. Isolated angiitis of the central nervous system in childhood. Can J Neurol Sci 1990;17:151.
147. Ganesan V, McShane MA, Liesner R, et al. Inherited prothrombotic states and ischaemic stroke in childhood. J Neurol Neurosurg Psychiatry 1998;65:508.
148. Fermo I, Vigano DS, Paroni R, et al. Prevalence of moderate hyperhomocysteinemia in patients with early-onset venous and arterial occlusive disease. Ann Intern Med 1995;123:747.
149. George BD, Neville BG, Lumley JS. Transcranial revascularisation in childhood and adolescence. Dev Med Child Neurol 1993;35:675.
150. Vernet O, Montes JL, O'Gorman AM, et al. Encephaloduroarterio-synangiosis in a child with sickle cell anemia and moyamoya disease. Pediatr Neurol 1996;14:226.
151. Miller DH, Robb SA, Ormerod IE, et al. Magnetic resonance imaging of inflammatory and demyelinating white-matter diseases of childhood. Dev Med Child Neurol 1990;32:97.
152. Kleiman M, Brunquell P. Acute disseminated encephalomyelitis: response to intravenous immunoglobulin. J Child Neurol 1995;10:481.
153. Kanter DS, Horensky D, Sperling RA, et al. Plasmapheresis in fulminant acute disseminated encephalomyelitis. Neurology 1995;45:824.
154. Korinthenberg R, Monting JS. Natural history and treatment effects in Guillain-Barré syndrome: a multicentre study. Arch Dis Child 1996;74:281.
155. Beausoleil JL, Nordgren RE, Modlin JF. Vaccine-associated paralytic poliomyelitis. J Child Neurol 1994;9:334.
156. Cochran DP, Appleton RE. Infant botulism—is it that rare? Dev Med Child Neurol 1997;37:274.

157. Gibbs TC, Payan J, Brett EM, et al. Peripheral neuropathy as the presenting feature of tyrosinaemia type I and effectively treated with an inhibitor of 4-hydroxyphenylpyruvate dioxygenase. J Neurol Neurosurg Psychiatry 1993;56:1129.
158. Coker SB. Leigh disease presenting as Guillain-Barré syndrome. Pediatr Neurol 1993;9:61.
159. Nicolaides P, Appleton RE. Immunoglobulin therapy in Guillain-Barré syndrome in children. Dev Med Child Neurol 1995;37:1110.
160. Jeffery DR, Mandler RN, Davis LE. Transverse myelitis. Retrospective analysis of 33 cases, with differentiation of cases associated with multiple sclerosis and parainfectious events. Arch Neurol 1993;50:532.
161. Janas JS, Barohn RJ. A clinical approach to the congenital myasthenic syndromes. J Child Neurol 1995;10:168.
162. Vajsar J, Sloane A, MacGregor DL, et al. Arthrogryposis multiplex congenita due to congenital myasthenic syndrome. Pediatr Neurol 1995;12:237.
163. Gilchrist JM, Massey JM, Sanders DB. Single fiber EMG and repetitive stimulation of the same muscle in myasthenia gravis. Muscle Nerve 1994;17:171.
164. Ichikawa M, Koh CS, Hata Y, et al. Immunoadsorption plasmapheresis for severe generalised myasthenia gravis. Arch Dis Child 1993;69:236.

Index

Note: Page numbers followed by *f* indicate figures; page numbers followed by *t* indicate tables.

Ventilation *(continued)*
    intermittent, hypotheses related
        to, 272
    positive-pressure, for chronic respiratory
        failure of neurogenic origin, 269
Ventilator(s), body, for chronic respiratory
        failure of neurogenic origin,
        270–271, 270f
Ventilatory support, for Guillain-Barré syn-
        drome, 39
Ventral medullary shell, respiratory control
        and, 3–4
Ventral respiratory group, respiratory con-
        trol and, 2
Vestibulo-ocular reflexes, in coma,
        102–104
Viral encephalitis, 303–309
Viral meningitis, 309–311
    clinical presentation of, 310
    diagnosis of, 310–311
    incidence of, 309–310
    pathophysiology of, 309–310
    treatment of, 311
Volume replacement, in acute ischemic
        stroke, 170
Voluntary control, of respiration,
        254–255, 255f

Warfarin
    for cerebral venous thrombosis, 202t, 203
    resistance to, in antiphospholipid syn-
        drome, 213–214

Weakness
    acute, in intensive care unit, causes of,
        69–89
        hepatic porphyrias, acute, 83–85
        quadriplegic myopathy, acute, 74t,
            75–78, 77f, 78f. *See also*
            Quadriplegic myopathy,
            acute
        animal toxins, 85, 86t
        botulism, 81–82
        clinical features of, 71, 71t
        muscle inexcitability and, 79–80
        neuromuscular complications of criti-
            cal illness, 72–75. *See also*
            Critical illness, neuromuscular
            complications of
        rabies, 82–83
        tetanus, 80–81
    bulbar, in myasthenia gravis, 54–55
    clinical evaluation of, 70–72
        diagnostic tests for, 71–72
    differential diagnosis of, 69, 70t
    focal, acute, in neonates and children,
        367–370
    generalized, acute, in neonates and chil-
        dren, 371–372
    muscle, fatigable, in myasthenia gravis, 54
    pharyngeal, in bulbar dysfunction,
        23–24
Wegener's granulomatosis
    cerebral venous thrombosis and, 193
    criteria for, 215t

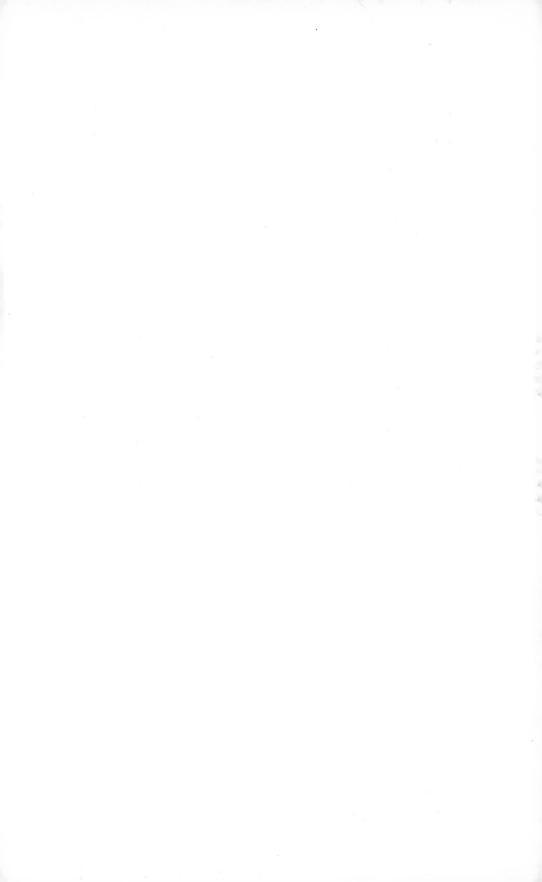